CURREN'S
MATH
for
MEDS

DOSAGES & SOLUTIONS

ELEVENTH EDITION

CURREN'S
MATH
for
MEDS

DOSAGES & SOLUTIONS
ELEVENTH EDITION

Anna M. Curren, RN, MA
Former Associate Professor of Nursing
Long Beach City College
Long Beach, California

Margaret H. Witt, BSN, MPT, DPT
Major USAF, Retired
Rehabilitation Coordinator
VA Medical Center
Spokane, Washington

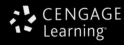

Australia • Brazil • Japan • Korea • Mexico • Singapore • Spain • United Kingdom • United States

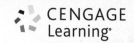
CENGAGE
Learning·

Curren's Math for Meds: Dosages and Solutions, Eleventh Edition
Anna M. Curren, RN, MA, and Margaret Witt, BSN, MPT, DPT

Publisher: Stephen Helba

Senior Product Manager: Maureen Rosener

Director, Development: Marah Bellegarde

Product Development Manager: Juliet Steiner

Senior Content Developer: Elisabeth Williams

Editorial Assistant: Jennifer Wheaton

Senior Production Director: Wendy Troeger

Production Manager: Andrew Crouth

Senior Content Project Manager: Kenneth McGrath

Senior Art Director: Jack Pendleton

Cover Image(s): Shutterstock.com/Ozernia Anna

For product information and technology assistance, contact us at
Cengage Learning Customer & Sales Support, 1-800-354-9706
For permission to use material from this text or product, submit all requests online at **www.cengage.com/permissions.**
Further permissions questions can be e-mailed to
permissionrequest@cengage.com

Library of Congress Control Number: 2013947483

ISBN-13: 978-1-1115-4091-3

Cengage Learning
200 First Stamford Place, 4th Floor
Stamford, CT 06902
USA

Cengage Learning is a leading provider of customized learning solutions with office locations around the globe, including Singapore, the United Kingdom, Australia, Mexico, Brazil, and Japan. Locate your local office at:
www.cengage.com/global

Cengage Learning products are represented in Canada by Nelson Education, Ltd.

To learn more about Cengage Learning, visit **www.cengage.com**
Purchase any of our products at your local college store or at our preferred online store **www.cengagebrain.com**

Printed in the United States of America
1 2 3 4 5 6 7 16 15 14 13

CONTENTS

SECTION **1** *Refresher Math*

CHAPTER 1
Relative Value, Addition, and Subtraction of Decimals ▶ 2

CHAPTER 2
Multiplication and Division of Decimals ▶ 11

CHAPTER 3
Solving Common Fraction Equations ▶ 22

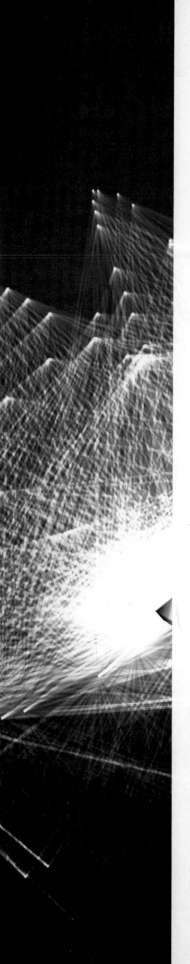

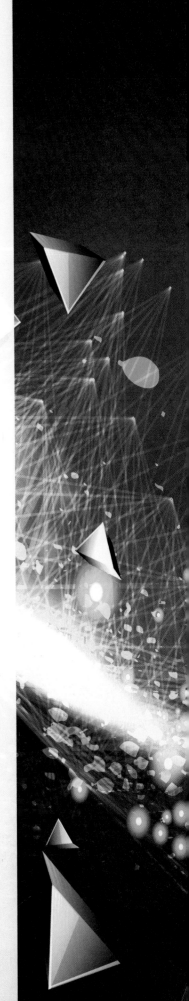

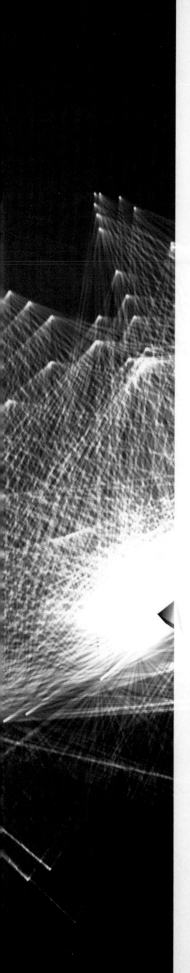

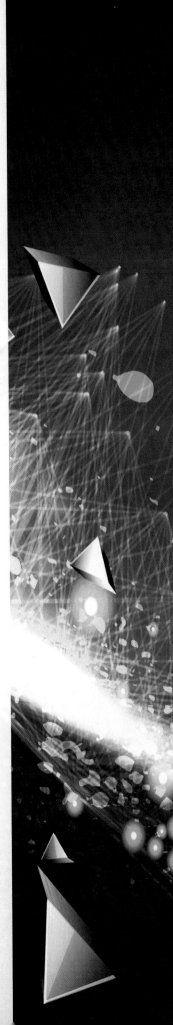

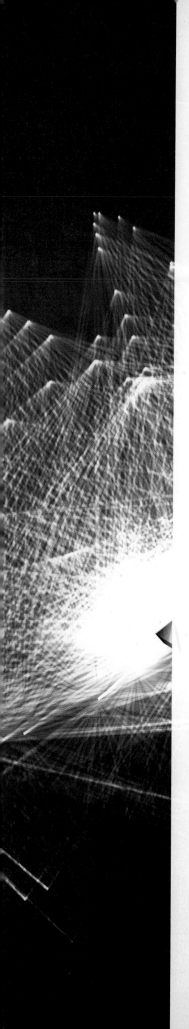

PREFACE

Curren's Math for Meds: Dosages & Solutions, eleventh edition, is your best partner for success in the dosage calculations arena. With a growing record of positive instruction with hundreds of thousands of users, its fully self-instructional approach fosters achievement and confidence as the ideal choice for both learners and instructors.

A large part of the credit for this successful journey lies in the fact that *Curren's Math for Meds,* eleventh edition, has kept up with the times, while never losing sight of the beginning students it was designed to teach. *Curren's Math for Meds* is the only calculations text of its kind that is completely focused to teach from simple to complex. It eliminates the unnecessary, keeps instruction consistently geared toward clinical realities, and offers a solid and seamless learning process from day one until program completion.

ORGANIZATION

Curren's Math for Meds allows for self-paced study, progressing from basic to more complex information. All learners are invited to complete the Refresher Math Pretest on page xvii to determine their competence in basic math skills. Section 1, Refresher Math, is also recommended for all learners, as the numerous shortcuts and memory cues included in this section are used in examples throughout the text. Calculators are used routinely in clinical facilities and on the NCLEX exam, and their use is encouraged in this text. Bear in mind that fractional variations in answers due to rounding of numbers may occur and should be considered correct.

Once the fundamental skills are mastered, the learner will move on to the basics needed for calculating dosages and administering medications; metric system units and milliequivalent dosages; reading dosage labels and syringe calibrations; and working with reconstituted drugs and insulin. Hundreds of sample dosage problems will cement these learnings.

With these basic skills solidified, students are prepared for the advanced calculations presented in the second half of the text. Body weight and body surface area dosage calculations, as well as intravenous and heparin calculations, are thoroughly covered and tested. Pediatric medication calculations round out the learner's education.

FEATURES

Curren's Math for Meds, eleventh edition, offers examples and review tests throughout to enhance comprehension, and running answers allow the learner to receive immediate feedback on deficits and strengths. An icon 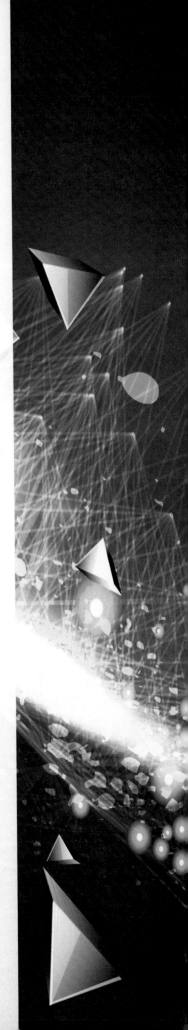 is used throughout the chapters to allow learners to easily identify important information. The most up-to-date equipment and safety devices are depicted in color, and real, full-color drug labels and syringes are included with explanations and dosage problems. With the goal of helping students become safe and effective practitioners, *Curren's Math for Meds* works through basic and advanced calculations in detail, including intravenous and pediatric calculations, so that students are fully equipped to safely prepare and administer medications in a clinical setting.

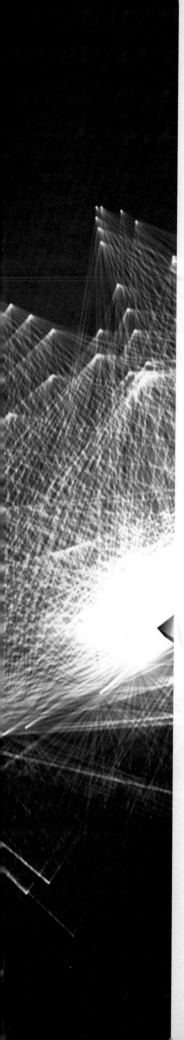

NEW TO THIS EDITION

▶ Many new, current drug labels have been added to reflect the most up-to-date information on the market. Medications nurses are likely to encounter in practice are included throughout.

▶ Content related to apothecary measurement has been placed in an appendix to offer more discussion space for current measurement systems.

▶ New online tools and interactive resources, as described below, have been added to enhance the student's experience and develop stronger dosage calculation skills.

Learning Package for the Student

Premium Website

The **Premium Website** is available to purchasers of the text, and is accessed at **www.CengageBrain.com**. Enter your passcode, found on the card in the front of the book, and the Premium Website will be added to your bookshelf. Here you can access the Student Practice Software, which includes tutorials, practice questions, and tests for every chapter in the text, as well as interactive syringe exercises.

Teaching Package for the Instructor

Instructor Companion Website

The **Instructor Companion Website** is a complete teaching tool to aid instructors in preparing lessons, creating lectures, developing quizzes, and outlining presentations. The following components are included in this resource, which is complementary to adopters of *Curren's Math for Meds*, eleventh edition:

▶ **Lecture Slides**, created in PowerPoint®, facilitate classroom instruction by offering ready-made presentation outlines, tools, and procedures.

▶ A **Test Bank** offers several hundred new questions designed for testing and evaluation.

▶ A **Solutions Manual** includes step-by-step solutions to all problems and self-tests included in the text.

INTRODUCTION FOR THE LEARNER

Welcome to what we anticipate will be one of the more enjoyable texts in your bookbag. *Curren's Math for Meds: Dosages & Solutions,* eleventh edition, is about to reassure you that math is nothing to be afraid of, and that on completion of your instruction you will have the calculation skills you need to practice safely in your profession. You don't have to be a math expert to be successful in dosage calculations; what you do need is a desire for accuracy and a motivation to learn. If you have not used your math skills for a number of years, Section 1, Refresher Math, will quickly bring you up to date. *Curren's Math for Meds* is fully self-instructional and lets you move at your own pace through the content. Hundreds of examples and problems will keep your learning on track. Here are some tips to help you get started.

1. Gather a calculator, pencil or pen, and plenty of scratch paper.

2. Start by completing the Refresher Math Pretest on page xvii. This will alert you to those areas in Section 1, Refresher Math, that will need your particular attention. Some of the items in the Pretest and Refresher Math section were designed to be completed without using a calculator, but the choice is entirely yours; when you need a calculator, use one. You must remember, however, that calculator settings vary. All answers in this text were checked with a calculator set to hundredths. If you use one with a different setting, you may experience small differences in your answers in the tenths or hundredths.

3. Record the answers to calculations on the scratch paper as well as in your text. This makes checking your answers against those we provide much easier.

4. As you work your way through the chapters, do exactly as you are instructed to do. Programmed learning proceeds in small steps, and jumping ahead may cause confusion. All chapters are designed to let you move at your own speed, and if you already know some of the basics, you will move through them more quickly than you can imagine.

5. Once you have completed your instruction, keep *Curren's Math for Meds* in your personal library. As you move to different clinical areas during your career, you will encounter different types of calculations. A quick refresher with *Curren's Math for Meds* will be invaluable when that occurs.

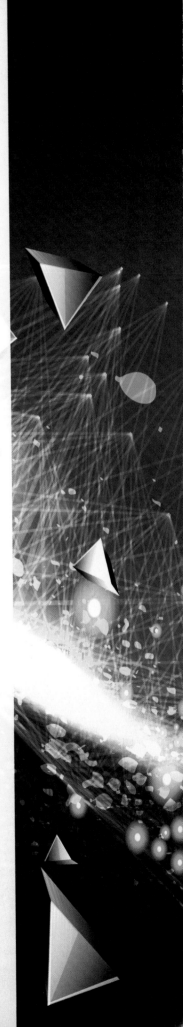

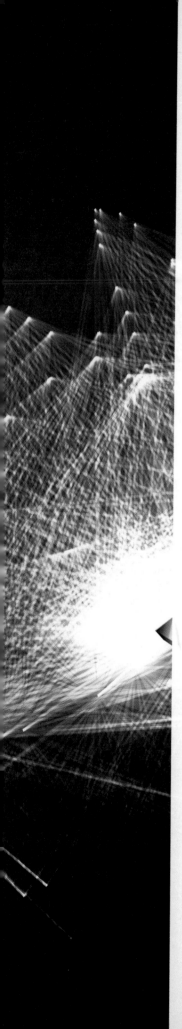

INTRODUCTION FOR THE INSTRUCTOR

Welcome to the eleventh edition of *Curren's Math for Meds*. Whether you are a seasoned user of this text or are becoming acquainted with it for the first time, we would like to share a few ideas on how to most effectively incorporate this bestselling text into your curriculum. *Curren's Math for Meds* is designed to be used starting early in the students' beginning semester. Many instructors assign the entire Section 1, Refresher Math, to be completed before the semester starts, and test on it within the first two weeks. Or, chapters can be assigned on a weekly basis at a pace fitting your students' profiles.

Students have many pressures on their time, and experience has shown that they learn best when their progress is routinely both encouraged and monitored. A short weekly test of about ten questions on the content assigned is the ideal way to do this. If a student struggles with the first test, provide a makeup opportunity. If a second test is unsuccessful, you will need to delve more deeply to determine the exact problem and help the student establish a study plan. The content in Section 1 is ideally suited to bring students up to the level of math skills required for success in dosage calculations.

Because testing and reinforcement are such vital components of learner success, encourage learners to use the Student Practice Software available on the Premium Website. Each module in this valuable electronic resource opens with a short tutorial designed to reinforce text concepts. Interactive problems and self-tests for each module reinforce accuracy and offer feedback as the student works at an individual pace.

As an instructor, you will also have access to valuable electronic resources that will enhance your students' success. Lecture slides created in PowerPoint®, calculation solutions, and a test bank are all included on our Instructor Companion Website, with the goal of facilitating classroom preparation and allowing you to focus as much time as possible on student interaction and competence. With *Curren's Math for Meds*, both you and your students are prepared for success!

USING THE LEARNING PACKAGE

▶ An **icon** designates important reminders to help with calculations and to highlight important safety considerations. As you study for your exams, locate these **Keys** and make sure you know and understand them. Consider making flash cards of the Keys to be certain you know them.

 KEYpoint: Volumes larger than 3 mL are difficult for a single IM injection site to absorb, and the 0.5 to 3 mL volume can be used as a guideline for accuracy of calculations in IM and subcutaneous dosages.

▶ **Example** icons walk you through each concept in a step-by-step manner, showing the calculation and mathematical processes. Focus on these areas to be sure you understand how to do each different type of calculation.

EXAMPLE 2 A dosage strength of **40 mEq in 5 mL** is available. You are to prepare **30 mEq**.

$$\frac{30 \text{ mEq}}{40 \text{ mEq}} \times 5 \text{ mL} = X \text{ mL}$$

$$\frac{30}{40} \times 5 = 3.75 = \mathbf{3.8 \text{ mL}}$$

A volume of 3.8 mL is necessary to prepare a 30 mEq dosage.

The dosage ordered, 30 mEq, is less than the 40 mEq dosage strength available. It must be contained in a smaller volume than 5 mL, and the answer, 3.8 mL, indicates that it is.

▶ **Problems** are sprinkled throughout each chapter. This is your opportunity to put your skills to the test, to identify your areas of strength, and to also acknowledge those areas where you need additional study. Answers to all problems are printed in the accompanying shaded box. Double-check your calculations if you have difficulty, or talk to your instructor for additional help.

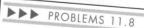 ▶▶▶ PROBLEMS 11.8

For each of the following combined Regular and NPH insulin dosages, indicate the total volume of the combined dosage and the smallest capacity syringe you can use to prepare it; 30, 50, and 100 unit capacity syringes are available.

	Total Volume	Syringe Size
1. 28 units Regular, 64 units NPH	_____	_____
2. 16 units NPH, 6 units Regular	_____	_____
3. 33 units Regular, 41 units NPH	_____	_____
4. 21 units Regular, 52 units NPH	_____	_____
5. 13 units Regular, 27 units NPH	_____	_____

Answers 1. 92 units; 100 unit **2.** 22 units; 30 unit **3.** 74 units; 100 unit **4.** 73 units; 100 unit
5. 40 units; 50 unit

Actual **full-color labels** are used to support the problems and examples. Challenge yourself to read the labels carefully and accurately; are you able to understand the quantity, strength, form, dosing, and administration guidelines for every label you encounter?

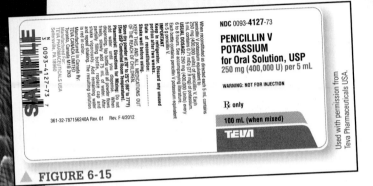

▲ FIGURE 6-15

Photos of syringes are depicted in actual size so that you can gain confidence in perfecting the real-life skill of accurately reading and interpreting syringe calibrations and medication levels.

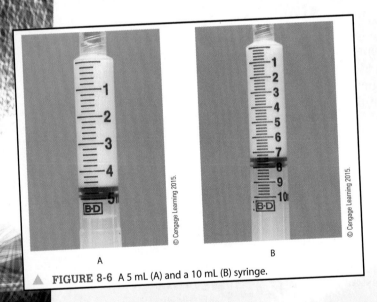

▲ FIGURE 8-6 A 5 mL (A) and a 10 mL (B) syringe.

▶ **Summary Self-Tests** round out each chapter. Complete these as you finish studying the material, identify areas where you need to focus, and review the content again until you are confident in your calculating ability. Many of these tests include combined label and syringe questions, where you must calculate a dosage and then measure the dosage on a syringe. This is an excellent tool to test how well you apply your knowledge.

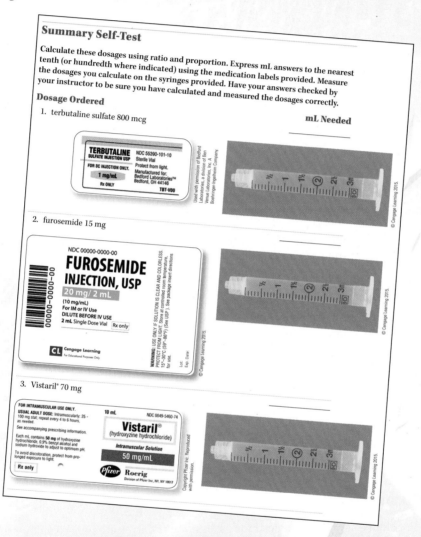

▶ **Online Resources** are available at your fingertips. Visit the Premium Website for valuable course content, including the Student Practice Software and additional quizzing.

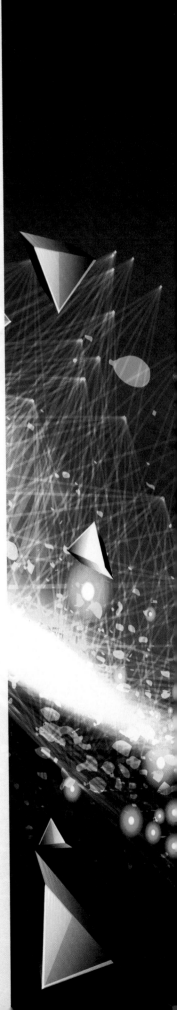

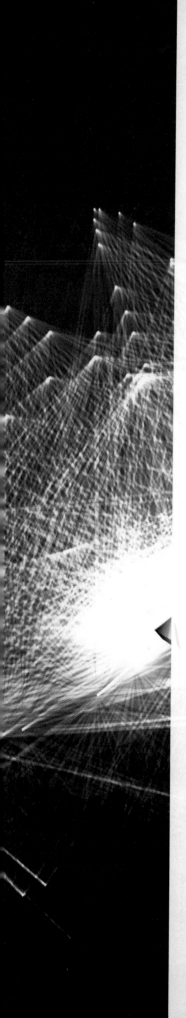

USING THE ONLINE STUDENT PRACTICE SOFTWARE

The **Online Student Practice Software** is a built-in learning tutor. After studying each chapter, be sure to also work with the online software. This valuable resource will help cement understanding of key rules and math explanations, and continuously expand skills and confidence in performing dosage calculations.

ORGANIZATION AND FEATURES

Main Menu

The main menu is organized by units and chapters that correspond to the units and chapters in the core book.

Tutorials

Tutorials open each chapter. These provide a quick review of the text content to ensure complete understanding of the material in these first few screens before moving on to the problems and self-tests.

Problems

Each chapter includes practice problems that incorporate labels and syringes for the most realistic and challenging practice experience. Practice problems allow two tries to obtain the correct answer. If the correct answer is not obtained on the second try, the answer and solution will appear on the screen.

Scoring

Problem answers are scored for assessment of strengths and weaknesses and to determine which topics need further study.

Interactive Syringes

Some questions include the use of interactive syringes. The computer mouse can be used to click and drag the syringe plunger to the correct syringe measurement. All syringes are duplicated in actual size.

Summary Self-Tests

Comprehensive tests follow each chapter, providing a single opportunity to correctly answer to simulate a true testing environment. Answers and solutions are provided.

A LETTER FROM THE AUTHOR

Dear Educators:

The first edition of *Math for Meds* was welcomed as the text that "eliminates the unnecessary." It did just that, and it introduced the **clinically focused approach** to dosage calculation instruction that is now the standard in the field. The first edition had only 56 pages. Adoption and support from appreciative educators made *Math for Meds* the leading text on dosage calculations continent-wide, a distinction it still holds.

The explosion of relevant information in subsequent years makes *Math for Meds'* original 56-page count seem like a myth. But more is not necessarily better. In fact, "more" has reached a competitive stage where the slogan "eliminates the unnecessary" is again a critical issue in dosage calculations instruction.

Math for Meds has never lost sight of the beginning students it is designed to teach. What is really needed is a clear presentation of the solid basics that students can build on throughout their programs and in their clinical experience. The size and depth of this new eleventh edition makes it the perfect vehicle for accomplishing this.

Curren's Math for Meds: Dosages & Solutions, eleventh edition, is the only text that teaches first to the over 90% of average dosages that the beginning student will learn from. It THEN introduces the advanced calculations that require the use of ratio and proportion, dimensional analysis, or the formula method. All three calculation methods are presented in the new *Curren's Math for Meds*, eleventh edition.

Refresher math is limited to the essentials needed. Metric and other dosage measures are succinct yet complete; hundreds of dosage label and syringe calibration photos are incorporated into clinically realistic calculations. The more advanced calculations are properly positioned to build on basic calculation skills as instruction moves to its logical completion.

The format and content of *Curren's Math for Meds* is not an accident. It is the result of the combined close working relationship between the author and educators over more than a 40-year period. More than a million students can attest to its effectiveness.

I thank you for choosing *Curren's Math for Meds*, eleventh edition, and invite you to evaluate its content and clarity. Suggestions from educators continue to be my most important revision tool; I solicit ongoing input from both educators and learners, sent care of Cengage Learning, in continuing to make future editions even more fitting to your needs.

Margaret Witt

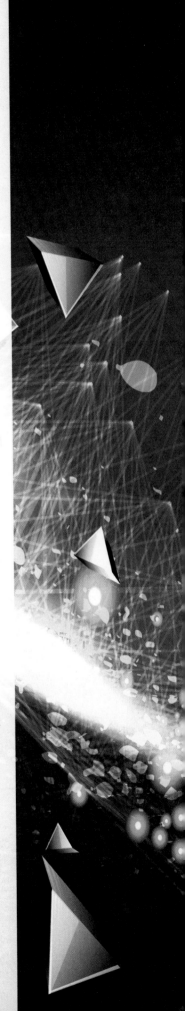

HONORARIUM

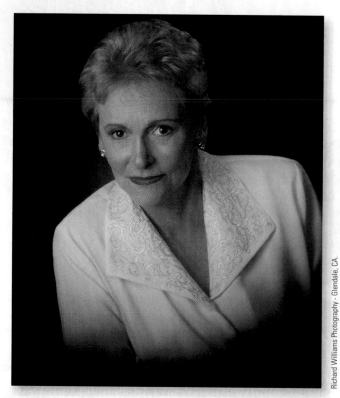

Richard Williams Photography - Glendale, CA.

Anna M. Curren, BN, MA

With this edition of *Curren's Math for Meds*, Cengage Learning honors **Anna M. Curren**'s 40 years of inspired authorship of her texts. By permanently identifying *Math for Meds* as "Curren's," Anna will experience what she calls her "*Gray's Anatomy* moment," referencing British author Henry Gray's 1858 authorship and ongoing identification with his first anatomy text.

Anna's authorship began when, as an Associate Professor of Nursing at Long Beach City College in California, she was assigned to teach from a programmed math text that bore no relationship to her students' clinical needs. Anna, who was pursuing an MA in Instructional Design, immediately enrolled in a Programmed Instruction course and began to write her own clinically focused text. Testing her text step by step with her students resulted in an immediate and dramatic improvement in her students' clinical math skills. At her students' insistence, Anna decided to submit her text to a national publisher. Undeterred by the rejection of her manuscript, and already recognizing the need for vital instructional products for injection skill training, Anna began exploring both self-publication of her text as well as production possibilities for these products.

The result was Anna's founding, in 1972, of **Wallcur, Inc.**, now known throughout North America for its outstanding line of **Practi-Products**. Anna named her company Wallcur to honor her father, **Wall**ace **Cur**ren, whose financial gift made her entrepreneurship possible. In its first year Wallcur introduced **Injecta-Pad** and **Practi-Amp**, shortly followed by Anna's first edition of *Math for Meds*. In a few short years, *Math for Meds* not only became the most adopted programmed text in its subject area, but the definitive content and format guide now adopted by many other authors in this subject area. Under Anna's direction, Wallcur enlarged its line of instructional products to include **Practi-Insulin Training Pack**, **Practi-Vial**, **Practi-Powder Vial**, **Practi-Mini Vial**, and **Practi-Oral Med Pack**.

In 1998 Anna authored her second dosage calculations text, *Dimensional Analysis for Meds,* in which she introduced a simplified formula for the units conversion calculations method used in the physical sciences, which has also now been adopted by other authors in this subject area.

In 2000 Anna moved her authorship of both texts to Cengage Learning. At the same time, to ensure the future availability of Wallcur's essential nursing skill products, Anna gifted the product line of her company to a nurse educator who had helped her build the company during the late '80s and '90s. In doing so, she secured the availability of her vital instructional products for several decades.

Anna, a proud native of St. John's, Newfoundland, became a U.S. citizen in 1970. She lives in San Diego, California. She wishes to take this final opportunity to thank the many students and instructors who have contacted her with suggestions and feedback throughout her career.

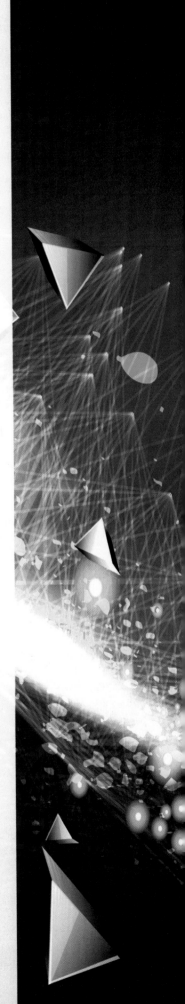

REFRESHER MATH PRETEST

If you can complete the Pretest with 100% accuracy, you are off to an exceptional start. However, don't be alarmed if you make some errors because the Refresher Math section that follows is designed to bring your math skills up to date. **Regardless of your proficiency, it's important that you complete the entire Refresher Math section.** It includes memory cues and shortcuts for simplifying and solving many of the clinical calculations that are included in the entire text, and you will need to be familiar with these.

Identify the decimal fraction with the greatest value in each set.

1. a) 4.4   b) 2.85   c) 5.3   _____
2. a) 6.3   b) 5.73   c) 4.4   _____
3. a) 0.18   b) 0.62   c) 0.35   _____
4. a) 0.2   b) 0.125   c) 0.3   _____
5. a) 0.15   b) 0.11   c) 0.14   _____
6. a) 4.27   b) 4.31   c) 4.09   _____

Add these decimals.

7. $0.2 + 2.23 =$ _____
8. $1.5 + 0.07 =$ _____
9. $6.45 + 12.1 + 9.54 =$ _____
10. $0.35 + 8.37 + 5.15 =$ _____

Subtract these decimals.

11. $3.1 - 0.67 =$ _____
12. $12.41 - 2.11 =$ _____
13. $2.235 - 0.094 =$ _____
14. $4.65 - 0.7 =$ _____
15. If tablets with a strength of 0.2 mg are available and 0.6 mg is ordered, how many tablets must you give? _____
16. If tablets are labeled 0.8 mg and 0.4 mg is ordered, how many tablets must you give? _____
17. If the available tablets have a strength of 1.25 mg and 2.5 mg is ordered, how many tablets must you give? _____
18. If 0.125 mg is ordered and the tablets available are labeled 0.25 mg, how many tablets must you give? _____

Express these to the nearest tenth.

19. $2.17 =$ _____
20. $0.15 =$ _____
21. $3.77 =$ _____
22. $4.62 =$ _____
23. $11.74 =$ _____
24. $5.26 =$ _____

Express these to the nearest hundredth.

25. $1.357 =$ _____
26. $7.413 =$ _____
27. $10.105 =$ _____
28. $3.775 =$ _____
29. $0.176 =$ _____
30. Define "product." _____

Multiply these decimals. Express your answers to the nearest tenth.

31. $0.7 \times 1.2 =$ _____
32. $1.8 \times 2.6 =$ _____
33. $5.1 \times 0.25 \times 1.1 =$ _____
34. $3.3 \times 3.75 =$ _____

Divide these fractions. Express your answers to the nearest hundredth.

35. $16.3 \div 3.2 =$ _____
36. $15.1 \div 1.1 =$ _____
37. $2 \div 0.75 =$ _____
38. $4.17 \div 2.7 =$ _____
39. Define "numerator."
_____
_____
40. Define "denominator."
_____
_____
41. Define "highest common denominator."
_____
_____

Solve these equations. Express your answers to the nearest tenth.

42. $\dfrac{1}{4} \times \dfrac{2}{3} =$ _____
43. $\dfrac{240}{170} \times \dfrac{135}{300} =$ _____
44. $\dfrac{0.2}{1.75} \times \dfrac{1.5}{0.2} =$ _____
45. $\dfrac{2.1}{3.6} \times \dfrac{1.7}{1.3} =$ _____
46. $\dfrac{0.26}{0.2} \times \dfrac{3.3}{1.2} =$ _____
47. $\dfrac{750}{1} \times \dfrac{300}{50} \times \dfrac{7}{2} =$ _____
48. $\dfrac{50}{1} \times \dfrac{60}{240} \times \dfrac{1}{900} \times \dfrac{400}{1} =$ _____
49. $\dfrac{35,000}{750} \times \dfrac{35}{1} =$ _____
50. $\dfrac{50}{40} \times \dfrac{450}{40} \times \dfrac{1}{900} \times \dfrac{114}{1} =$ _____

Answers

1. c
2. a
3. b
4. c
5. a
6. b
7. 2.43
8. 1.57
9. 28.09
10. 13.87
11. 2.43
12. 10.3
13. 2.141
14. 3.95
15. 3 tab
16. 1/2 tab
17. 2 tab
18. 1/2 tab
19. 2.2
20. 0.2
21. 3.8
22. 4.6
23. 11.7
24. 5.3
25. 1.36
26. 7.41
27. 10.11
28. 3.78
29. 0.18
30. The answer obtained from multiplication of two or more numbers
31. 0.8
32. 4.7
33. 1.4
34. 12.4
35. 5.09
36. 13.73
37. 2.67
38. 1.54
39. The top number in a common fraction
40. The bottom number in a common fraction
41. The greatest number that can be divided into two numbers to reduce them to their lowest terms (values)
42. 0.2
43. 0.6
44. 0.9
45. 0.8
46. 3.6
47. 15,750
48. 5.6
49. 1633.3
50. 1.8

SECTION

1

Refresher Math

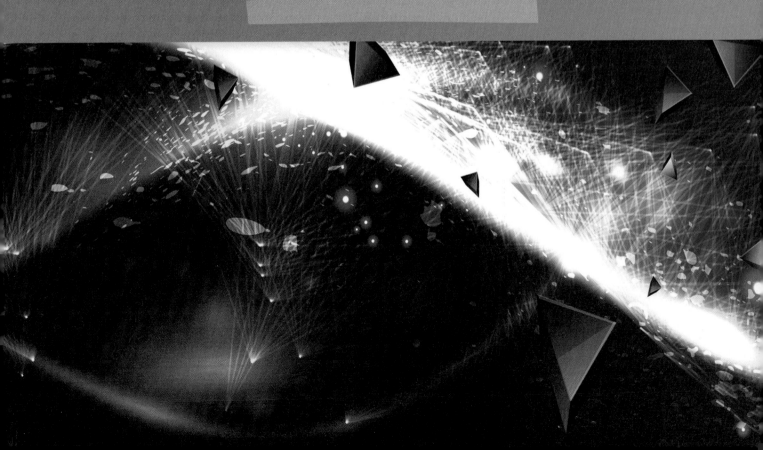

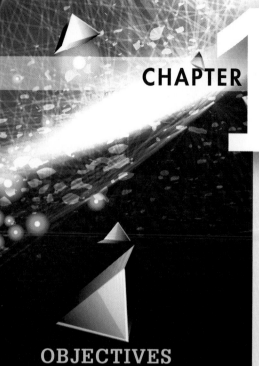

CHAPTER 1

RELATIVE VALUE, ADDITION, AND SUBTRACTION OF DECIMALS

OBJECTIVES

The learner will:

1. identify the relative value of decimals.

2. add decimals.

3. subtract decimals.

PREREQUISITES

Recognize the abbreviations mg, for milligram, and g, for gram, as drug measures.

In the course of administering medications, you will be dealing with decimal fraction dosages on a daily basis. The first two chapters of this text provide a complete refresher on everything you need to know about decimals, including safety measures when you do calculations both manually and with a calculator. We'll start with a review of the range of decimal values you will see in dosages. This will enable you to recognize which of two or more numbers has the greater (or lesser) value–a skill you will use constantly in your professional career.

RELATIVE VALUE OF DECIMALS

The most helpful fact to remember about decimals is that **our monetary system of dollars and cents is a decimal system**. The whole numbers in dosages have the same relative value as dollars, and decimal fractions have the same value as cents: **the greater the number, the greater the value**. If you keep this in mind, you will have already learned the most important safety measure of dealing with decimals in dosages.

The range of drug dosages, which includes decimal fractions, stretches from millions on the whole number side, to thousandths on the decimal side. Refer to the decimal scale in Figure 1-1, and locate the decimal point, which is slightly to the right on this scale. Notice the whole numbers on the left of the scale, which rise increasingly in value from ones (units) to millions, which is the largest whole-number drug dosage in current use.

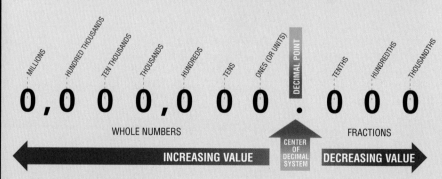

▲ FIGURE 1-1

KEY *point:* The first determiner of the relative value of decimals is the presence of whole numbers. The greater the whole number, the greater the value.

EXAMPLE 1 ▶	10.1 is greater than 9.15
EXAMPLE 2 ▶	3.2 is greater than 2.99
EXAMPLE 3 ▶	7.01 is greater than 6.99

▶▶▶ PROBLEMS 1.1

Choose the greatest value in each set.

1. a) 3.5	b) 2.7	c) 4.2	_____
2. a) 6.15	b) 5.95	c) 4.54	_____
3. a) 12.02	b) 10.19	c) 11.04	_____
4. a) 2.5	b) 1.75	c) 0.75	_____
5. a) 4.3	b) 2.75	c) 5.1	_____
6. a) 6.15	b) 7.4	c) 5.95	_____
7. a) 7.25	b) 8.1	c) 9.37	_____
8. a) 4.25	b) 5.1	c) 3.75	_____
9. a) 9.4	b) 8.75	c) 7.4	_____
10. a) 5.1	b) 6.33	c) 4.2	_____

Answers 1. c **2.** a **3.** a **4.** a **5.** c **6.** b **7.** c **8.** b **9.** a **10.** b

If, however, the whole numbers are the same—for example, **10**.2 and **10**.7—or there are no whole numbers—for example, **0**.25 and **0**.35—**then the fraction will determine the relative value**. Let's take a closer look at the fractional side of the scale (refer to Figure 1-2).

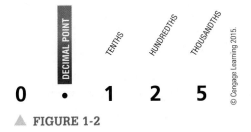

▲ **FIGURE 1-2**

It is necessary to **consider only three figures after the decimal point on the fractional side**, because drug dosages measured as decimal fractions do not contain more than three digits; for example, 0.125 mg. Notice that a **zero is used to replace the whole number** in this decimal fraction and in all dosages that do not contain a whole number.

 KEY *point:* If a decimal fraction is not preceded by a whole number, a zero is used in front of the decimal point to emphasize that the number is a fraction.

EXAMPLE   0.125   0.1   0.45

Look again at Figure 1-2. The numbers to the right of the decimal point represent **tenths**, **hundredths**, and **thousandths**, in that order. When you see a decimal fraction in which the **whole numbers are the same**, or there are **no whole numbers**, stop and look first at the number representing **tenths**.

 KEYpoint: The fraction with the greater number representing tenths has the greater value.

EXAMPLE 1   0.3 is greater than 0.27

EXAMPLE 2   0.4 is greater than 0.29

EXAMPLE 3   1.2 is greater than 1.19

EXAMPLE 4   3.5 is greater than 3.2

▶▶▶ PROBLEMS 1.2

Choose the greatest value in each set.

1. a) 0.4   b) 0.2   c) 0.5   _____
2. a) 2.73   b) 2.61   c) 2.87   _____
3. a) 0.19   b) 0.61   c) 0.34   _____
4. a) 3.5   b) 3.75   c) 3.25   _____
5. a) 0.3   b) 0.25   c) 0.4   _____
6. a) 1.35   b) 1.29   c) 1.4   _____
7. a) 2.5   b) 2.7   c) 2.35   _____
8. a) 4.51   b) 4.75   c) 4.8   _____
9. a) 0.8   b) 0.3   c) 0.4   _____
10. a) 2.1   b) 2.05   c) 2.15   _____

Answers **1.** c.   **2.** c   **3.** b   **4.** b   **5.** c   **6.** c   **7.** b   **8.** c   **9.** a   **10.** c

If in decimal fractions the numbers representing **the tenths are identical**—for example, 0.25 and 0.27—then **the number representing the hundredths will determine the relative value**.

 KEYpoint: When the tenths are identical, the fraction with the greater number representing hundredths will have the greater value.

EXAMPLE 1   0.2**7** is greater than 0.2**5**

EXAMPLE 2   0.1**5** is greater than 0.1 (0.1 is the same as 0.1**0**)

KEY *point:* Extra zeros on the end of decimal fractions are omitted in drug dosages because they can easily be misread and lead to errors.

EXAMPLE 1   2.25 is greater than 2.2 (same as 2.20)

EXAMPLE 2   9.77 is greater than 9.7 (same as 9.70)

▶▶▶ PROBLEMS 1.3

Choose the greatest value in each set.

1. a) 0.12	b) 0.15	c) 0.17	_____
2. a) 1.2	b) 1.24	c) 1.23	_____
3. a) 0.37	b) 0.3	c) 0.36	_____
4. a) 3.27	b) 3.25	c) 3.21	_____
5. a) 0.16	b) 0.11	c) 0.19	_____
6. a) 4.23	b) 4.2	c) 4.09	_____
7. a) 3.27	b) 3.21	c) 3.29	_____
8. a) 2.75	b) 2.73	c) 2.78	_____
9. a) 0.31	b) 0.37	c) 0.33	_____
10. a) 0.43	b) 0.45	c) 0.44	_____

Answers   **1.** c   **2.** b   **3.** a   **4.** a   **5.** c   **6.** a   **7.** c   **8.** c   **9.** b   **10.** b

▶▶▶ PROBLEMS 1.4

Which fraction has the greater value?

a) 0.125   b) 0.25

Answers   If you chose 0.125, you have just made a serious drug dosage error. Look again at the numbers representing the tenths, and you will see that 0.**2**5 is greater than 0.**1**25. Remember that extra zeros are omitted in decimal fraction dosages because they can lead to errors. In this fraction, 0.25 is the same as 0.250, which is exactly double the value of 0.125. **Check the tenths carefully, regardless of the total of numbers after the decimal point.**

EXAMPLE 1   0.15 (same as 0.150) is greater than 0.125

EXAMPLE 2   0.3 (same as 0.30) is greater than 0.15

EXAMPLE 3   0.75 (same as 0.750) is greater than 0.325

EXAMPLE 4   0.8 (same as 0.80) is greater than 0.16

KEY_point:_ The number of figures on the right of the decimal point is not an indication of relative value. Always look at the figure representing the tenths first, and if these are identical, check the hundredths to determine which has the greater value.

This completes your introduction to the relative value of decimals. The key points just reviewed will cover all situations in dosage calculations in which you will have to recognize greater and lesser values. Test yourself more extensively on this information in the following problems.

▶▶▶ PROBLEMS 1.5

Choose the greatest value in each set.

1. a) 0.24	b) 0.5	c) 0.125	_____
2. a) 0.4	b) 0.45	c) 0.5	_____
3. a) 7.5	b) 6.25	c) 4.75	_____
4. a) 0.3	b) 0.25	c) 0.35	_____
5. a) 1.125	b) 1.75	c) 1.5	_____
6. a) 4.5	b) 4.75	c) 4.25	_____
7. a) 0.1	b) 0.01	c) 0.04	_____
8. a) 5.75	b) 6.25	c) 6.5	_____
9. a) 0.6	b) 0.16	c) 0.06	_____
10. a) 3.55	b) 2.95	c) 3.7	_____

Answers **1.** b **2.** c **3.** a **4.** c **5.** b **6.** b **7.** a **8.** c **9.** a **10.** c

ADDITION AND SUBTRACTION OF DECIMALS

Complex addition and subtraction of decimals should be done with a calculator, but, on occasion, time can be saved by doing simple calculations without one. Let's start by looking at a few key points that will make manual solution safer.

 KEY_point:_ When you write down the numbers, line up the decimal points.

EXAMPLE   To add 0.25 and 0.27

0.25
+0.27 is safe

0.25
+0.27 is unsafe; it could lead to errors.

 KEY_point:_ Always add or subtract from right to left.

If you decide to write down the numbers, **do not confuse yourself by trying to "eyeball" the answer**. Also, write any numbers carried or rewrite those reduced by borrowing if you find this helpful.

EXAMPLE 1 When adding 0.25 and 0.27

$$
\begin{array}{r}
1 \\
0.25 \\
+\ 0.27 \\
\hline
0.52
\end{array}
$$

Add the 5 and 7 first, then the 2, 2, and the 1 you carried; work from right to left

EXAMPLE 2 When subtracting 0.63 from 0.71

$$
\begin{array}{r}
61 \\
0.71 \\
-\ 0.63 \\
\hline
0.08
\end{array}
$$

Borrow 1 from 7 and rewrite as 6
Write the borrowed 1; subtract 3 from 11
Subtract 6 from 6; work from right to left

 KEYpoint: Add zeros as necessary to make the fractions of equal length.

Adding zeros to make the fractions of equal length does not alter the value of the fractions, and it helps prevent confusion and mistakes.

EXAMPLE When subtracting 0.125 from 0.25

$$
\begin{array}{lll}
0.25 & \text{becomes} & 0.250 \\
-\ 0.125 & \text{becomes} & -\ 0.125
\end{array}
$$

Answer = **0.125**

If you follow these simple rules and make them a habit, you will automatically reduce calculation errors. The following problems will give you an excellent opportunity to practice addition and subtraction.

▶▶▶ PROBLEMS 1.6

Add decimals.

1. $0.25 + 0.55 =$ _____

2. $0.1 + 2.25 \ \ =$ _____

3. $1.74 + 0.76 =$ _____

4. $1.4 + 0.02 \ \ =$ _____

5. $2.3 + 1.45 \ \ =$ _____

6. $3.75 + 1.05 =$ _____

7. $6.35 + 2.05 =$ _____

8. $5.57 + 4.03 =$ _____

9. $0.33 + 2.42 =$ _____

10. $1.44 + 3.06 =$ _____

Subtract decimals.

11. $1.25 - 1.125 =$ _____

12. $3.25 - 0.65 \;\;\; =$ _____

13. $2.3 - 1.45 \;\;\;\; =$ _____

14. $0.02 - 0.01 \;\; =$ _____

15. $5.5 - 2.5 \;\;\;\;\; =$ _____

16. $7.33 - 4.03 \;\; =$ _____

17. $4.25 - 1.75 \;\; =$ _____

18. $0.07 - 0.035 =$ _____

19. $0.235 - 0.12 =$ _____

20. $5.75 - 0.95 \;\; =$ _____

Answers 1. 0.8 **2.** 2.35 **3.** 2.5 **4.** 1.42 **5.** 3.75 **6.** 4.8 **7.** 8.4 **8.** 9.6 **9.** 2.75 **10.** 4.5
11. 0.125 **12.** 2.6 **13.** 0.85 **14.** 0.01 **15.** 3 **16.** 3.3 **17.** 2.5 **18.** 0.035 **19.** 0.115 **20.** 4.8

Note: If you did not add a zero before the decimal point in answers that do not contain a whole number, or failed to eliminate
unnecessary zeros from the end of decimal fractions, your answers are incorrect.

Summary

This concludes the refresher on relative value, addition, and subtraction of simple decimal fractions. The important points to remember from this chapter are:

▼ If a decimal fraction contains a whole number, the value of the whole number is the first determiner of relative value.

▼ If a fraction does not include a whole number, a zero is placed in front of the decimal point to emphasize that it is a fractional dosage.

▼ If there is no whole number, or if the whole numbers are the same, the number representing the tenths in the decimal fraction will be the next determiner of relative value.

▼ If the tenths in decimal fractions are identical, the number representing hundredths will determine relative value.

▼ When manually adding or subtracting decimal fractions, first line up the decimal points, then add or subtract from right to left.

▼ Extra zeros on the end of decimal fractions can be a source of error in drug dosages, and are routinely eliminated.

Summary Self-Test

Choose the decimal with the greatest value.

1. a) 2.45   b) 2.57   c) 2.19   _____

2. a) 3.07   b) 3.17   c) 3.71   _____

3. a) 0.12   b) 0.02   c) 0.01   _____

4. a) 5.31   b) 5.35   c) 6.01   _____

5. a) 4.5   b) 4.51   c) 4.15   _____

6. a) 0.015   b) 0.15   c) 0.1   _____

7. a) 1.3   b) 1.25   c) 1.35   _____

8. a) 0.1   b) 0.2   c) 0.25   _____

9. a) 0.125   b) 0.1   c) 0.05   _____

10. a) 13.7   b) 13.5   c) 13.25   _____

Use critical thinking to choose the best answer.

11. If you have medication tablets whose strength is 0.1 mg and you must give 0.3 mg, you will need

    a) 1 tab.   b) less than 1 tab.   c) more than 1 tab.   _____

12. If you have tablets with a strength of 0.25 mg and you must give 0.125 mg, you will need

    a) 1 tab.   b) less than 1 tab.   c) more than 1 tab.   _____

13. If you have an order to give a dosage of 7.5 mg and the tablets have a strength of 3.75 mg, you will need

    a) 1 tab.   b) less than 1 tab.   c) more than 1 tab.   _____

14. If the order is to give 0.5 mg and the tablet strength is 0.5 mg, you will give

    a) 1 tab.   b) less than 1 tab.   c) more than 1 tab.   _____

15. The order is to give 0.5 mg and the tablets have a strength of 0.25 mg. You must give

    a) 1 tab.   b) less than 1 tab.   c) more than 1 tab.   _____

Add the decimals manually.

16. 1.31 + 0.4 = _____   20. 1.3 + 1.04 = _____

17. 0.15 + 0.25 = _____   21. 4.7 + 3.03 = _____

18. 2.5 + 0.75 = _____   22. 0.5 + 0.5 = _____

19. 3.2 + 2.17 = _____   23. 5.4 + 2.6 = _____

Use critical thinking to answer the following.

24. You have just given 2 tab with a dosage strength of 3.5 mg each. What was the total dosage administered?   _____

25. You are to give your patient 1 tab labeled 0.5 mg and one labeled 0.25 mg. What is the total dosage of these two tablets?   _____

26. If you give 2 tab labeled 0.02 mg, what total dosage will you administer?   _____

27. You are to give 1 tab labeled 0.8 mg and 2 tab labeled 0.4 mg. What is the total dosage?   _____

28. You have two tablets: one is labeled 0.15 mg and the other 0.3 mg. What is the total dosage of these two tablets?   _____

Subtract the decimals manually.

29. 4.32 − 3.1 = _____   33. 1.3 − 0.02 = _____

30. 2.1 − 1.91 = _____   34. 0.2 − 0.07 = _____

31. 3.73 − 1.93 = _____   35. 3.95 − 0.35 = _____

32. 5.75 − 4.05 = _____   36. 1.9 − 0.08 = _____

Use critical thinking to answer the following.

37. Your patient is to receive a dosage of 7.5 mg and you have only 1 tab labeled 3.75 mg. How many more milligrams must you give? _____

38. You have a tablet labeled 0.02 mg and your patient is to receive 0.06 mg. How many more milligrams must you give? _____

39. The tablet available is labeled 0.5 mg, but you must give a dosage of 1.5 mg. How many more milligrams will you need to obtain the correct dosage? _____

40. Your patient is to receive a dosage of 1.2 mg and you have 1 tab labeled 0.6 mg. What additional dosage in milligrams will you need? _____

41. You must give your patient a dosage of 2.2 mg, but you have only 2 tab labeled 0.55 mg. What additional dosage in milligrams will you need? _____

Determine how many tablets will be needed to give the dosages.

42. Tablets are labeled 0.01 mg. You must give 0.02 mg. _____

43. Tablets are labeled 2.5 mg. You must give 5 mg. _____

44. Tablets are labeled 0.25 mg. Give 0.125 mg. _____

45. Tablets are 0.5 mg. Give 1.5 mg. _____

46. A dosage of 1.8 mg is ordered. Tablets are 0.6 mg. _____

47. Tablets available are 0.04 mg. You are to give 0.02 mg. _____

48. The dosage ordered is 3.5 mg. The tablets available are 1.75 mg. _____

49. Prepare a dosage of 3.2 mg using tablets with a strength of 1.6 mg. _____

50. You have tablets labeled 0.25 mg and a dosage of 0.375 mg is ordered. _____

Answers	11. c	22. 1	33. 1.28	44. ½ tab
1. b	12. b	23. 8	34. 0.13	45. 3 tab
2. c	13. c	24. 7 mg	35. 3.6	46. 3 tab
3. a	14. a	25. 0.75 mg	36. 1.82	47. ½ tab
4. c	15. c	26. 0.04 mg	37. 3.75 mg	48. 2 tab
5. b	16. 1.71	27. 1.6 mg	38. 0.04 mg	49. 2 tab
6. b	17. 0.4	28. 0.45 mg	39. 1 mg	50. 1½ tab
7. c	18. 3.25	29. 1.22	40. 0.6 mg	
8. c	19. 5.37	30. 0.19	41. 1.1 mg	
9. a	20. 2.34	31. 1.8	42. 2 tab	
10. a	21. 7.73	32. 1.7	43. 2 tab	

Note: If you did not add a zero before the decimal point in answers that did not contain a whole number, or failed to eliminate unnecessary zeros from the end of decimal fractions, your answers are incorrect.

CHAPTER 2

MULTIPLICATION AND DIVISION OF DECIMALS

Multiplication and division are integral parts of dosage calculations. As is the case with addition and subtraction, some multiplication and division problems involving dosages can be done manually, so the basic steps in multiplication and division are reviewed in this chapter. In addition, a number of shortcuts will be introduced that can make numbers easier to work with, especially those containing decimal fractions. And for those calculations that are more safely handled with a calculator, safety in calculator use will be discussed.

MULTIPLICATION OF DECIMALS

The main precaution in multiplication of decimals is the **placement of the decimal point in the answer**, which is called the **product**.

 KEY*point:* The decimal point in the product of decimal fractions is placed the same number of places to the left in the product as the total of numbers following the decimal points in the fractions multiplied.

EXAMPLE 1   Multiply 0.35 by 0.5

It is safer to begin by lining up the numbers to be multiplied on the right side. Then, disregard the decimals during multiplication.

$$\begin{array}{r} 0.35 \\ \times\ 0.5 \\ \hline 175 \end{array}$$

The product/answer is 175; 0.35 has two numbers after the decimal and 0.5 has one. Place the decimal point three places to the left in the product to make it .175, then add a zero (0) in front of the decimal to emphasize the fraction.

$$\text{Answer} = \mathbf{0.175}$$

OBJECTIVES

The learner will:

1. define product, numerator, and denominator.
2. multiply decimal fractions.
3. divide decimal fractions.
4. simplify common fractions containing decimal numbers.
5. reduce fractions using common denominators.
6. reduce common fractions that end in zeros.
7. express answers to the nearest tenth and hundredth.
8. use a calculator to multiply and divide.

PREREQUISITE

Chapter 1

EXAMPLE 2 ▸   Multiply 1.61 by 0.2

$$
\begin{array}{r}
1.61 \\
\times\ \ 0.2 \\
\hline
322
\end{array}
$$
     Line up the numbers on the right

The product is 322; 1.61 has two numbers after the decimal point and 0.2 has one. Place the decimal point three places to the left in the product so that 322 becomes .322, then add a zero in front of the decimal to emphasize the fraction.

Answer = **0.322**

 KEY_point:_ If the product contains insufficient numbers for correct placement of the decimal point, add as many zeros as necessary to the left of the product to correct this.

EXAMPLE 3 ▸   Multiply 1.5 by 0.06

$$
\begin{array}{r}
1.5 \\
\times\ 0.06 \\
\hline
90
\end{array}
$$
     Line up the numbers on the right

The product is 90; 1.5 has one number after the decimal point and 0.06 has two. To place the decimal three places to the left in the product, a zero must be added, making it .090. Eliminate the excess zero from the end of the fraction, and add a zero in front of the decimal point.

Answer = **0.09**

EXAMPLE 4 ▸   Multiply 0.21 by 0.32

$$
\begin{array}{r}
0.21 \\
\times\ 0.32 \\
\hline
42\ \ \\
63\ \ \ \\
\hline
672\ \ \\
\end{array}
$$
     Indent second number multiplication
     Add the totals

In this example, 0.21 has two numbers after the decimal point and 0.32 also has two. Add a zero in front of 672 to allow correct placement of the decimal point, making it .0672, then add a zero in front of the fraction to emphasize it.

Answer = **0.0672**

EXAMPLE 5 ▸   Multiply 0.12 by 0.2

$$
\begin{array}{r}
0.12 \\
\times\ \ 0.2 \\
\hline
24
\end{array}
$$

In this example, there are a total of three numbers after the decimal points in 0.12 and 0.2. Add a zero in front of 24 for correct decimal placement, making it .024, then add a zero in front of .024 to emphasize the fraction.

Answer = **0.024**

▶▶▶ PROBLEMS 2.1

Multiply the decimal fractions without using a calculator.

1. 0.45 × 0.2 = _____

2. 0.35 × 0.12 = _____

3. 1.3 × 0.05 = _____

4. 0.7 × 0.04 = _____

5. 0.4 × 0.17 = _____

6. 2.14 × 0.03 = _____

7. 1.4 × 0.4 = _____

8. 3.3 × 1.2 = _____

9. 2.7 × 2.2 = _____

10. 2.1 × 0.3 = _____

Answers 1. 0.09 **2.** 0.042 **3.** 0.065 **4.** 0.028 **5.** 0.068 **6.** 0.0642 **7.** 0.56 **8.** 3.96
9. 5.94 **10.** 0.63

DIVISION OF DECIMAL FRACTIONS

A calculator may also be used for division of complex decimal fractions. However, let's start by reviewing the terminology of common fraction division, and **three important precalculator** steps that may make final manual division easier: **elimination of decimal points, reduction of the fractions**, and **reduction of numbers ending in zero**. The following is a sample of a common fraction division seen in dosages.

EXAMPLE 1 ▶ $\dfrac{0.25}{0.125} = \dfrac{\text{numerator}}{\text{denominator}}$

You'll recall that the **top number** in a common fraction is called the **numerator**, whereas the **bottom number** is called the **denominator**. If you have trouble remembering which is which, think of **D**, for **down**, for **denominator**. The denominator is on the bottom. With this basic terminology reviewed, we are now ready to look at preliminary math steps that can be used to simplify a fraction or actually solve an equation and eliminate the need for calculator division.

ELIMINATION OF DECIMAL POINTS

Decimal points can be eliminated from numbers in a decimal fraction without changing its value, if they are moved the same number of places in one numerator and one denominator.

KEY*point:* To eliminate the decimal points from decimal fractions, move them the same number of places to the right in a numerator and a denominator until they are eliminated from both. Zeros may have to be added to accomplish this.

EXAMPLE 1 ▶ $\dfrac{0.25}{0.125}$ becomes $\dfrac{250}{125}$

The decimal point must be moved three places to the right in the denominator 0.125 to make it 125. Therefore, it must be moved three places to the right in the numerator 0.25, which requires the addition of one zero to make it 250.

EXAMPLE 2 $\dfrac{0.3}{0.15}$ becomes $\dfrac{30}{15}$

The decimal point must be moved two places in 0.15 to make it 15, so it must be moved two places in 0.3, which requires the addition of one zero to become 30.

EXAMPLE 3 $\dfrac{1.5}{2}$ becomes $\dfrac{15}{20}$

Move the decimal point one place in 1.5 to make it 15; add one zero to 2 to make it 20.

EXAMPLE 4 $\dfrac{4.5}{0.95}$ becomes $\dfrac{450}{95}$

 KEYpoint: Eliminating the decimal points from a decimal fraction before final division does not alter the value of the fraction, or the answer obtained in the final division.

▶▶▶ PROBLEMS 2.2

Eliminate the decimal points from these common fractions.

1. $\dfrac{17.5}{2}$ = _____

2. $\dfrac{0.5}{25}$ = _____

3. $\dfrac{6.3}{0.6}$ = _____

4. $\dfrac{3.76}{0.4}$ = _____

5. $\dfrac{8.4}{0.7}$ = _____

6. $\dfrac{0.1}{0.05}$ = _____

7. $\dfrac{0.9}{0.03}$ = _____

8. $\dfrac{10.75}{2.5}$ = _____

9. $\dfrac{0.4}{0.04}$ = _____

10. $\dfrac{1.2}{0.4}$ = _____

Answers 1. $\dfrac{175}{20}$ 2. $\dfrac{5}{250}$ 3. $\dfrac{63}{6}$ 4. $\dfrac{376}{40}$ 5. $\dfrac{84}{7}$ 6. $\dfrac{10}{5}$ 7. $\dfrac{90}{3}$ 8. $\dfrac{1075}{250}$ 9. $\dfrac{40}{4}$ 10. $\dfrac{12}{4}$

REDUCTION OF FRACTIONS

Once the decimals are eliminated, a second simplification step is to reduce the numbers as far as possible using common denominators/divisors, the largest number that will divide both a numerator and a denominator.

 KEYpoint: To further reduce fractions, divide numbers by their greatest common denominator (the largest number that will divide into both a numerator and a denominator).

The **greatest common denominator** is usually **2, 3, 4, 5, or multiples of these numbers**, such as 6, 8, 25, and so on.

EXAMPLE 1 $\dfrac{175}{20}$ The greatest common denominator is 5

$$\dfrac{\cancel{175}}{\cancel{20}} = \dfrac{35}{4}$$

EXAMPLE 2 $\dfrac{63}{6}$ The greatest common denominator is 3

$$\dfrac{\cancel{63}}{\cancel{6}} = \dfrac{21}{2}$$

EXAMPLE 3 $\dfrac{1075}{250}$ The greatest common denominator is 25

$$\dfrac{\cancel{1075}}{\cancel{250}} = \dfrac{43}{10}$$

There is a second way you could have reduced the fraction in Example 3, and it is equally as correct. Divide by 5, then by 5 again.

$$\dfrac{\cancel{1075}}{\cancel{250}} = \dfrac{\cancel{215}}{\cancel{50}} = \dfrac{43}{10}$$

 KEY*point:*   If the greatest common denominator is difficult to determine, reduce several times by using smaller common denominators.

EXAMPLE 4 $\dfrac{376}{40} = \dfrac{47}{5}$ Divide by 8

Or divide by 4, then 2 $\dfrac{\cancel{376}}{\cancel{40}} = \dfrac{\cancel{94}}{\cancel{10}} = \dfrac{47}{5}$

Or divide by 2, then 2, then 2 $\dfrac{\cancel{376}}{\cancel{40}} = \dfrac{\cancel{188}}{\cancel{20}} = \dfrac{\cancel{94}}{\cancel{10}} = \dfrac{47}{5}$

Remember that **simple numbers are easiest to work with**, and the time spent in extra reductions may be well worth the payoff in safety.

▶▶▶ PROBLEMS 2.3

Reduce the fractions in preparation for final division.

1. $\dfrac{84}{8}$ = _____

2. $\dfrac{20}{16}$ = _____

3. $\dfrac{250}{325}$ = _____

4. $\dfrac{96}{34}$ = _____

5. $\dfrac{175}{20}$ = _____

6. $\dfrac{40}{14}$ = _____

7. $\dfrac{82}{28}$ = _____

8. $\dfrac{100}{75}$ = _____

9. $\dfrac{50}{75}$ = _____

10. $\dfrac{60}{88}$ = _____

Answers **1.** $\dfrac{21}{2}$ **2.** $\dfrac{5}{4}$ **3.** $\dfrac{10}{13}$ **4.** $\dfrac{48}{17}$ **5.** $\dfrac{35}{4}$ **6.** $\dfrac{20}{7}$ **7.** $\dfrac{41}{14}$ **8.** $\dfrac{4}{3}$ **9.** $\dfrac{2}{3}$ **10.** $\dfrac{15}{22}$

REDUCTION OF NUMBERS ENDING IN ZERO

The third type of simplification is not solely related to decimal fractions but is best covered at this time. This concerns reductions in a common fraction when both a numerator and a denominator end with zeros.

 KEYpoint: Numbers that end in a zero or zeros may be reduced by crossing off the same number of zeros in both a numerator and a denominator.

EXAMPLE 1 ◧ $\dfrac{800}{250}$

In this fraction, the numerator, 800, has two zeros, but the denominator, 250, has one zero. The number of zeros crossed off must be the same in both numerator and denominator, so only one zero can be eliminated from each.

$$\frac{80\cancel{0}}{25\cancel{0}} = \frac{80}{25} \qquad \text{Reduce by 5} = \frac{16}{5}$$

EXAMPLE 2 ◧ $\dfrac{2400}{2000} = \dfrac{24}{20}$ Reduce by 4 $= \dfrac{6}{5}$

Two zeros can be eliminated from the denominator and the numerator in this fraction.

EXAMPLE 3 ◧ $\dfrac{15{,}000}{30{,}000} = \dfrac{15}{30}$ Reduce by 15 $= \dfrac{1}{2}$

In this fraction, three zeros can be eliminated.

PROBLEMS 2.4

Reduce the fractions to their lowest terms.

1. $\dfrac{50}{250}$ = _____

2. $\dfrac{120}{50}$ = _____

3. $\dfrac{2500}{1500}$ = _____

4. $\dfrac{1,000,000}{750,000}$ = _____

5. $\dfrac{800}{150}$ = _____

6. $\dfrac{110}{100}$ = _____

7. $\dfrac{200,000}{150,000}$ = _____

8. $\dfrac{1000}{800}$ = _____

9. $\dfrac{60}{40}$ = _____

10. $\dfrac{150}{200}$ = _____

Answers 1. $\dfrac{1}{5}$ 2. $\dfrac{12}{5}$ 3. $\dfrac{5}{3}$ 4. $\dfrac{4}{3}$ 5. $\dfrac{16}{3}$ 6. $\dfrac{11}{10}$ 7. $\dfrac{4}{3}$ 8. $\dfrac{5}{4}$ 9. $\dfrac{3}{2}$ 10. $\dfrac{3}{4}$

USING A CALCULATOR

Calculators vary in how addition, subtraction, division, and multiplication must be entered, and in the number of fractional numbers displayed after the decimal point. The first precaution in calculator use is to ensure you **know how to use the one available to you**. If you must do frequent calculations, it would be wise to buy and use your own. The next precaution—and this is critical—is to enter decimal numbers correctly, which includes **entering the decimal points**. This is not as easy to remember as it sounds, and this is a step where dosage calculation errors can occur.

 KEYpoint: Calculator entry errors tend to be repetitive, so visually check each entry before entering the next.

EXPRESSING TO THE NEAREST TENTH

When a fraction is reduced as much as possible, it is ready for final division. If necessary, this is done using a calculator to **divide the numerator by the denominator**. Dosage answers are most frequently rounded off and expressed as decimal fractions to the nearest tenth.

 KEYpoint: To express an answer to the nearest tenth, the division is carried to hundredths (two places after the decimal). When the number representing hundredths is 5 or larger, the number representing tenths is increased by one. If the number representing hundredths is less than 5, the number representing tenths remains unchanged.

EXAMPLE 1 $\dfrac{0.35}{0.4} = 0.35 \div 0.4 = 0.87$

Answer = **0.9**

The number representing hundredths is 7, so the number representing tenths is increased by one: 0.87 becomes 0.9.

EXAMPLE 2 ▶ $\dfrac{0.5}{0.3} = 0.5 \div 0.3 = 1.66 = \mathbf{1.7}$

The number representing hundredths, 6, is larger than 5, so 1.66 becomes 1.7.

EXAMPLE 3 ▶ $\dfrac{0.16}{0.3} = 0.53 = \mathbf{0.5}$

The number representing hundredths, 3, is less than 5, so the number representing tenths, 5, remains unchanged.

EXAMPLE 4 ▶ $\dfrac{0.2}{0.3} = 0.66 = \mathbf{0.7}$

EXAMPLE 5 ▶ An answer of 1.42 remains **1.4**

EXAMPLE 6 ▶ An answer of 1.86 becomes **1.9**

▶▶▶ PROBLEMS 2.5

Use a calculator to divide the common fractions. Express answers to the nearest tenth.

1. $\dfrac{5.1}{2.3} = $ _____

2. $\dfrac{0.9}{0.7} = $ _____

3. $\dfrac{3.7}{2} = $ _____

4. $\dfrac{6}{1.3} = $ _____

5. $\dfrac{1.5}{2.1} = $ _____

6. $\dfrac{2.7}{1.1} = $ _____

7. $\dfrac{4.2}{5} = $ _____

8. $\dfrac{0.5}{2.5} = $ _____

9. $\dfrac{5.2}{0.91} = $ _____

10. $\dfrac{2.4}{2.7} = $ _____

Answers 1. 2.2 2. 1.3 3. 1.9 4. 4.6 5. 0.7 6. 2.5 7. 0.8 8. 0.2 9. 5.7 10. 0.9

EXPRESSING TO THE NEAREST HUNDREDTH

Some drugs are administered in dosages carried to the nearest hundredth. This is common in pediatric dosages, and in drugs that alter a vital function of the body, for example, heart rate.

 KEY *point:* To express an answer to the nearest hundredth, the division is carried to thousandths (three places after the decimal point). When the number representing thousandths is 5 or larger, the number representing hundredths is increased by one.

| EXAMPLE 1 | 0.736 | becomes | **0.74** |

The number representing thousandths, 6, is larger than 5, so the number representing hundredths, 3, is increased by one to become 4.

| EXAMPLE 2 | 0.777 | becomes | **0.78** |

| EXAMPLE 3 | 0.373 | remains | **0.37** |

The number representing thousandths, 3, is less than 5, so the number representing hundredths, 7, remains unchanged.

| EXAMPLE 4 | 0.934 | remains | **0.93** |

▶▶▶ PROBLEMS 2.6

Express the numbers to the nearest hundredth.

1. 0.175 = _____

2. 0.344 = _____

3. 1.853 = _____

4. 0.306 = _____

5. 3.015 = _____

6. 2.154 = _____

7. 1.081 = _____

8. 1.327 = _____

9. 0.739 = _____

10. 0.733 = _____

11. 2.072 = _____

12. 0.089 = _____

Answers **1.** 0.18 **2.** 0.34 **3.** 1.85 **4.** 0.31 **5.** 3.02 **6.** 2.15 **7.** 1.08 **8.** 1.33 **9.** 0.74
10. 0.73 **11.** 2.07 **12.** 0.09

Summary

This concludes the chapter on multiplication and division of decimals. The important points to remember from this chapter are:

▼ When decimal fractions are multiplied manually, the decimal point is placed the same number of places to the left in the product as the total of numbers after the decimal points in the fractions multiplied.

▼ Zeros must be placed in front of a product if it contains insufficient numbers for the correct placement of the decimal point.

▼ Excess trailing zeros are eliminated in dosages.

▼ To simplify fractions for final division, the preliminary steps of eliminating decimal points, reducing the numbers by common denominators, and reducing numbers ending in zeros can be used.

▼ To express to tenths, increase the answer by one if the number representing the hundredths is 5 or larger.

▼ To express to hundredths, increase the answer by one if the number representing the thousandths is 5 or larger.

▼ Practice using a calculator until proficiency is achieved.

▼ All calculator entries and answers must be double-checked.

▼ Calculator running totals should be disregarded because they can cause confusion.

▼ A personal calculator is a must if frequent calculations are necessary.

Summary Self-Test

Multiply the decimals. A calculator may be used.

1. $1.49 \times 0.05 =$ _____

2. $0.15 \times 3.04 =$ _____

3. $0.025 \times 3.5 =$ _____

4. $0.55 \times 2.5 \ =$ _____

5. $1.31 \times 2.07 =$ _____

6. $5.3 \times 1.02 \ =$ _____

7. $0.35 \times 1.25 =$ _____

8. $4.32 \times 0.05 =$ _____

9. $0.2 \times 0.02 \ =$ _____

10. $0.4 \times 1.75 \ =$ _____

Use critical thinking to answer the following.

11. You are to administer 4 tab with a dosage strength of 0.04 mg each. What total dosage are you giving? _____

12. You have given 2½ (2.5) tab with a strength of 1.25 mg per tablet. What total dosage is this? _____

13. The tablets your patient is to receive are labeled 0.1 mg, and you are to give 3½ (3.5) tab. What total dosage is this? _____

14. You gave your patient 3 tab labeled 0.75 mg each, and he was to receive a total of 2.25 mg. Did he receive the correct dosage? _____

15. The tablets available for your patient are labeled 12.5 mg, and you are to give 4½ (4.5) tab. What total dosage will this be? _____

16. Your patient is to receive a dosage of 4.5 mg. The tablets available are labeled 3.5 mg, and there are 2½ tab in his medication drawer. Is this a correct dosage? _____

Divide the fractions. Express answers to the nearest tenth. A calculator may be used.

17. $\dfrac{1.3}{0.7}$ = _____

18. $\dfrac{1.9}{3.2}$ = _____

19. $\dfrac{32.5}{9}$ = _____

20. $\dfrac{0.04}{0.1}$ = _____

21. $\dfrac{1.45}{1.2}$ = _____

22. $\dfrac{250}{1000}$ = _____

23. $\dfrac{0.8}{0.09}$ = _____

24. $\dfrac{2,000,000}{1,500,000}$ = _____

25. $\dfrac{4.1}{2.05}$ = _____

26. $\dfrac{7.3}{12}$ = _____

27. $\dfrac{150,000}{120,000}$ = _____

28. $\dfrac{0.15}{0.08}$ = _____

29. $\dfrac{2700}{900}$ = _____

30. $\dfrac{0.25}{0.15}$ = _____

Divide the fractions. Express answers to the nearest hundredth. A calculator may be used.

31. $\dfrac{900}{1700}$ = _____

32. $\dfrac{0.125}{0.3}$ = _____

33. $\dfrac{1450}{1500}$ = _____

34. $\dfrac{65}{175}$ = _____

35. $\dfrac{0.6}{1.35}$ = _____

36. $\dfrac{0.04}{0.12}$ = _____

37. $\dfrac{750}{10,000}$ = _____

38. $\dfrac{0.65}{0.8}$ = _____

39. $\dfrac{3.01}{4.2}$ = _____

40. $\dfrac{4.5}{6.1}$ = _____

41. $\dfrac{0.13}{0.25}$ = _____

42. $\dfrac{0.25}{0.7}$ = _____

43. $\dfrac{3.3}{5.1}$ = _____

44. $\dfrac{0.19}{0.7}$ = _____

45. $\dfrac{1.1}{1.3}$ = _____

46. $\dfrac{3}{4.1}$ = _____

47. $\dfrac{62}{240}$ = _____

48. $\dfrac{280,000}{300,000}$ = _____

49. $\dfrac{115}{255}$ = _____

50. $\dfrac{10}{14.3}$ = _____

Answers					
	9. 0.004	18. 0.6	27. 1.3	36. 0.33	45. 0.85
1. 0.0745	10. 0.7	19. 3.6	28. 1.9	37. 0.08	46. 0.73
2. 0.456	11. 0.16 mg	20. 0.4	29. 3	38. 0.81	47. 0.26
3. 0.0875	12. 3.125 mg	21. 1.2	30. 1.7	39. 0.72	48. 0.93
4. 1.375	13. 0.35 mg	22. 0.3	31. 0.53	40. 0.74	49. 0.45
5. 2.7117	14. yes	23. 8.9	32. 0.42	41. 0.52	50. 0.7
6. 5.406	15. 56.25 mg	24. 1.3	33. 0.97	42. 0.36	
7. 0.4375	16. no	25. 2	34. 0.37	43. 0.65	
8. 0.216	17. 1.9	26. 0.6	35. 0.44	44. 0.27	

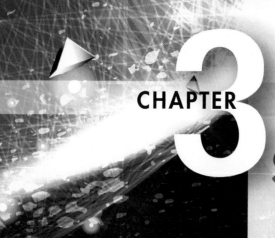

SOLVING COMMON FRACTION EQUATIONS

OBJECTIVES

The learner will solve equations containing:

1. whole numbers.
2. decimal numbers.
3. multiple numbers.

PREREQUISITES

Chapters 1 and 2

The majority of clinical drug dosage calculations involve solving an equation containing one to five common fractions. Two examples are:

$$\frac{2}{5} \times \frac{3}{4} \quad \text{and} \quad \frac{20}{1} \times \frac{1000}{60,000} \times \frac{1200}{1} \times \frac{1}{60}$$

Two options are available to solve common fraction equations: calculator use throughout, or initial fraction reduction followed by calculator use for final division. Both options are presented in this chapter, and you may use whichever you wish, or whichever your instructor requires.

 KEYpoint: Common fraction equations are solved by dividing the numerators by the denominators.

It is important that you do the calculations for each example and then compare them with the math provided. Just reading the examples will not teach you the calculation skills you need. The examples and problems provided incorporate all the content covered in the first two chapters. They represent the full range of calculations you will be doing on a continuing basis.

 KEYpoint: Calculator solution of equations is most safely done by concentrating only on the entries being made, not the numbers that register and change throughout the calculation.

WHOLE-NUMBER EQUATIONS

EXAMPLE 1 **Option 1: Calculator Use Throughout**

$$\frac{2}{5} \times \frac{3}{4}$$

$2 \times 3 \div 5 \div 4$ 　　Multiply the numerators, 2 and 3, and then divide by the denominators, 5 then 4, in continuous entries

$= 0.3$

Answer $= \mathbf{0.3}$ **(tenth)**

Option 2: Initial Reduction of Fractions

$$\frac{2}{5} \times \frac{3}{4}$$

$$\frac{\overset{1}{\cancel{2}}}{5} \times \frac{3}{\underset{2}{\cancel{4}}}$$ Divide the numerator, 2, and the denominator, 4, by 2 (to become 1 and 2)

$$3 \div 5 \div 2$$ Use the calculator to divide the remaining numerator, 3, by the remaining denominators, 5 and 2

$$= 0.3$$

Answer = **0.3 (tenth)**

 KEY_point:_ Initial reduction of fractions in an equation can simplify final calculator entries, especially if the numbers are large, or contain decimal fractions or zeros.

EXAMPLE 2   **Option 1: Calculator Use Throughout**

$$\frac{250}{175} \times \frac{150}{325}$$

$$250 \times 150 \div 175 \div 325$$ Multiply the numerators, 250 and 150, then divide by the denominators, 175 and 325

$$= 0.659$$

Answer = **0.7 (tenth)** or **0.66 (hundredth)**

Option 2: Initial Reduction of Fractions

$$\frac{250}{175} \times \frac{150}{325}$$

$$\frac{\overset{10}{\cancel{250}}}{\underset{7}{\cancel{175}}} \times \frac{\overset{6}{\cancel{150}}}{\underset{13}{\cancel{325}}}$$ Divide the numerator, 250, and the denominator, 175, by 25 (to become 10 and 7); divide the numerator, 150, and the denominator, 325, by 25 (to become 6 and 13)

$$10 \times 6 \div 7 \div 13$$ Use the calculator to multiply the numerators, 10 and 6, then divide by the denominators, 7 and 13

$$= 0.659$$

Answer = **0.7 (tenth)** or **0.66 (hundredth)**

EXAMPLE 3   **Option 1: Calculator Use Throughout**

$$\frac{7}{50} \times \frac{25}{3} \times \frac{120}{32}$$

$7 \times 25 \times 120 \div 50 \div 3 \div 32$ Multiply the numerators, 7, 25, and 120, then divide by the denominators, 50, 3, and 32

$= 4.375$

Answer $= $ **4.4 (tenth)** or **4.38 (hundredth)**

Option 2: Initial Reduction of Fractions

$$\frac{7}{50} \times \frac{25}{3} \times \frac{120}{32}$$

$$\frac{7}{\cancel{50}_{2}} \times \frac{\cancel{25}^{1}}{3} \times \frac{\cancel{120}^{15}}{\cancel{32}_{4}}$$ Divide 25 and 50 by 25, then divide 120 and 32 by 8

$7 \times 15 \div 2 \div 3 \div 4$

$= 4.375$

Answer $= $ **4.4 (tenth)** or **4.38 (hundredth)**

EXAMPLE 4

Option 1: Calculator Use Throughout

$$\frac{20}{1} \times \frac{1000}{60,000} \times \frac{1200}{1} \times \frac{1}{60}$$

$20 \times 1000 \times 1200 \div 60,000 \div 60$

$= 6.666$

Answer $= $ **6.7 (tenth)** or **6.67 (hundredth)**

Option 2: Initial Reduction of Fractions

$$\frac{20}{1} \times \frac{1000}{60,000} \times \frac{1200}{1} \times \frac{1}{60}$$

$$\frac{\cancel{20}^{1}}{1} \times \frac{\cancel{1000}^{1}}{\cancel{60,000}_{3}} \times \frac{\cancel{1200}^{20}}{1} \times \frac{1}{\cancel{60}_{1}}$$

$20 \div 3$

$= 6.666$

Answer $= $ **6.7 (tenth)** or **6.67 (hundredth)**

EXAMPLE 5

Option 1: Calculator Use Throughout

$$\frac{2000}{1500} \times \frac{2500}{3000}$$

$2000 \times 2500 \div 1500 \div 3000$

$= 1.111$

Answer $= $ **1.1 (tenth)** or **1.11 (hundredth)**

Option 2: Initial Reduction of Fractions

$$\frac{2000}{1500} \times \frac{2500}{3000}$$

$$\frac{\overset{2}{\cancel{2000}}}{\underset{3}{\cancel{1500}}} \times \frac{\overset{5}{\cancel{2500}}}{\underset{3}{\cancel{3000}}}$$

$$2 \times 5 \div 3 \div 3$$

$$= 1.111$$

Answer = **1.1 (tenth)** or **1.11 (hundredth)**

▶▶▶ PROBLEMS 3.1

Solve the equations. Express answers to the nearest tenth and hundredth. A calculator may be used.

1. $\dfrac{3}{8} \times \dfrac{6}{3}$　　　　= _____ _____

2. $\dfrac{3}{4} \times \dfrac{10}{2}$　　　　= _____ _____

3. $\dfrac{3}{5} \times \dfrac{1050}{40}$　　　= _____ _____

4. $\dfrac{10}{1} \times \dfrac{750}{40,000} \times \dfrac{1000}{1} \times \dfrac{1}{60}$ = _____ _____

5. $\dfrac{12}{1} \times \dfrac{500}{2700} \times \dfrac{2000}{1} \times \dfrac{1}{60}$ = _____ _____

6. $\dfrac{1500}{750} \times \dfrac{350}{600}$　　= _____ _____

7. $\dfrac{1000}{2700} \times \dfrac{1300}{500} \times \dfrac{70}{50}$ = _____ _____

8. $\dfrac{15}{1} \times \dfrac{2500}{20,000} \times \dfrac{1000}{1} \times \dfrac{1}{60}$ = _____ _____

9. $\dfrac{8}{1} \times \dfrac{1000}{5000} \times \dfrac{100}{1} \times \dfrac{1}{60}$ = _____ _____

10. $\dfrac{750}{500} \times \dfrac{250}{300}$　　= _____ _____

Answers **1.** 0.8; 0.75　**2.** 3.8; 3.75　**3.** 15.8; 15.75　**4.** 3.1; 3.13　**5.** 74.1; 74.07　**6.** 1.2; 1.17　**7.** 1.3; 1.35　**8.** 31.3; 31.25　**9.** 2.7; 2.67　**10.** 1.3; 1.25

SECTION 1

DECIMAL FRACTION EQUATIONS

Decimal fraction equations raise an instant warning flag in calculations, because it is here that most dosage errors occur. As with whole-number equations, simplifying the numbers by eliminating decimal points and reducing the numbers is an optional first step. If you elect to do the entire calculation with a calculator, be sure to enter the decimal points carefully. Double-check all calculator entries and answers.

 KEY_point:_ Particular care must be taken with calculator entry of decimal numbers to include the decimal point. Each entry and answer must be routinely double-checked.

EXAMPLE 1

Option 1: Calculator Use Throughout

$$\frac{0.3}{1.65} \times \frac{2.5}{1}$$

$0.3 \times 2.5 \div 1.65$ Multiply 0.3 by 2.5, then divide by 1.65

$= 0.454$

Answer = **0.5 (tenth)** or **0.45 (hundredth)**

Option 2: Initial Elimination of Decimal Points and Reduction of Fractions

$$\frac{0.3}{1.65} \times \frac{2.5}{1}$$

$$\frac{30}{165} \times \frac{25}{10}$$ Move the decimal point two places in 0.3 and 1.65 (to become 30 and 165) and one place in 2.5 and 1 (to become 25 and 10)

$$\frac{\overset{3}{\cancel{30}}}{\underset{33}{\cancel{165}}} \times \frac{\overset{5}{\cancel{25}}}{\underset{1}{\cancel{10}}}$$ Divide 30 and 10 by 10, then divide 25 and 165 by 5

$$\frac{\overset{1}{\cancel{3}}}{\underset{11}{\cancel{33}}} \times \frac{5}{1}$$ Divide 3 and 33 by 3

$5 \div 11$ Divide the remaining numerator, 5, by the denominator, 11

$= 0.454$

Answer = **0.5 (tenth)** or **0.45 (hundredth)**

EXAMPLE 2

Option 1: Calculator Use Throughout

$$\frac{0.3}{1.2} \times \frac{2.1}{0.15}$$

$0.3 \times 2.1 \div 1.2 \div 0.15$ Multiply 0.3 by 2.1, then divide by 1.2 and 0.15

$= 3.5$

Answer = **3.5 (tenth)** or **3.5 (hundredth)**

Option 2: Initial Elimination of Decimal Points and Reduction of Fractions

$$\frac{0.3}{1.2} \times \frac{2.1}{0.15}$$

$$\frac{3}{12} \times \frac{210}{15}$$ Eliminate the decimal points by moving them one place in 0.3 and 1.2 (to become 3 and 12) and two places in 2.1 and 0.15 (to become 210 and 15)

$$\frac{\overset{1}{\cancel{3}}}{\underset{4}{\cancel{12}}} \times \frac{\overset{42}{\cancel{210}}}{\underset{3}{\cancel{15}}}$$ Divide 3 and 12 by 3, then divide 210 and 15 by 5

$$\frac{1}{\underset{2}{\cancel{4}}} \times \frac{\overset{21}{\cancel{42}}}{3}$$ Divide 42 and 4 by 2

$21 \div 2 \div 3$ Use a calculator to divide the numerator, 21, by 2 and then by 3

$= 3.5$

Answer = **3.5 (tenth)** or **3.5 (hundredth)**

EXAMPLE 3

Option 1: Calculator Use Throughout

$$\frac{0.15}{0.17} \times \frac{3.1}{2}$$

$0.15 \times 3.1 \div 0.17 \div 2$ Multiply 0.15 by 3.1, divide by 0.17, and then divide by 2

$= 1.367$

Answer = **1.4 (tenth)** or **1.37 (hundredth)**

Option 2: Initial Elimination of Decimal Points and Reduction of Fractions

$$\frac{0.15}{0.17} \times \frac{3.1}{2}$$

$$\frac{15}{17} \times \frac{31}{20}$$ Move the decimal point two places in 0.15 and 0.17 and one place in 3.1 and 2 (requires adding a zero to 2)

$$\frac{\overset{3}{\cancel{15}}}{17} \times \frac{31}{\underset{4}{\cancel{20}}}$$ Divide 15 and 20 by 5

$3 \times 31 \div 17 \div 4$ Complete this with a calculator

$= 1.367$

Answer = **1.4 (tenth)** or **1.37 (hundredth)**

EXAMPLE 4   **Option 1: Calculator Use Throughout**

$$\frac{2.5}{1.5} \times \frac{1.2}{1.1}$$

$$2.5 \times 1.2 \div 1.5 \div 1.1$$

$$= 1.818$$

Answer = **1.8 (tenth)** or **1.82 (hundredth)**

Option 2: Initial Elimination of Decimal Points and Reduction of Fractions

$$\frac{2.5}{1.5} \times \frac{1.2}{1.1}$$

$$\frac{25}{15} \times \frac{12}{11}$$

$$\frac{\overset{5}{\cancel{25}}}{\underset{3}{\cancel{15}}} \times \frac{12}{11}$$

$$\frac{5}{\underset{1}{\cancel{3}}} \times \frac{\overset{4}{\cancel{12}}}{11}$$

$$5 \times 4 \div 11$$

$$= 1.818$$

Answer = **1.8 (tenth)** or **1.82 (hundredth)**

▶▶▶ PROBLEMS 3.2

Solve the equations. Express answers to the nearest tenth and hundredth. A calculator may be used.

1. $\dfrac{2.1}{1.15} \times \dfrac{0.9}{1.2} = $ _____ _____

2. $\dfrac{3.1}{2.7} \times \dfrac{2.2}{1.4} = $ _____ _____

3. $\dfrac{0.3}{1.2} \times \dfrac{3}{2.1} = $ _____ _____

4. $\dfrac{0.17}{0.3} \times \dfrac{2.5}{1.5} = $ _____ _____

5. $\dfrac{1.75}{0.95} \times \dfrac{1.5}{2} = $ _____ _____

6. $\dfrac{0.75}{1.15} \times \dfrac{3}{1.25} = $ _____ _____

7. $\dfrac{10.2}{1.5} \times \dfrac{2}{5.1} = $ _____ _____

8. $\dfrac{0.125}{0.25} \times \dfrac{2.5}{1.5} = $ _____ _____

9. $\dfrac{0.9}{0.3} \times \dfrac{1.2}{1.4} = $ _____ _____

10. $\dfrac{0.35}{1.7} \times \dfrac{2.5}{0.7} = $ _____ _____

Answers 1. 1.4; 1.37 **2.** 1.8; 1.8 **3.** 0.4; 0.36 **4.** 0.9; 0.94 **5.** 1.4; 1.38 **6.** 1.6; 1.57
7. 2.7; 2.67 **8.** 0.8; 0.83 **9.** 2.6; 2.57 **10.** 0.7; 0.74

MULTIPLE-NUMBER EQUATIONS

The calculation steps just practiced are also used for multiple-number equations, which occur frequently in advanced clinical calculations. **Reduction of numbers may be of particular benefit here because calculations of this type sometimes have numbers that cancel and/or reduce dramatically.** Answers are expressed to the nearest whole number in the examples and problems that follow to replicate actual clinical calculations.

EXAMPLE 1

Option 1: Calculator Use Throughout

$$\frac{60}{1} \times \frac{1000}{4} \times \frac{1}{1000} \times \frac{6}{1}$$

$60 \times 1000 \times 6 \div 4 \div 1000$ Multiply 60 by 1000, then by 6; divide by 4 and 1000

$= 90$

Answer $= $ **90**

Option 2: Initial Reduction of Fractions

$$\frac{60}{1} \times \frac{1000}{4} \times \frac{1}{1000} \times \frac{6}{1}$$

$$\frac{60}{1} \times \frac{\overset{1}{\cancel{1000}}}{\underset{2}{\cancel{4}}} \times \frac{1}{\underset{1}{\cancel{1000}}} \times \frac{\overset{3}{\cancel{6}}}{1}$$ Eliminate 1000 from a numerator and denominator, then divide 6 and 4 by 2

$60 \times 3 \div 2$ Multiply 60 by 3, then divide by 2

$= 90$

Answer $= $ **90**

EXAMPLE 2

Option 1: Calculator Use Throughout

$$\frac{20}{1} \times \frac{75}{1} \times \frac{1}{60}$$

$20 \times 75 \div 60$ Multiply 20 by 75, then divide by 60

$= 25$

Answer $= $ **25**

Option 2: Initial Reduction of Fractions

$$\frac{20}{1} \times \frac{75}{1} \times \frac{1}{60}$$

$$\frac{\overset{1}{\cancel{20}}}{1} \times \frac{\overset{25}{\cancel{75}}}{1} \times \frac{1}{\underset{3_1}{\cancel{60}}}$$ Divide 20 and 60 by 20 to become 1 and 3, then divide 75 and 3 by 3 to become 25 and 1

$= 25$

Answer $= $ **25**   The answer is obtained by cancellation alone

EXAMPLE 3

Option 1: Calculator Use Throughout

$$\frac{2}{0.5} \times \frac{1}{100} \times \frac{275}{1}$$

$2 \times 275 \div 0.5 \div 100$ Multiply 2 by 275, then divide by 0.5 and 100

$= 11$

Answer $= \mathbf{11}$

Option 2: Initial Reduction of Fractions

$$\frac{2}{0.5} \times \frac{1}{100} \times \frac{275}{1}$$

$$\frac{20}{5} \times \frac{1}{100} \times \frac{275}{1}$$ Eliminate the decimal point by moving it one place in 0.5 and one place in 2, which requires adding a zero to 2 (to become 5 and 20)

$$\frac{\overset{1}{\cancel{20}}}{\underset{1}{\cancel{5}}} \times \frac{1}{\underset{5}{\cancel{100}}} \times \frac{\overset{55}{\cancel{275}}}{1}$$ Divide 20 and 100 by 20, then divide 275 and 5 by 5

$$\frac{1}{\underset{1}{\cancel{5}}} \times \frac{\overset{11}{\cancel{55}}}{1}$$ Divide 5 and 55 by 5

$= 11$

Answer $= \mathbf{11}$ The answer is obtained by cancellation alone

EXAMPLE 4

Option 1: Calculator Use Throughout

$$\frac{1}{60} \times \frac{1}{12} \times \frac{10}{1} \times \frac{750}{1}$$

$10 \times 750 \div 60 \div 12$

$= 10.4$

Answer $= \mathbf{10}$

Option 2: Initial Reduction of Fractions

$$\frac{1}{60} \times \frac{1}{12} \times \frac{10}{1} \times \frac{750}{1}$$

$$\frac{1}{\underset{6}{\cancel{60}}} \times \frac{1}{\underset{6}{\cancel{12}}} \times \frac{\overset{1}{\cancel{10}}}{1} \times \frac{\overset{375}{\cancel{750}}}{1}$$

$375 \div 6 \div 6$

$= 10.4$

Answer $= \mathbf{10}$

▶▶▶ PROBLEMS 3.3

Solve the equations. Express answers to the nearest whole number.

1. $\dfrac{15}{1} \times \dfrac{350}{5} \times \dfrac{1}{60}$ = _____

2. $\dfrac{1}{32} \times \dfrac{60}{1} \times \dfrac{7.5}{3.1}$ = _____

3. $\dfrac{10}{1} \times \dfrac{2500}{24} \times \dfrac{1}{60}$ = _____

4. $\dfrac{1.7}{2.3} \times \dfrac{15.3}{12.1} \times \dfrac{6.2}{0.3}$ = _____

5. $\dfrac{20}{1} \times \dfrac{1200}{16} \times \dfrac{1}{60}$ = _____

6. $\dfrac{5}{1} \times \dfrac{320}{1.5} \times \dfrac{1}{60}$ = _____

7. $\dfrac{100}{1} \times \dfrac{1750}{200} \times \dfrac{1}{60}$ = _____

8. $\dfrac{60}{1} \times \dfrac{1150}{200} \times \dfrac{1}{100}$ = _____

9. $\dfrac{25}{4} \times \dfrac{1000}{8} \times \dfrac{1}{60}$ = _____

10. $\dfrac{18}{10} \times \dfrac{120}{7} \times \dfrac{9}{17}$ = _____

Answers **1.** 18 **2.** 5 **3.** 17 **4.** 19 **5.** 25 **6.** 18 **7.** 15 **8.** 3 **9.** 13 **10.** 16

Summary

This concludes the chapter on solving common fraction equations. The important points to remember from this chapter are:

▽ Most clinical calculations consist of an equation containing one to five common fractions.

▽ In solving equations, all the numerators are multiplied, then divided by the denominators.

▽ Numbers in an equation may initially be reduced using common denominators/ divisors to simplify final multiplication and division.

▽ Zeros may be eliminated from the same number of numerators and denominators without altering the value.

▽ Double-check all calculator entries and answers.

▽ Answers may be expressed as whole numbers, or to the nearest tenth or hundredth, depending on the calculation being done.

Summary Self-Test

Solve the equations. Express answers to the nearest tenth and hundredth. A calculator may be used.

1. $\dfrac{0.8}{0.65} \times \dfrac{1.2}{1}$ = _____ _____

2. $\dfrac{350}{1000} \times \dfrac{4.4}{1}$ = _____ _____

3. $\dfrac{0.35}{1.3} \times \dfrac{4.5}{1}$ = _____ _____

4. $\dfrac{0.4}{1.5} \times \dfrac{2.3}{1}$ = _____ _____

5. $\dfrac{1}{75} \times \dfrac{500}{1}$ = _____ _____

6. $\dfrac{0.15}{0.12} \times \dfrac{1.45}{1}$ = _____ _____

7. $\dfrac{100,000}{80,000} \times \dfrac{1.7}{1}$ = _____ _____

8. $\dfrac{1.45}{2.1} \times \dfrac{1.5}{1}$ = _____ _____

9. $\dfrac{1550}{500} \times \dfrac{0.5}{1}$ = _____ _____

10. $\dfrac{4}{0.375} \times \dfrac{0.25}{1}$ = _____ _____

11. $\dfrac{0.08}{0.1} \times \dfrac{2.1}{1}$ = _____ _____

12. $\dfrac{1.5}{1.25} \times \dfrac{1.45}{1}$ = _____ _____

13. $\dfrac{0.5}{0.15} \times \dfrac{0.35}{1}$ = _____ _____

14. $\dfrac{300,000}{200,000} \times \dfrac{1.7}{1}$ = _____ _____

15. $\dfrac{13.5}{10} \times \dfrac{1.8}{1}$ = _____ _____

16. $\dfrac{1,000,000}{800,000} \times \dfrac{1.4}{1}$ = _____ _____

17. $\dfrac{1.3}{0.2} \times \dfrac{0.25}{1}$ = _____ _____

18. $\dfrac{1.5}{0.1} \times \dfrac{0.25}{1}$ = _____ _____

19. $\dfrac{1.9}{3.5} \times \dfrac{3.2}{1.4}$ = _____ _____

20. $\dfrac{15,000}{7500} \times \dfrac{3.5}{1.2}$ = _____ _____

21. $\dfrac{4.7}{1.3} \times \dfrac{50}{20} \times \dfrac{4}{25} \times \dfrac{8.2}{2.1} =$ _____ _____

22. $\dfrac{40}{24} \times \dfrac{250}{5} \times \dfrac{0.375}{7.5} =$ _____ _____

23. $\dfrac{6.9}{21.6} \times \dfrac{250}{5} \times \dfrac{0.75}{2.1} =$ _____ _____

24. $\dfrac{1}{60} \times \dfrac{1}{25} \times \dfrac{10}{1} \times \dfrac{1000}{1} =$ _____ _____

25. $\dfrac{50.5}{22.75} \times \dfrac{4.7}{6.3} \times \dfrac{31.7}{10.2} =$ _____ _____

Solve the equations. Express answers to the nearest whole number. A calculator may be used.

26. $\dfrac{104}{95} \times \dfrac{20}{15} \times \dfrac{63}{1.6} =$ _____

27. $\dfrac{40,000}{10,000} \times \dfrac{30}{1} \times \dfrac{3.7}{12.5} =$ _____

28. $\dfrac{60}{1} \times \dfrac{500}{50} \times \dfrac{1}{1000} \times \dfrac{116}{1} =$ _____

29. $\dfrac{1.5}{0.6} \times \dfrac{10}{14} \times \dfrac{3.2}{5.3} \times \dfrac{100}{2} =$ _____

30. $\dfrac{60}{1} \times \dfrac{50}{250} \times \dfrac{1}{100} \times \dfrac{455}{1} =$ _____

31. $\dfrac{33.7}{15.9} \times \dfrac{19.2}{2.6} \times \dfrac{2.9}{3.85} =$ _____

32. $\dfrac{20}{4} \times \dfrac{100}{88} \times \dfrac{1200}{250} \times \dfrac{10}{30} =$ _____

33. $\dfrac{14}{7.9} \times \dfrac{88}{8} =$ _____

34. $\dfrac{10}{1} \times \dfrac{325}{1.5} \times \dfrac{1}{60} =$ _____

35. $\dfrac{60}{1} \times \dfrac{300}{400} \times \dfrac{1}{800} \times \dfrac{400}{1} =$ _____

36. $\dfrac{3.7}{1.3} \times \dfrac{12}{8} \times \dfrac{3.1}{7.4} \times \dfrac{5}{1} =$ _____

37. $\dfrac{20}{2} \times \dfrac{125}{25} \times \dfrac{2}{750} \times \dfrac{216}{1} =$ _____

38. $\dfrac{4}{3} \times \dfrac{45}{1} \times \dfrac{22.5}{37.8}$ = _____

39. $\dfrac{7.5}{12.3} \times \dfrac{55}{5} \times \dfrac{23.2}{1.2}$ = _____

40. $\dfrac{1000}{1} \times \dfrac{50}{250} \times \dfrac{20}{1} \times \dfrac{1}{60}$ = _____

41. $\dfrac{15}{1} \times \dfrac{1000}{4000} \times \dfrac{800}{1} \times \dfrac{1}{60}$ = _____

42. $\dfrac{15}{1} \times \dfrac{500}{3} \times \dfrac{1}{60}$ = _____

43. $\dfrac{25}{3} \times \dfrac{750}{8} \times \dfrac{0.1}{1}$ = _____

44. $\dfrac{40}{2} \times \dfrac{250}{50} \times \dfrac{1}{800} \times \dfrac{154}{1}$ = _____

45. $\dfrac{33}{4} \times \dfrac{75}{40} \times \dfrac{2}{150} \times \dfrac{432}{1}$ = _____

46. $\dfrac{22.5}{7} \times \dfrac{100}{5} \times \dfrac{1}{700} \times \dfrac{3}{80} \times \dfrac{3150}{1}$ = _____

47. $\dfrac{100}{250} \times \dfrac{50}{1} \times \dfrac{27.5}{1.375}$ = _____

48. $\dfrac{2.2}{0.25} \times \dfrac{3.6}{1} \times \dfrac{3.7}{7.1}$ = _____

49. $\dfrac{1.3}{0.21} \times \dfrac{0.3}{2} \times \dfrac{10.1}{0.75}$ = _____

50. $\dfrac{27.5}{10} \times \dfrac{40}{7} \times \dfrac{8.5}{1.9}$ = _____

Answers

1. 1.5; 1.48	**11.** 1.7; 1.68	**22.** 4.2; 4.17	**33.** 19	**44.** 19
2. 1.5; 1.54	**12.** 1.7; 1.74	**23.** 5.7; 5.7	**34.** 36	**45.** 89
3. 1.2; 1.21	**13.** 1.2; 1.17	**24.** 6.7; 6.67	**35.** 23	**46.** 11
4. 0.6; 0.61	**14.** 2.6; 2.55	**25.** 5.1; 5.15	**36.** 9	**47.** 400
5. 6.7; 6.67	**15.** 2.4; 2.43	**26.** 57	**37.** 29	**48.** 17
6. 1.8; 1.81	**16.** 1.8; 1.75	**27.** 36	**38.** 36	**49.** 13
7. 2.1; 2.13	**17.** 1.6; 1.63	**28.** 70	**39.** 130	**50.** 70
8. 1; 1.04	**18.** 3.8; 3.75	**29.** 54	**40.** 67	
9. 1.6; 1.55	**19.** 1.2; 1.24	**30.** 55	**41.** 50	
10. 2.7; 2.67	**20.** 5.8; 5.83	**31.** 12	**42.** 42	
	21. 5.6; 5.65	**32.** 9	**43.** 78	

SECTION

Introduction to Drug Measures

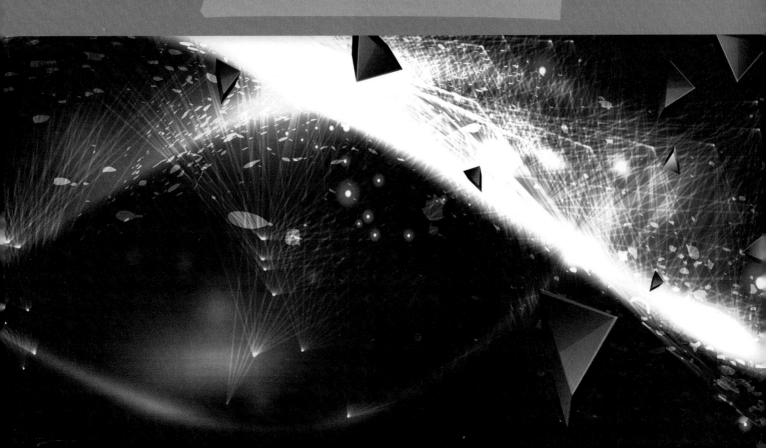

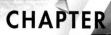

METRIC/ INTERNATIONAL (SI) SYSTEM

OBJECTIVES

The learner will:

1. list the commonly used units of measure in the metric system.

2. express metric weights and volumes using correct notation rules.

3. convert metric weights and volumes within the system.

PREREQUISITE

Familiarity with the metric system.

You are probably already familiar with the metric system, which is the major system of weights and measures used in medicine. The metric/international/SI (from the French Système International) system was invented in France in 1875, and takes its name from the meter, a length roughly equivalent to a yard, from which all other units of measure in the system are derived. The strength of the metric system lies in its simplicity, because all units of measure differ from each other in powers of ten (10). Conversions between units in the system are accomplished by simply moving a decimal point.

 KEYpoint: A major strength of the metric system is that all its units of measure differ from each other in powers of ten (10), and conversions between the units can be made by simply moving the decimal point.

This is also one of the metric system's greatest hazards. This is because a misplaced decimal point alters the value of a number by a multiple of at least 10. It is not necessary for you to know the entire metric system to administer medications safely, but you must understand its basic structure and become familiar with the units of measure you will be using in the clinical setting.

 KEYpoint: The greatest hazard of the metric system in drug dosages is that a misplaced decimal point will alter a dosage by a multiple of at least 10.

BASIC UNITS OF THE METRIC/SI SYSTEM

Three types of metric measures are in common clinical use: those for **length**, **volume** (or capacity), and **weight**. The basic units of these measures are:

length — meter
volume — liter
weight — gram

CHAPTER 4

Memorize the basic units if you do not already know them. In addition to the basic units, **there are both larger and smaller units of measure** for length, volume, and weight. Let's compare this concept with something familiar. The pound is a unit of weight that we use every day. A smaller unit of measure is the ounce; a larger, the ton. **However, all are units measuring weight**.

In the same way, there are smaller and larger units than the basic meter, liter, and gram. In the metric system, however, there is one very important advantage: **all other units, whether larger or smaller than the basic units, have the name of the basic unit incorporated in them**. So when you see a unit of metric measure, there is no doubt what it is measuring: **meter—length, liter—volume**, and **gram—weight**.

▶▶▶ PROBLEMS 4.1

Identify the metric measures with their appropriate category of weight, length, or volume.

1. milligram   _____

2. centimeter   _____

3. milliliter   _____

4. millimeter   _____

5. kilogram   _____

6. microgram   _____

7. kilometer   _____

8. kiloliter   _____

Answers 1. weight **2.** length **3.** volume **4.** length **5.** weight **6.** weight **7.** length **8.** volume

METRIC/SI PREFIXES

Prefixes are used in combination with the names of the basic units to identify larger and smaller units of measure. The same prefixes are used with all three measures. Therefore, there is a kilo**meter**, kilo**gram**, and a kilo**liter**.

KEY_point:_ Identical prefixes are used to identify units that are larger or smaller than the basic metric measures.

Prefixes also change the value of each of the basic units by the same amount. For example, the prefix "kilo" identifies a unit of measure that is larger than (or multiplies) the basic unit by 1000.

1 kilometer	=	1000 meters
1 kilogram	=	1000 grams
1 kiloliter	=	1000 liters

Kilo is the only prefix you will be using in the clinical setting that identifies a measure **larger** than the basic unit. Kilograms are frequently used as a measure for body weight, especially for infants and children.

You will see only three measures **smaller** than the basic unit in common clinical use. The prefixes for these are:

> **milli**—as in milligram—for weight
> **micro**—as in microgram—for weight
> **centi**—as in centimeter—for length

Therefore, you will actually be working with only four prefixes: **kilo**, which identifies a larger unit of measure than the basic; and **milli, micro,** and **centi**, which identify smaller units than the basic.

METRIC/SI ABBREVIATIONS

In clinical use, units of metric measure are abbreviated.

 KEY*point:* The basic units are abbreviated to their first initial and printed in small (lowercase) letters, with the exception of liter, which is capitalized (uppercase).

> meter is abbreviated **m**
> gram is abbreviated **g**
> liter is abbreviated **L**

 KEY*point:* The abbreviations for the prefixes used in combination with the basic units are all printed using small letters.

> kilo is **k** (as in kilogram—kg)
> milli is **m** (as in milligram—mg)
> micro is **mc** (as in microgram—mcg)
> centi is **c** (as in centimeter—cm)

Micro has an additional abbreviation, the symbol μ, but its use has been discontinued in medication dosages. This became necessary because medication errors were made when handwritten μg was misread as mg, a dosage 1000 times the mcg dosage ordered.

 KEY*point:* Micro is always abbreviated using the prefix mc rather than the symbol μ, which has an inherent safety risk.

In combination, liter remains capitalized. Therefore, milliliter is **mL** and kiloliter is **kL**.

▶ ▶ ▶ PROBLEMS 4.2

Abbreviate the following metric units.

1. microgram   _____
2. liter   _____
3. kilogram   _____
4. milliliter   _____
5. centimeter   _____

6. milligram   _____
7. meter   _____
8. kiloliter   _____
9. millimeter   _____
10. gram   _____

Answers **1.** mcg **2.** L **3.** kg **4.** mL **5.** cm **6.** mg **7.** m **8.** kL **9.** mm **10.** g

METRIC/SI NOTATION RULES

To remember the rules of metric **notations**, in which **a unit of measure is expressed with a quantity**, it is helpful to memorize some prototypes (examples) that incorporate all the rules. For the metric system, the notations for one-half, one, and one and one-half milliliters incorporate all the official notation rules.

Prototype Notations: 0.5 mL   1 mL   1.5 mL

RULE 1 ● The quantity is written in Arabic numerals: 1, 2, 3, 4, and so forth.
    Example: 0.5   1   1.5

RULE 2 ● The numerals representing the quantity are placed in front of the abbreviations.
    Example: 0.5 mL   1 mL   1.5 mL   (**not** mL 0.5, mL 1, mL 1.5)

RULE 3 ● A full space is used between the numeral and the abbreviation.
    Example: 0.5 mL   1 mL   1.5 mL   (**not** 0.5mL, 1mL, 1.5mL)

RULE 4 ● Fractional parts of a unit are expressed as decimal fractions.
    Example: 0.5 mL   1.5 mL   (**not** ½ mL, 1½ mL)

RULE 5 ● A zero is placed in front of the decimal when it is not preceded by a whole number, to emphasize the decimal point.
    Example: 0.5 mL (**not** .5 mL)

RULE 6 ● Excess zeros following a decimal fraction are eliminated.
    Example: 0.5 mL   1 mL   1.5 mL   (**not** 0.50 mL, 1.0 mL, 1.50 mL)

▶▶▶ PROBLEMS 4.3

Write the metric measures using official abbreviations and notation rules.

1. two grams   _____
2. five hundred milliliters   _____
3. five-tenths of a liter   _____
4. two-tenths of a milligram   _____
5. five-hundredths of a gram   _____
6. two and five-tenths kilograms   _____

7. one hundred micrograms   _____

8. two and three-tenths milliliters   _____

9. seven-tenths of a milliliter   _____

10. three-tenths of a milligram   _____

11. two and four-tenths liters   _____

12. seventeen and five-tenths kilograms   _____

13. nine-hundredths of a milligram   _____

14. ten and two-tenths micrograms   _____

15. four-hundredths of a gram   _____

Answers 1. 2 g **2.** 500 mL **3.** 0.5 L **4.** 0.2 mg **5.** 0.05 g **6.** 2.5 kg **7.** 100 mcg **8.** 2.3 mL **9.** 0.7 mL **10.** 0.3 mg **11.** 2.4 L **12.** 17.5 kg **13.** 0.09 mg **14.** 10.2 mcg **15.** 0.04 g

CONVERSION BETWEEN METRIC/SI UNITS

When you administer medications, you will be routinely **converting units of measure within the metric system**; for example, g to mg and mg to mcg. Learning the relative value of the units with which you will be working is the first prerequisite for accurate conversions.

There are only four metric **weights** commonly used in medicine. From **greater** to **lesser** value, these are:

kg	=	kilogram
g	=	gram
mg	=	milligram
mcg	=	microgram

Only two units of **volume** are frequently used. From **greater** to **lesser** value, these are:

L	=	liter
mL	=	milliliter

KEY*point:* Each of these clinical metric measures differs from the next by 1000.

1 kg	=	1000 g
1 g	=	1000 mg
1 mg	=	1000 mcg
1 L	=	1000 mL

Once again, from greater to lesser value, the units are, for weight: kg—g—mg—mcg; for volume: L—mL. Each unit differs in value from the next by 1000, and **all conversions will be between touching units of measure**; for example, g to mg, mg to mcg, and L to mL.

▶▶▶ PROBLEMS 4.4

Choose true (T) or false (F) for each conversion.

1. T F   1000 mL =   1000 L

2. T F   1000 mg =   1 g

3. T F   1000 g   =   1 kg

4. T F   1000 mg   =   1 mcg

5. T F   1000 mcg   =   1 g

6. T F   1 kg   =   1000 g

7. T F   1 mg   =   1000 g   9. T F   1 g   =   100 mcg

8. T F   1000 mcg =   1 mg   10. T F   1000 L =   1 kL

Answers **1.** F **2.** T **3.** T **4.** F **5.** F **6.** T **7.** F **8.** T **9.** F **10.** T

Because the metric system is a decimal system, **conversions between the units are accomplished by moving the decimal point**. Also, because each unit of measure in clinical use differs from the next by 1000, if you know one conversion, you know them all.

How far do you move the decimal point? There is an unforgettable memory cue that can be used with **all** metric conversions. There are **three zeros in 1000**. The decimal point moves **three places**, the **same number of places as the zeros** in the conversion.

KEYpoint: In metric conversions between touching units of clinical measures differing by 1000, the decimal point is moved three places, the same as the number of zeros in 1000.

This rule holds true for **all** decimal conversions in the metric system. If the difference in value was **10**, which has **one zero**, it would move **one place**. If the difference was **100**, which has **two zeros**, it would move **two places**. When the difference is **1000**, as in clinical conversions, which has **three zeros**, the decimal point moves **three places**.

Which way do you move the decimal point? If you are converting to a **smaller** unit of measure—for example, g to mg or L to mL—the **quantity must get larger**. The decimal point must move three places to the **right**.

EXAMPLE 1   0.5 g = _____ mg

You are converting to smaller units of measure, from **g to mg**, so the quantity will be **larger**. Move the decimal point **three places to the right**. To do this, you must **add two zeros** to the end of the quantity, and **eliminate the zero in front** of it. The larger 500 mg quantity indicates that you have moved the decimal point in the correct direction.

Answer **0.5 g = .500 mg**   Move the decimal three places to the right

EXAMPLE 2   2.5 L = _____ mL

You are converting to smaller units of measure, so the quantity will be **larger**. Move the decimal point **three places to the right**. To do this, you must **add two zeros**. The larger 2500 mL quantity indicates that you have moved the decimal point in the correct direction.

Answer **2.5 L = 2.500 mL**

▶▶▶ PROBLEMS 4.5

Convert the metric measures.

1. 7 mg = _____ mcg   4. 0.03 kg = _____ g

2. 1.7 L = _____ mL   5. 0.4 mg = _____ mcg

3. 3.2 g = _____ mg   6. 1.5 mg = _____ mcg

7. $0.7 \text{ g} = $ _____ mg   9. $7 \text{ kg} = $ _____ g

8. $0.3 \text{ L} = $ _____ mL   10. $0.01 \text{ mg} = $ _____ mcg

Answers 1. 7000 mcg **2.** 1700 mL **3.** 3200 mg **4.** 30 g **5.** 400 mcg **6.** 1500 mcg
7. 700 mg **8.** 300 mL **9.** 7000 g **10.** 10 mcg

In metric conversions from **smaller to larger units** of measurement, such as mL to L and mcg to mg, the quantity will be **smaller**. The decimal point is moved **three places to the left**.

EXAMPLE 1 $200 \text{ mL} = $ _____ L

You are converting to a larger unit of measure, **mL to L**, so the quantity will be **smaller**. Move the decimal point **three places to the left**.

$$.200, \text{ mL} = .200 \text{ L}$$

Eliminate the two unnecessary zeros at the end of the quantity (to make it .2), then add a zero in front of the decimal point to correctly write the dosage as 0.2 L.

Answer $.200, \text{ mL} = \textbf{0.2 L}$

EXAMPLE 2 $1500 \text{ mcg} = $ _____ mg

You are converting to a larger unit of measure, so the quantity will be smaller. Move the decimal point **three places to the left. Place a decimal point in front of** the 5, and **eliminate the two zeros** after the 5.

Answer $\textbf{1,500, mcg} = \textbf{1.5 mg}$

EXAMPLE 3 $300 \text{ mcg} = $ _____ mg

You are converting to a larger unit of measure, **mcg** to **mg**, so the quantity will be **smaller**. Move the decimal point **three places to the left**.

$$.300, \text{ mcg} = .300 \text{ mg}$$

Two zeros will need to be eliminated from the end of this decimal fraction (to make it .3), and a zero must be placed in front of the decimal point to complete the decimal fraction.

Answer   **300 mcg = 0.3 mg**

▶▶▶ PROBLEMS 4.6

Convert the metric measures.

1. $3500 \text{ mL} = $ _____ L   6. $250 \text{ mcg} = $ _____ mg

2. $520 \text{ mg} = $ _____ g   7. $1200 \text{ mg} = $ _____ g

3. $1800 \text{ mcg} = $ _____ mg   8. $600 \text{ mL} = $ _____ L

4. $750 \text{ mL} = $ _____ L   9. $100 \text{ mg} = $ _____ g

5. $150 \text{ mg} = $ _____ g   10. $950 \text{ mcg} = $ _____ mg

Answers 1. 3.5 L **2.** 0.52 g **3.** 1.8 mg **4.** 0.75 L **5.** 0.15 g **6.** 0.25 mg **7.** 1.2 g **8.** 0.6 L
9. 0.1 g **10.** 0.95 mg

COMMON ERRORS IN METRIC/SI DOSAGES

Most errors in the metric system occur because orders are not written using correct notation rules, or they are not transcribed correctly. **Errors usually involve decimal fractions**. Even though you have just finished learning metric notation rules, let's review the most common errors.

One error is the **failure to enter a zero in front of a decimal point**; for example, .2 mg instead of 0.2 mg. Regardless of the presence of a zero in front of the decimal in a written order, one must be added when the order is transcribed to a medication administration record.

 KEYpoint: Fractional dosages in the metric system are transcribed with a zero in front of the decimal point.

Another common error is to **include zeros where they should not be**; for example, 2.**0** mg instead of 2 mg or 0.2**0** mg instead of 0.2 mg. Each error can be misread as 20 mg, a dosage greatly in excess of the intended dosage.

 KEYpoint: Unnecessary zeros are eliminated when metric dosages are transcribed.

Errors are also more likely to occur in **calculations that include decimal fractions**. The presence of a decimal fraction in a calculation raises a warning flag to slow down and double-check all math. **Use your reasoning powers**. If a decimal is misplaced, the answer will be a minimum of 10 times too large or 10 times too small. **Question quantities that seem unreasonable**. A 1.5 mL IM injection dosage makes sense, but a 0.15 mL or 15 mL does not, and this is the type of error you might see.

 KEYpoint: Question orders and calculations that seem unreasonably large or small.

Additional errors to be aware of are in **conversions within the metric system**. Errors in conversions can be eliminated by thinking **three**. All conversions between the g, mg, mcg, mL, and L measures are accomplished by moving the decimal point **three** places. Always and forever. There are not many things for which you can use the words "always" and "forever," but converting between these units of measure in the metric system is one of those rare instances.

 KEYpoint: Conversions between g, mg, mcg, mL, and L units of measure in metric measures require moving the decimal point three places.

Be constantly mindful of these problem areas to become a safe clinical practitioner.

Summary

This concludes the refresher on the metric system. The important points to remember from this chapter are:

▼ The meter (m), liter (L), and gram (g) are the basic units of metric measure.

▼ Only liter is capitalized, L.

▼ Larger and smaller units than the basics are identified by the use of prefixes.

▼ The prefixes are printed using small (lowercase) letters.

▼ The one larger unit you will be seeing is the kilo, whose prefix is k.

▼ The smaller units you will be seeing are milli (m), micro (mc), and centi (c).

▼ Each prefix changes the value of a basic unit by the same amount.

▼ Converting from one unit to another within the system is accomplished by moving a decimal point.

▼ When you convert from larger to smaller units of measurement, the quantity will increase.

▼ To convert from larger to smaller units, the decimal point is moved to the right.

▼ When you convert from smaller to larger units of measurement, the quantity will get smaller.

▼ To convert from smaller to larger units, the decimal point is moved to the left.

▼ Conversions between g to mg, mg to mcg, and mL to L all require moving the decimal point three places.

▼ Fractional dosages are transcribed with a zero in front of the decimal point.

▼ Unnecessary zeros are eliminated from dosages.

Summary Self-Test

List the basic units of measure of the metric system and the measure they are used for.

1. _____   _____

   _____   _____

   _____   _____

Which of the following are official metric/SI abbreviations?

2. a) L   e) mg
   b) g   f) kg
   c) kL   g) ml
   d) mgm   h) G

   _____

Use official metric abbreviations and notation rules to express these as numerals.

3. six-hundredths of a milligram _____

4. three hundred and ten milliliters _____

5. three-tenths of a kilogram _____

6. four-tenths of a milliliter _____

7. one and five-tenths grams _____

8. one-hundredths of a gram _____

9. four thousand milliliters _____

10. one and two-tenths milligrams _____

List the four commonly used clinical units of weight and the two of volume from greater to lesser value.

11. Weight _____ _____ _____ _____

    Volume _____ _____

Convert the following metric measures.

12. 160 mg = _____ g	27. 300 mg = _____ g
13. 10 kg = _____ g	28. 2.5 mg = _____ mcg
14. 1500 mcg = _____ mg	29. 1 kL = _____ L
15. 750 mg = _____ g	30. 3 L = _____ mL
16. 200 mL = _____ L	31. 2 L = _____ mL
17. 0.3 g = _____ mg	32. 0.7 mg = _____ mcg
18. 0.05 g = _____ mg	33. 4 g = _____ mg
19. 0.15 g = _____ mg	34. 1000 mL = _____ L
20. 1.2 L = _____ mL	35. 2500 mL = _____ L
21. 1800 mL = _____ L	36. 1000 mg = _____ g
22. 2 mg = _____ mcg	37. 0.2 mg = _____ mcg
23. 900 mcg = _____ mg	38. 2000 g = _____ kg
24. 2.1 L = _____ mL	39. 1.4 g = _____ mg
25. 475 mL = _____ L	40. 2.5 L = _____ mL
26. 0.9 L = _____ mL	

Answers

1. gram-weight; liter-volume; meter-length
2. a, b, c, e, f
3. 0.06 mg
4. 310 mL
5. 0.3 kg
6. 0.4 mL
7. 1.5 g
8. 0.01 g
9. 4000 mL
10. 1.2 mg
11. kg, g, mg, mcg, L, mL
12. 0.16 g
13. 10,000 g
14. 1.5 mg
15. 0.75 g
16. 0.2 L
17. 300 mg
18. 50 mg
19. 150 mg
20. 1200 mL
21. 1.8 L
22. 2000 mcg
23. 0.9 mg
24. 2100 mL
25. 0.475 L
26. 900 mL
27. 0.3 g
28. 2500 mcg
29. 1000 L
30. 3000 mL
31. 2000 mL
32. 700 mcg
33. 4000 mg
34. 1 L
35. 2.5 L
36. 1 g
37. 200 mcg
38. 2 kg
39. 1400 mg
40. 2500 mL

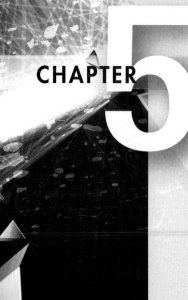

UNIT, PERCENTAGE, MILLIEQUIVALENT, RATIO, AND HOUSEHOLD MEASURES

OBJECTIVES

The learner will recognize dosages:

1. measured in units.
2. measured as percentages.
3. using ratio strengths.
4. in milliequivalents.
5. in household measures.

Although metric measures predominate in medications, there are several other measures frequently used, particularly in parenteral (injectable) solutions, that are important for you to know. In addition, you must be familiar with several measures in the household system because you may occasionally see these.

INTERNATIONAL UNITS (units)

A number of drugs are measured in International Units. Insulin, penicillin, and heparin are commonly seen examples. Antibiotics, such as penicillin, have dosages in the hundredths, thousandths, and millionths, and heparin has dosages in the thousandths. A unit **measures a drug in terms of its action**, not its physical weight. The word "units" is **not abbreviated; it is written in lowercase using Arabic numerals in front of the measure, with a space between**; for example, 2000 units or 1,000,000 units. **Commas are not usually used in a quantity unless it has at least five numbers**; for example, 45,000 units.

▶▶▶ PROBLEMS 5.1

Express the unit dosages in numerals.

1. two hundred and fifty thousand units   _____
2. ten units   _____
3. five thousand units   _____
4. forty-four units   _____
5. forty thousand units   _____

6. one million units _____

7. one thousand units _____

8. twenty-five hundred units _____

9. thirty-four units _____

10. one hundred units _____

Answers **1.** 250,000 units **2.** 10 units **3.** 5000 units **4.** 44 units **5.** 40,000 units **6.** 1,000,000 units **7.** 1000 units **8.** 2500 units **9.** 34 units **10.** 100 units

PERCENTAGE (%) MEASURES

Percentage strengths are used extensively in intravenous solutions, and somewhat less commonly for a variety of other medications, including eye and topical (for external use) ointments. **Percentage (%) means parts per hundred. The greater the percentage strength, the stronger the solution or ointment**; for example, 3% is stronger than 1%. Fractional percentages are expressed as decimal fractions; for example, 0.45%. Notice that, unlike other written dosages, percentages are generally written with **no space between the quantity and percentage sign**.

 KEYpoint: In solutions, percent represents the number of grams of drug per 100 mL of solution.

EXAMPLE 1   100 mL of a 1% solution will contain 1 g of drug.

EXAMPLE 2   100 mL of a 2.5% solution will contain 2.5 g of drug.

EXAMPLE 3   100 mL of a 10% solution will contain 10 g of drug.

EXAMPLE 4   100 mL of a 0.9% solution will contain 0.9 g of drug.

 KEYpoint: These examples are included to point out that percentage solutions contain a significant amount of drug or other solute, and that reading percentage labels requires the same care as that used with other drug dosages.

MILLIEQUIVALENT (mEq) MEASURES

Milliequivalents (**mEq**) is **an expression of the number of grams of a drug contained in 1 mL of a normal solution**. This is a definition that is quite understandable to a pharmacist or chemist, but you need not memorize it. Milliequivalent dosages are also written using **Arabic numerals**, with a space between the **abbreviation that follows**, for example, 30 mEq. You will see milliequivalents used in a variety of oral and parenteral solutions, potassium chloride being a common intravenous example.

▶▶▶ PROBLEMS 5.2

Express the milliequivalent dosages in numerals.

1. sixty milliequivalents   _____
2. fifteen milliequivalents   _____
3. forty milliequivalents   _____
4. one milliequivalent   _____
5. fifty milliequivalents   _____
6. eighty milliequivalents   _____
7. fifty-five milliequivalents   _____
8. seventy milliequivalents   _____
9. thirty milliequivalents   _____
10. twenty milliequivalents   _____

Answers 1. 60 mEq **2.** 15 mEq **3.** 40 mEq **4.** 1 mEq **5.** 50 mEq **6.** 80 mEq **7.** 55 mEq **8.** 70 mEq
9. 30 mEq **10.** 20 mEq

RATIO MEASURES

Ratio strengths are used primarily in solutions. They represent **parts of drug per parts of solution**; for example, 1 : 1000 (one part drug to 1000 parts solution).

EXAMPLE 1 A 1 : 100 strength solution has 1 part drug in 100 parts solution.

EXAMPLE 2 A 1 : 5 solution contains 1 part drug in 5 parts solution.

EXAMPLE 3 A solution that is 1 part drug in 2 parts solution would be written 1 : 2.

 KEYpoint: The less solution a drug is dissolved in, the stronger the solution.

For example, a ratio strength of 1 : 10 (1 part drug to 10 parts solution) is much stronger than a 1 : 100 (1 part drug in 100 parts solution).

Ratio strengths are always expressed in their **simplest terms**. For example, 2 : 10 would be incorrect because it can be reduced to 1 : 5. Notice that ratio dosages are written separated by a colon, with a space between both numbers and the colon. Dosages using ratio strengths are not common, but you do need to know what they represent.

▶▶▶ PROBLEMS 5.3

Express as ratios.

1. 1 part drug to 200 parts solution   _1 : 200_
2. 1 part drug to 4 parts solution   _____
3. 1 part drug to 7 parts solution   _____

Identify the strongest solution.

4 a) 1 : 20   b) 1 : 200   c) 1 : 2   _____

5 a) 1 : 50   b) 1 : 20   c) 1 : 100   _____

6 a) 1 : 1000   b) 1 : 5000   c) 1 : 2000   _____

Answers 1. 1 : 200 **2.** 1 : 4 **3.** 1 : 7 **4.** c **5.** b **6.** a

HOUSEHOLD MEASURES

Household measures are rarely used. They are only used in the home care setting, and their clinical use is becoming less frequent. The measures you may occasionally see include the **ounce, tablespoon, teaspoon, dram,** and **drop**. Abbreviations and/or names for all of these measures, except the drop, **still appear on many disposable medication cups**, and care must be taken not to confuse them with metric dosages. It is quite possible that these measures will be eliminated in the future because the health care industry has been moving rapidly to improve dosage labeling and medication abbreviation guidelines to reduce the possibility of errors.

The various abbreviations for household dosages and their metric equivalents are as follows:

Household Measure	Abbreviation	Metric Equivalent
ounce	oz	30 mL
tablespoon	T, TBS, tbs	15 mL
teaspoon	t, TSP, tsp	5 mL
dram	dr	4 mL
drop	gtt	1 mL

KEYpoint: The volume of a drop depends on the size of the dropper being used.

A drop is such an inaccurate and variable measure that medication droppers are now often included with small-volume liquid medication preparations; the dropper is specific to that medication. The use of drops is largely restricted to eye and ear drop use. One exception is in small-volume pediatric liquid medications, which are prepared with **integral (included with the medication) medicine droppers that are calibrated by volume, or by actual dosage**.

APOTHECARY MEASURES

Apothecary measures are officially obsolete. In Chapter 6 on oral medication labels it will be pointed out that the labels of a few very, very old drugs, aspirin and nitroglycerine, may still contain the apothecary abbreviation "gr" for grains. The grain was originally based on the weight of a grain of wheat, which exposes its inaccuracy, and why this measure is now obsolete. As drug manufacturers begin to adopt updated official abbreviations and drug measures, "gr" will be deleted from the few remaining medication labels where it still appears. Appendix A includes some additional information on this obsolete system, in the event your instructor feels it necessary for you to learn.

Summary

This concludes your introduction to the additional measures you will see used in dosages and in solutions. The important points to remember from this chapter are:

▼ International units measure a drug by its action rather than its weight.

▼ There is no abbreviation for units, which is written in full, units, in lowercase letters.

▼ Percentage (%) strengths are frequently used in solutions and ointments.

▼ Percent represents grams of drug per 100 mL of solution.

▼ The greater the percentage strength, the stronger the solution.

▼ Milliequivalent is abbreviated mEq and is frequently used in solution measurements.

▼ Ratio strengths represent parts of drug per parts of solution.

▼ The smaller the volume of solution, the greater the ratio strength.

▼ T or tbs is the abbreviation for tablespoon (15 mL), and t or tsp for teaspoon (5 mL).

▼ The abbreviation gtt is used for drop, and oz for ounce.

Summary Self-Test

Express the dosages using the official symbols/abbreviations.

1. three hundred thousand units   _____

2. forty-five units   _____

3. ten percent   _____

4. two and a half percent   _____

5. forty milliequivalents   _____

6. a one in two thousand ratio   _____

7. a one in ten ratio   _____

8. one percent   _____

9. one drop   _____

10. two thousand units   _____

11. five milliequivalents   _____

12. nine-tenths percent   _____

13. ten units   _____

14. a one in two ratio   _____

15. five percent   _____

16. twenty milliequivalents   _____

17. fourteen units   _____

18. twenty percent   _____

19. two million units   _____

20. one hundred thousand units   _____

Answers

1. 300,000 units	**5.** 40 mEq	**10.** 2000 units	**15.** 5%	**20.** 100,000 units
2. 45 units	**6.** 1 : 2000	**11.** 5 mEq	**16.** 20 mEq	
3. 10%	**7.** 1 : 10	**12.** 0.9%	**17.** 14 units	
4. 2.5%	**8.** 1%	**13.** 10 units	**18.** 20%	
	9. 1 gtt	**14.** 1 : 2	**19.** 2,000,000 units	

SECTION

Reading Medication Labels and Syringe Calibrations

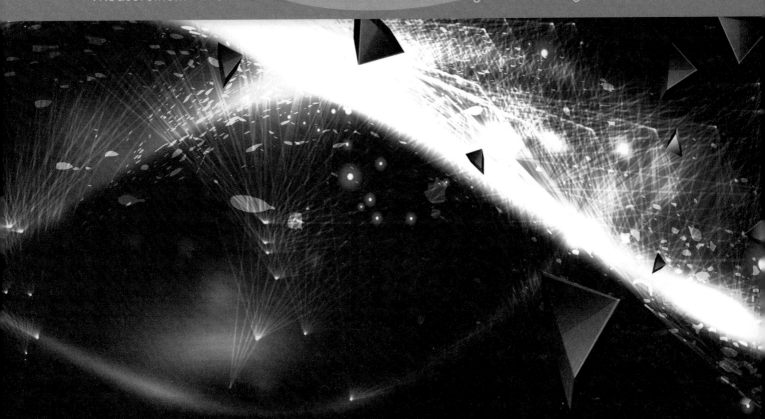

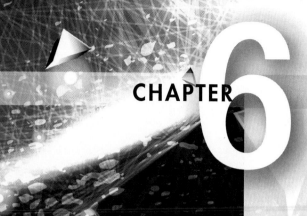

6

ORAL MEDICATION LABELS AND DOSAGE CALCULATION

OBJECTIVES

The learner will:

1. identify scored tablets, unscored tablets, and capsules.

2. read drug labels to identify trade and generic names.

3. locate dosage strengths and calculate average dosages.

4. measure oral solutions using a medicine cup.

In this chapter, you will be introduced to labels of oral medications for both solid (tablet and capsule) and liquid (mL) medications. Medication label information includes trade and generic drug names, metric dosage strengths, manufacturer's name, and other details you need to be aware of, primarily so that you can quickly locate the correct dosage strength to calculate ordered dosages. You will then use actual drug labels to calculate a full range of oral medication dosages. **Average dosage calculations require only the information you have already learned on the metric system and in the Refresher Math Section on addition and subtraction.** They are routinely done mentally. Advanced calculations are needed primarily in clinical specialty areas, and they will be covered in later chapters.

 KEYpoint: Most oral dosages consist of one-half to three tablets or capsules, or one-half to double the milliliter volume of liquid medications, and are done mentally.

We will begin with labels for solid drug preparations. These include tablets, scored tablets (which contain an indented marking to make breakage for partial dosages possible), enteric-coated tablets (which delay absorption until the drug reaches the small intestine), capsules (powdered or oily drugs in a gelatin cover), and sustained or controlled-release capsules (action spread over a prolonged period of time; for example, 12 hours). See Figure 6-1.

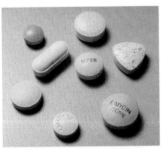
Tabelts

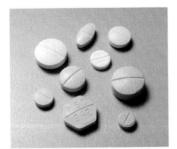
Scored Tablets

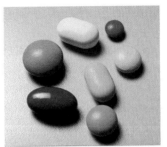
Enteric-Coated Tablets

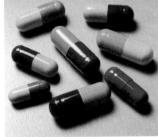
Capsules

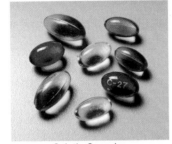
Gelatin Capsules

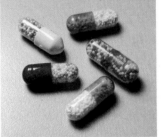
Controlled-Release Capsules

© Cengage Learning 2015.

▲ FIGURE 6-1

TABLET AND CAPSULE LABELS

The most common type of label you will see in the clinical setting is the **unit dosage label**, in which each tablet or capsule is packaged separately. However, the dosage information on both unit and multiple dose labels is identical.

EXAMPLE 1 ▶

Look at the Synthroid® label in Figure 6-2. The first thing to notice is that this drug has two names. The first, **Synthroid**, is its **trade name**, which is identified by the ® registration symbol. Trade names are usually **capitalized** and **printed first** on the label. The name in smaller print, **levothyroxine sodium**, is the **generic** or **official name** of the drug. Each drug has only **one** official name but may have **several trade names**, each for the exclusive use of the company that manufactures it. It is important to remember, however, that most labels do contain **both** names. Drugs may be ordered by either name depending on hospital policy or prescriber preference. You will frequently need to cross-check trade and generic names for accurate drug identification.

Next on the label is the **dosage strength,** 100 mcg or 0.1 mg. The prepared dosage often represents the **average dosage strength; the dosage given to the average**

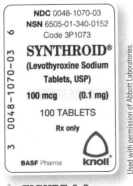

▲ FIGURE 6-2

patient at one time. This label also identifies the **manufacturer** of this drug, Knoll Pharmaceuticals.

Notice that **100 TABLETS** is printed near the **bottom** of the label. This is the **total number** of tablets in the bottle. Be careful not to confuse the quantity of tablets or capsules with the dosage strength. **The dosage strength always has a unit of measure associated with it**; in this case, mcg and mg. Because label designs vary widely, this is an important point to remember.

EXAMPLE 2

The **Percocet®** label in Figure 6-3 is an example of a medication that contains not one but **two drugs**: 5 mg of the narcotic oxycodone and 325 mg of acetaminophen, an analgesic. The dosages in multiple drug products are routinely written in the same order as the drugs listed in the product. Oxycodone and acetaminophen are generic names, and Percocet is the manufacturer's trade name for this product. Medications that contain more than one drug are usually **ordered by trade name and number of tablets or capsules** to be given rather than by dosage.

The balance of the label information includes the total number of tablets near the bottom, 100; average dosage considerations; a bar code; and a space where the manufacturer would enter the drug lot number and expiration date. Expiration dates are carefully monitored by clinical pharmacies, but you must also make checking them a habit.

 KEY *point:* Tablets and capsules that contain more than one drug are usually ordered by trade name and number of tablets or capsules to be given, rather than by dosage.

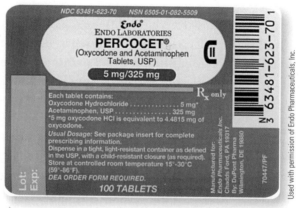

▲ **FIGURE 6-3**

EXAMPLE 3

The small unit dosage label in Figure 6-4 bears only one name, **phenobarbital**, which is actually the **generic** name of the drug. Generic labeling is common with drugs that have been in use for generations. The official (generic) name was so well established that drug manufacturers did not try to promote their own trade names. Also notice that following the drug name are the initials **U.S.P.** This is the abbreviation for **U**nited **S**tates **P**harmacopeia, one of the two official national listings of drugs. The other is the **N**ational **F**ormulary, **NF**. You will see U.S.P. and NF on drug labels and must not confuse them with other initials that identify additional drugs or specific action of drugs in a preparation. Also notice that the label contains the dosage strength in both the metric, **15 mg**, and apothecary, **1/4 gr**, measures. Finally, on the right of the label, printed sideways, is Exp 6-6-16, which identifies the last date when the drug should be used.

 KEY*point:* You may still see the obsolete apothecary abbreviation for grain ("gr"), on a few drug labels, as in Figures 6-4 and Figure 6-5. The apothecary system is gradually being eliminated from use in health care. In addition, not all medication labels have been updated to reflect The Joint Commission standards of leaving a space between the dosage and unit of measure, for example "500mg" instead of "500 mg"; or the use of "u" instead of "units." These also will continue to be corrected by the manufacturers.

Next, refer to Figure 6-5. Notice that this label also contains the dosage strength of nitroglycerin in both the **0.3 mg metric** and the **1/200 gr (grains)** of the obsolete **apothecary** system units of measure. As with phenobarbital, the inclusion of apothecary dosages on this label relates to the age and historic use of this drug. Relabeling is already well under way by manufacturers to remove apothecary dosages completely from their products.

 KEY*point:* For safety in medication administration, focus on the drug name and its dosage strength.

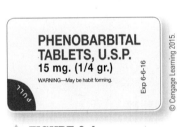

▲ **FIGURE 6-4**

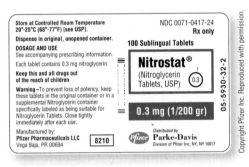

▲ **FIGURE 6-5**

▶▶▶ PROBLEMS 6.1

Refer to the label in Figure 6-5 and answer the questions about this drug.

1. What is the generic name?   _____

2. What is the trade name?   _____

3. What is the dosage strength in metric units?   _____

4. What is the dosage strength in the obsolete apothecary measure?   _____

5. If nitroglycerin 0.3 mg is ordered, how many tablets will be required?   _____

6. Read the information above the Nitrostat name. What kind of tablets are these?   _____

7. How must the drug be administered?   _____

8. Who is the manufacturer of this drug? _____

9. How many tablets will be needed to give a
0.6 mg dosage of nitroglycerin? _____

Answers **1.** nitroglycerin **2.** Nitrostat® **3.** 0.3 mg **4.** 1/200 gr **5.** 1 tab **6.** sublingual
7. under the tongue **8.** Parke-Davis, a division of Pfizer Pharmaceuticals LLC **9.** 2 tab

---

▶▶▶ PROBLEMS 6.2

Refer to the label in Figure 6-6 and answer the questions about this drug.

1. What is the generic name? _____

2. What is the trade name? _____

3. What is the dosage strength? _____

4. What company manufactured this drug? _____

5. How many tablets are in this container? _____

6. If Prinivil 5 mg is ordered, how many tablets will you give? _____

7. If lisinopril 10 mg is ordered, how many tablets will you give? _____

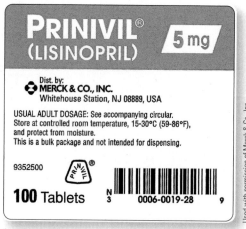

▲ **FIGURE 6-6**

Answers **1.** lisinopril **2.** Prinivil® **3.** 5 mg **4.** Merck & Co., Inc. **5.** 100 tablets **6.** 1 tab **7.** 2 tab

---

Refer to the Sinemet® label in Figure 6-7. Sinemet is another example of a combined drug tablet. The **generic** names of the drugs it contains are **carbidopa** and **levodopa**. These are listed on the label in several places: directly under the trade name and with the **amount** of each drug in the fine print near the bottom of the label. Also, notice the box to the right of the trade name, which contains the numbers 25–100. This again is the amount of carbidopa—25 mg—and levodopa—100 mg. Contrast this label with the Sinemet labels in Figure 6-8 and Figure 6-9.

In Figure 6-8, the dosage strengths are different. A blue box to the right of the Sinemet trade name identifies the strengths of carbidopa and levodopa as **10 mg** and **100 mg**, respectively, which are actually lower dosages. And, finally, Figure 6-9 is a label for Sinemet® **CR**, a controlled-release or sustained-release tablet, with yet another dosage strength of 50–200: **carbidopa 50 mg** and **levodopa 200 mg.** Unlike the previous combined drug tablet discussed, an order for Sinemet **must** include the dosage strength because it is available in several strengths.

KEY*point:* Extra numbers after a drug name may be used to identify the dosage strengths of more than one drug in a preparation, and extra initials may be used to identify a special drug action.

NDC 0056-0650-68

DU PONT PHARMACEUTICALS

DUPONT MFG. U.S. PAT. & TM OFF.

SINEMET® 25-100
(CARBIDOPA-LEVODOPA)

Each tablet contains:
Carbidopa . . . . 25 mg*
*(Anhydrous equivalent)
Levodopa . . . . .100 mg
Marketed by:
Du Pont Pharmaceuticals
Wilmington, Delaware 19880
100 TABLETS

CAUTION: Federal (USA) law prohibits dispensing without prescription. SINEMET is a registered trademark of MERCK & CO., Inc.

Manufactured by:
MERCK SHARP & DOHME
DIVISION OF MERCK & CO., Inc.
WEST POINT, PA 19486, USA

3365/7668301
7783/DB

USUAL ADULT DOSAGE:
See accompanying circular.

Dispense in a well-closed container. This is a bulk package and not intended for dispensing.

Used with permission of Merck & Co., Inc.

▲ FIGURE 6-7

NDC 0056-0647-68

DU PONT PHARMACEUTICALS

DUPONT MFG. U.S. PAT. & TM OFF.

SINEMET® 10-100
(CARBIDOPA-LEVODOPA)

Each tablet contains:
Carbidopa . . . . 10 mg*
*(Anhydrous equivalent)
Levodopa . . . . 100 mg
Marketed by:
Du Pont Pharmaceuticals
Wilmington, Delaware 19880
100 TABLETS

Used with permission of Merck & Co., Inc.

▲ FIGURE 6-8

DUPONT **SINEMET® CR** **50-200**
(CARBIDOPA-LEVODOPA, SUSTAINED-RELEASE)

Each tablet contains:
Carbidopa . . . . 50 mg*
*(Anhydrous equivalent)
Levodopa . . . . 200 mg
USUAL ADULT DOSAGE: See accompanying circular.
Tablets should be swallowed without chewing or crushing.
Avoid temperatures above 30°C (86°F).
CAUTION: Federal (USA) law prohibits dispensing without prescription.
This is a bulk package and not intended for dispensing.   3570/7753703
SINEMET is a registered trademark of MERCK & CO., Inc.   7859/EB
100 TABLETS

NDC 0056-0521-28   NSN 6505-01-343-3483

Used with permission of Merck & Co., Inc.

▲ FIGURE 6-9

TABLET/CAPSULE DOSAGE CALCULATION

When the time comes for you to administer medications, you will have to read a **M**edication **A**dministration **R**ecord, abbreviated MAR, to prepare the dosage. This will tell you the name and amount of drug to be given, but it will not tell you how many tablets or capsules contain this dosage. This you must calculate yourself. However, remember that most tablets/capsules are prepared in average dosage strengths, and most orders will involve giving one-half to three tablets (or one to three capsules, because capsules cannot be broken in half). **Learn to question orders for more than 3 tablets or capsules.** Although some drugs require multiple tablets, most do not. Some clinical pharmacies do carry a limited quantity of a particular medication as a cost-saving factor, so if a drug came in 25 mg, 50 mg, 100 mg, and 200 mg dosages and that facility's pharmacy only carried 25 mg tablets, an order for 200 mg would translate into 8 tablets, which would seem unreasonable. In the 100 or 200 mg supply, the order results in 1 or 2 tablets, which is reasonable. Always question an order of more than 3 tablets, and double-check your calculations.

KEY*point:* An unusual number of tablets or capsules could be a warning of an error in prescribing, transcribing, or calculating.

Let's now look at some sample orders and do some actual dosage calculations. **Assume that tablets are scored and can be broken in half.**

▶▶▶ PROBLEMS 6.3

Refer to the Inderal® LA label in Figure 6-10 to answer these questions.

1. What is the dosage strength? _____
2. If you have an order for 120 mg, give _____
3. If you have an order for 60 mg, give _____
4. What is the generic name of this drug? _____
5. What is the total number of capsules in this package? _____

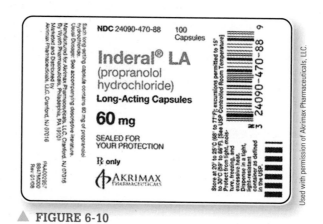

▲ **FIGURE 6-10**

Answers **1.** 60 mg **2.** 2 cap **3.** 1 cap **4.** propranolol hydrochloride **5.** 100 capsules

▶▶▶ PROBLEMS 6.4

Refer to the Glucotrol® label in Figure 6-11 to answer these questions.

1. What is the dosage strength? _____
2. If 10 mg is ordered, give _____
3. If 2.5 mg is ordered, give _____
4. If 5 mg is ordered, give _____
5. What is the generic name of this drug? _____
6. What is the total number of tablets in this package? _____

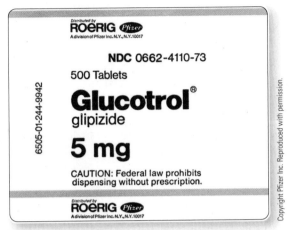

▲ **FIGURE 6-11**

Answers **1.** 5 mg **2.** 2 tab **3.** ½ tab **4.** 1 tab **5.** glipizide **6.** 500 tablets

It is not uncommon to have a drug **ordered** in one unit of metric measure—**for example, mg**—and discover that it is **labeled** in another measure—**for example, g**. It will then be necessary to **convert the metric units to calculate the dosage**. Conversions will always be between touching units of measure: g and mg or mg and mcg. **Converting involves moving the decimal point three places**.

EXAMPLE 1

Refer to the Halcion® label in Figure 6-12. A dosage of 250 mcg has been ordered. The label reads 0.25 mg. Convert the mg to mcg by moving the decimal point three places to the right, and you can mentally verify that these dosages are identical. Give 1 tablet.

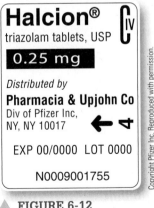

▲ **FIGURE 6-12**

EXAMPLE 2

Refer to the Xanax® label in Figure 6-13. A dosage of 500 mcg is ordered. The label reads 0.25 mg, so you must give 2 tablets (1 tab = 250 mcg, so 500 mcg requires 2 tab). The decimal moves three places to the right in this conversion from mg to mcg.

Rx only
See package insert for complete product information.
Keep container tightly closed.
Dispense in tight, light-resistant container.
Store at controlled room temperature 20° to 25° C (68° to 77° F) [see USP].

Pharmacia & Upjohn Company
Kalamazoo, MI 49001, USA

NDC 0009-0029-01
6505-01-143-9269

Xanax® C IV
alprazolam tablets, USP

0.25 mg

812 004 712

LOT
EXP

100 Tablets

0009-0029-01

Copyright Pfizer Inc. Reproduced with permission.

▲ FIGURE 6-13

▶▶▶ PROBLEMS 6.5

Locate the appropriate labels for the following dosages, and indicate how many tablets or capsules are needed to give them. Assume all tablets are scored and can be broken in half. Labels may be used in more than one problem.

1. verapamil HCl 0.12 g _____ cap

2. Terbutaline® 10 mg _____ tab

3. Ritalin® HCl 7.5 mg _____ tab

4. methylphenidate HCl 2500 mcg _____ tab

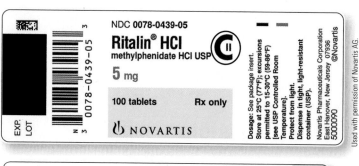

NDC 0078-0439-05

Ritalin® HCl
methylphenidate HCl USP C II

5 mg

100 tablets   Rx only

🔱 NOVARTIS

0078-0439-05

EXP.
LOT

Dosage: See package insert.
Store at 25°C (77°F); excursions permitted to 15-30°C (59-86°F) [see USP Controlled Room Temperature].
Protect from light.
Dispense in tight, light-resistant container (USP).

Novartis Pharmaceuticals Corporation
East Hanover, New Jersey 07936 ©Novartis
5000090

Used with permission of Novartis AG.

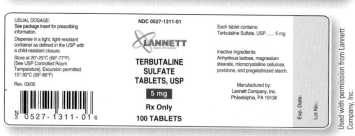

USUAL DOSAGE:
See package insert for prescribing information.
Dispense in a tight, light-resistant container as defined in the USP with a child-resistant closure.
Store at 20°-25°C (68°-77°F) [See USP Controlled Room Temperature]. Excursion permitted 15°-30°C (59°-86°F)
Rev. 03/05

NDC 0527-1311-01

✕ LANNETT

TERBUTALINE SULFATE TABLETS, USP

5 mg

Rx Only

100 TABLETS

3 0527-1311-01 6

Each tablet contains:
Terbutaline Sulfate, USP ...... 5 mg

Inactive Ingredients:
Anhydrous lactose, magnesium stearate, microcrystalline cellulose, povidone, and pregelatinized starch.

Manufactured by:
Lannett Company, Inc.
Philadelphia, PA 19136

Exp. Date:

Lot No.:

Used with permission from Lannett Company, Inc.

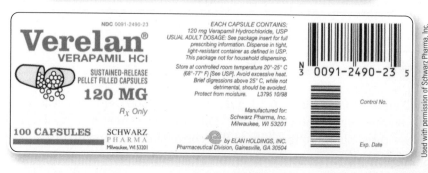

NDC 0091-2490-23

Verelan®
VERAPAMIL HCl

SUSTAINED-RELEASE PELLET FILLED CAPSULES

120 MG

Rx Only

100 CAPSULES SCHWARZ PHARMA
Milwaukee, WI 53201

EACH CAPSULE CONTAINS:
120 mg Verapamil Hydrochloride, USP
USUAL ADULT DOSAGE: See package insert for full prescribing information. Dispense in tight, light-resistant container as defined in USP. This package not for household dispensing.
Store at controlled room temperature 20°-25° C (68°-77° F) [See USP]. Avoid excessive heat. Brief digressions above 25° C, while not detrimental, should be avoided. Protect from moisture.   L3795 10/98

Manufactured for:
Schwarz Pharma, Inc.
Milwaukee, WI 53201

by ELAN HOLDINGS, INC.
Pharmaceutical Division, Gainesville, GA 30504

0091-2490-23

Control No.

Exp. Date

Used with permission of Schwarz Pharma, Inc.

Answers 1. 1 cap **2.** 2 tab **3.** 1½ tab **4.** ½ tab

CHAPTER 6

▶▶▶ PROBLEMS 6.6

Locate the appropriate labels for the following drug orders, and indicate the number of tablets/capsules that will be required to administer the dosages ordered. Assume that all tablets are scored and can be broken in half. Notice that both generic and trade names are used for the orders and that a label may be used in more than one problem.

1. isosorbide dinitrate 80 mg   _____ cap

2. sulfasalazine 0.5 g   _____ tab

3. Azulfidine® 1 g   _____ tab

4. terbutaline sulfate 2500 mcg   _____ tab

5. chlordiazepoxide HCl 50 mg   _____ cap

6. Librium® 25 mg   _____ cap

7. Dilatrate®–SR 80 mg   _____ cap

8. Synthroid® 0.2 mg   _____ tab

9. levothyroxine Na 0.2 mg   _____ tab

10. terbutaline sulfate 3.75 mg   _____ tab

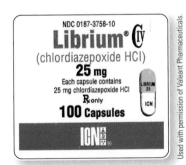

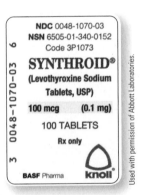

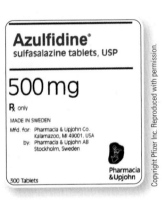

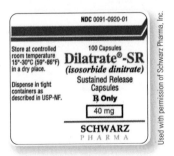

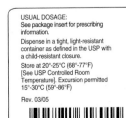

Answers   1. 2 cap   **2.** 1 tab   **3.** 2 tab   **4.** 1 tab   **5.** 2 cap   **6.** 1 cap   **7.** 2 cap   **8.** 2 tab
9. 2 tab   **10.** 1½ tab

ORAL SOLUTION LABELS

In liquid drug preparations, the dosage is contained in a certain mL **volume of solution**. Let's review dosages in some solid and liquid drug preparations to illustrate the difference.

EXAMPLE 1   **Solid:** 250 mg in **1 tablet**   **Liquid:** 250 mg in **5 mL**

EXAMPLE 2   **Solid:** 100 mg in **1 capsule**   **Liquid:** 100 mg in **10 mL**

EXAMPLE 3

Refer to the Lomotil® label in Figure 6-14. The information it contains will be familiar. **Lomotil** is the **trade** name and **diphenoxylate** is the **generic** or official name. The dosage strength is **2.5 mg per 5 mL**. As with solid drugs, the medication administration record, MAR, will tell you the **dosage of the drug** to be administered, but it **will not specify the volume that contains this dosage**.

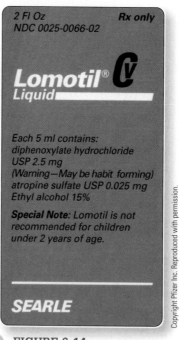

▲ **FIGURE 6-14**

▶▶▶   PROBLEMS 6.7

Refer to the Lomotil® label in Figure 6-14 to calculate these dosages.

1. The order is for diphenoxylate 2.5 mg. Give _____

2. The order is for Lomotil 5 mg. Give _____

Answers   1. 5 mL   **2.** 10 mL

Note: If you did not express your answers as mL, they are incorrect. Numbers have no meaning unless they are expressed with a unit of measure.

▶▶▶ PROBLEMS 6.8

Refer to the penicillin V label in Figure 6-15 to calculate these dosages.

1. The order is for penicillin V 400,000 units. _____

2. penicillin V 125 mg has been ordered. _____

3. penicillin V 375 mg has been ordered. _____

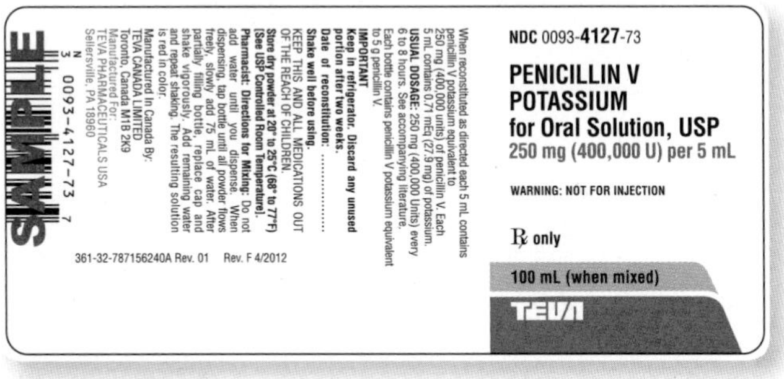

NDC 0093-**4127**-73

PENICILLIN V POTASSIUM
for Oral Solution, USP
250 mg (400,000 U) per 5 mL

WARNING: NOT FOR INJECTION

℞ only

100 mL (when mixed)

TEVA

Used with permission from Teva Pharmaceuticals USA.

▲ **FIGURE 6-15**

Answers **1.** 5 mL   **2.** 2.5 mL   **3.** 7.5 mL

Note: Your answers are incorrect unless they include mL as the unit of volume measure.

▶▶▶ PROBLEMS 6.9

Refer to the solution labels in Figure 6-16 and Figure 6-17 to calculate these dosages.

1. oxycodone soln. 10 mg   _____

2. cefaclor susp. 187 mg   _____

3. cefaclor susp. 374 mg   _____

4. oxycodone soln. 30 mg   _____

5. oxycodone soln. 20 mg   _____

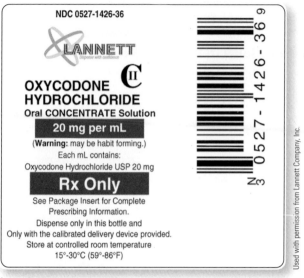

▲ FIGURE 6-16

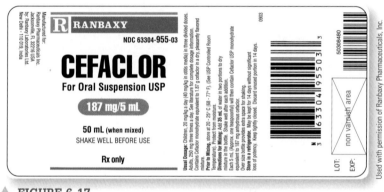

▲ FIGURE 6-17

Answers **1.** 0.5 mL **2.** 5 mL **3.** 10 mL **4.** 1.5 mL **5.** 1 mL

MEASUREMENT OF ORAL SOLUTIONS

Oral solutions are most commonly measured using a disposable **calibrated medication cup**. Take a close look at the schematic drawing of the medication cup calibrations in Figure 6-18. Many disposable medication cups, like this one, still contain the TSP (teaspoon), TBS (tablespoon), and OZ (ounce) calibrations of the household system and the obsolete DR (for dram) of the apothecary system. Some also contain the increasingly disused cc (cubic centimeter) calibration, which is identical to a mL (milliliter). Oral solutions are **most safely poured at eye level**. Because of the number of units of measure on these cups, **always read calibrations very carefully**.

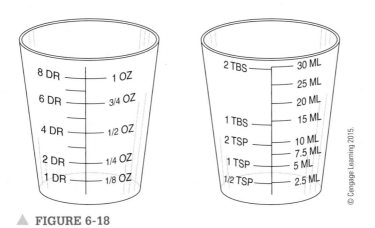

▲ FIGURE 6-18

Small-volume solution dosages can also be measured using specially calibrated **oral syringes** such as those illustrated in Figure 6-19 and Figure 6-20. Oral syringes have safety features built into their design to prevent their being mistaken for hypodermic syringes. One of these features is **color**, as illustrated in Figure 6-19. Hypodermic syringes are not colored, although their packaging and needle covers are colored to aid in identification. A second feature is the syringe tip, which is a **different size and shape** and is often **off center** (termed **eccentric**). Figure 6-20 illustrates an eccentric oral syringe tip. Hypodermic syringes **without a needle** can also be used to measure and administer oral dosages.

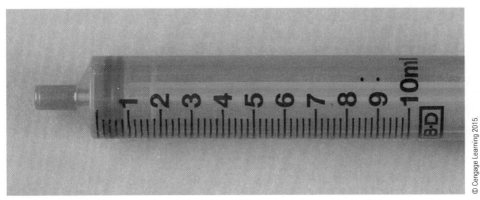

▲ FIGURE 6-19

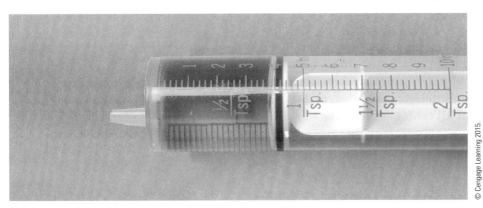

▲ FIGURE 6-20

The main concern with correct syringe identification is that **oral syringes, which are not sterile**, should not be confused and used for **hypodermic medications, which are sterile**. This mistake **has** been made in spite of the fact that hypodermic needles do not fit correctly on oral syringes. The precaution, therefore, does need to be stressed.

Oral solutions may also be ordered as drops (gtt), and when this is the case, the dropper is attached to the bottle stopper. Medicine droppers are often calibrated in mL or by actual dosage, such as 125 mg, and so forth. (Refer to Chapter 22 for more information on droppers.)

Summary

This concludes the chapter on reading oral medication labels. The important points to remember from this chapter are:

▼ Most labels contain both generic and trade names.

▼ Dosages are clearly printed on the label, including preparations containing multiple drugs.

▼ Combined dosage tablets and capsules may be ordered by trade name and number of tablets/capsules to be given and may include dosages.

▼ The letters U.S.P. (United States Pharmacopeia) and NF (National Formulary) on drug labels identify their official generic listings.

▼ Additional letters that follow a drug name are used to identify additional drugs in the preparation or a special action of the drug.

▼ Most dosages of tablets or capsules consist of ½ to 3 tablets (1-3 capsules, which cannot be broken in half). An unusual number of tablets or capsules may indicate an error.

▼ Check expiration dates on labels before use.

▼ For accurate measurement, solutions are poured at eye level when a medicine cup is used.

▼ Liquid oral medications may be measured and administered using an oral medication syringe or a hypodermic syringe without a needle.

▼ Care must be taken not to use oral syringes for hypodermic medication preparation because these are not sterile.

Summary Self-Test

Locate the appropriate label for each of the following drug orders, and indicate the number of tablets, capsules, or mL that will be required to administer them. Assume that all tablets are scored and can be broken in half. Labels may be used more than once in each problem set.

PART I

1. Glucotrol® 15 mg _____
2. dexamethasone 4 mg _____
3. Dilatrate®-SR 80 mg _____
4. morphine sulfate 20 mg _____

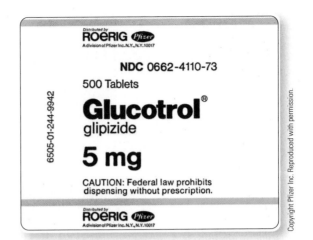

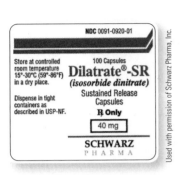

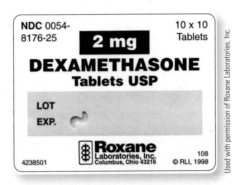

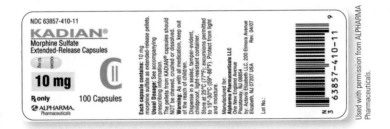

PART II

5. piroxicam 20 mg   _____

6. cefaclor susp. 250 mg   _____

7. Lortab® 5/500 2 tab   _____

8. Halcion® 250 mcg   _____

9. alprazolam 750 mcg   _____

10. gabapentin 0.2 g   _____

11. Biaxin® 1 g   _____

12. Xanax® 500 mcg   _____

13. clarithromycin 0.5 g   _____

14. triazolam 500 mcg   _____

Store below 86°F (30°C)

Dispense in tight, light-resistant containers (USP).

DOSAGE AND USE
See accompanying prescribing information. One capsule per day.

Each capsule contains 20 mg piroxicam.

IMPORTANT: This closure is not child-resistant.

CAUTION: Federal law prohibits dispensing without prescription.

NDC 0069-3230-66

100 Capsules

Feldene®
(piroxicam)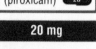

20 mg

 **Pfizer** **Pfizer Labs**
Division of Pfizer Inc, NY, NY 10017

6505-01-137-4628
05-4300-00-5
MADE IN USA
1292

©Abbott

0074258660

Store tablets at 15° to 30°C (59° to 86°F).

Exp Lot 03-2126-2/R4

NDC 0074-2586-60
60 Tablets

BIAXIN®
FILMTAB®
clarithromycin
tablets

500 mg

Caution: Federal (U.S.A.) law prohibits dispensing without prescription.

6505-01-354-8581
Do not accept if break-away ring on cap is broken or missing.
Dispense in a USP tight, light-resistant container.
Each tablet contains:
500 mg clarithromycin.
Each yellow tablet bears the and Abbo-Code KL for product identification.
Usual Adult Dose: One tablet every twelve hours. See enclosure for full prescribing information.
Filmtab—Film-sealed tablets, Abbott.
Abbott Laboratories
North Chicago, IL60064, U.S.A.

---

ucb Pharma

PHARMACIST: Dispense in a tight, light-resistant container with a child-resistant closure.

Store at controlled room temperature, 15°-30°C (59°-86°F).

Lot No.:
Exp. Date:

Manufactured for
UCB Pharma, Inc.
Smyrna, GA 30080
by Mallinckrodt Inc.
Hobart, NY 13788

NDC 50474-902-01   **100 TABLETS**

LORTAB® 5/500

**HYDROCODONE BITARTRATE
AND ACETAMINOPHEN
TABLETS, USP
5 mg/500 mg**

Each scored, white with blue specks tablet contains:
Hydrocodone Bitartrate . . . . 5 mg
Acetaminophen . . . . 500 mg

Rx only

USUAL DOSAGE: See package insert for complete dosage recommendations.

N 3 50474-902-01 1

Rev. 6/01
P/N 1003723

Manufactured for:
Ranbaxy Pharmaceuticals Inc.
Jacksonville, FL 32216 USA
by: Ranbaxy Laboratories Ltd.
New Delhi - 110 019, India

R RANBAXY

NDC 63304-**954**-01

CEFACLOR
For Oral Suspension USP

125 mg/5 mL

75 mL (when mixed)

SHAKE WELL BEFORE USE

Rx only

Usual Dosage: Children, 20 mg/kg a day (40 mg/kg in otitis media) in three divided doses.
Adults, 250 mg three times a day. See literature for complete dosage information.
Contains Cefaclor monohydrate equivalent to 1.875 g cefaclor in a dry, pleasantly flavored mixture.
Prior to Mixing, store at 20 - 25° C (68 - 77° F). (See USP Controlled Room Temperature). Protect from moisture.
Directions for Mixing: Add **53 mL** of water in two portions to dry mixture in the bottle. Shake well after each addition.
Each 5 mL (Approx. one teaspoonful) will then contain Cefaclor USP monohydrate equivalent to 125 mg anhydrous cefaclor.
Over size bottle provides extra space for shaking.
Store in a refrigerator. May be kept for 14 days without significant loss of potency. Keep tightly closed. Discard unused portion in 14 days.

0903

N 3 63304 19540 2

50509460

LOT:
EXP:

non varnish area

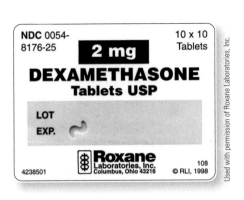

NDC 0054-
8176-25

2 mg

10 x 10
Tablets

DEXAMETHASONE
Tablets USP

LOT
EXP.

Roxane
Laboratories, Inc.
Columbus, Ohio 43216

4238501

108
© RLI, 1998

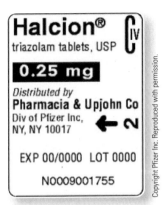

Halcion® C|IV

triazolam tablets, USP

0.25 mg

Distributed by
Pharmacia & Upjohn Co
Div of Pfizer Inc,
NY, NY 10017

EXP 00/0000 LOT 0000

N0009001755

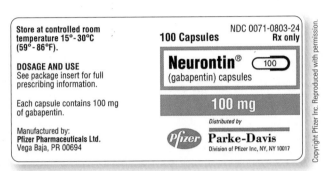

Store at controlled room
temperature 15°-30°C
(59°-86°F).

DOSAGE AND USE
See package insert for full
prescribing information.

Each capsule contains 100 mg
of gabapentin.

Manufactured by:
Pfizer Pharmaceuticals Ltd.
Vega Baja, PR 00694

100 Capsules

NDC 0071-0803-24
Rx only

Neurontin® 〔 100 〕
(gabapentin) capsules

100 mg

Distributed by
Pfizer **Parke-Davis**
Division of Pfizer Inc, NY, NY 10017

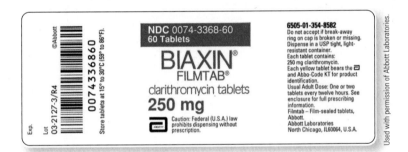

©Abbott

03-2127-3/R4

0074336860

Store tablets at 15° to 30°C (59° to 86°F).

Exp.

Lot

NDC 0074-3368-60
60 Tablets

BIAXIN®
FILMTAB®
clarithromycin tablets
250 mg

Caution: Federal (U.S.A.) law
prohibits dispensing without
prescription.

6505-01-354-8582
Do not accept if break-away
ring on cap is broken or missing.
Dispense in a USP tight, light-
resistant container.
Each tablet contains:
250 mg clarithromycin.
Each yellow tablet bears the ⊇
and Abbo-Code KT for product
identification.
Usual Adult Dose: One or two
tablets every twelve hours. See
enclosure for full prescribing
information.
Filmtab – Film-sealed tablets,
Abbott.
Abbott Laboratories
North Chicago, IL60064, U.S.A.

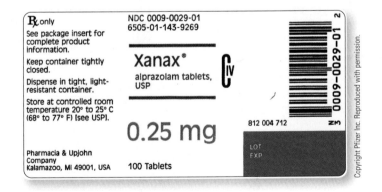

Rx only
See package insert for
complete product
information.

Keep container tightly
closed.

Dispense in tight, light-
resistant container.

Store at controlled room
temperature 20° to 25° C
(68° to 77° F) [see USP].

Pharmacia & Upjohn
Company
Kalamazoo, MI 49001, USA

NDC 0009-0029-01
6505-01-143-9269

Xanax® C|IV

alprazolam tablets,
USP

0.25 mg

100 Tablets

812 004 712

0009-0029-01

LOT
EXP

PART III

15. acetaminophen 650 mg   _____

16. Aldactone® 75 mg   _____

17. meclizine HCl 50 mg   _____

18. Kadian® 20 mg   _____

19. ciprofloxacin HCl 0.375 g   _____

20. metoprolol tartrate 0.15 g   _____

21. nifedipine 10 mg   _____

22. piroxicam 20 mg   _____

23. Feldene® 40 mg   _____

24. Lomotil® 2.5 mg   _____

25. Librium® 75 mg   _____

26. codeine 45 mg   _____

27. Aldactone® 50 mg   _____

28. Synthroid® 225 mcg   _____

29. nitroglycerin 600 mcg   _____

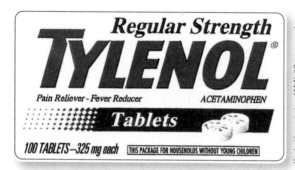

Used with permission of McNeil Consumer and Specialty Pharmaceuticals.

Used with permission of Valeant Pharmaceuticals.

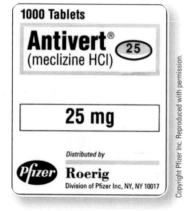

Copyright Pfizer Inc. Reproduced with permission.

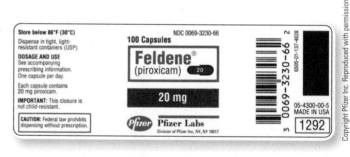

Copyright Pfizer Inc. Reproduced with permission.

Copyright Pfizer Inc. Reproduced with permission.

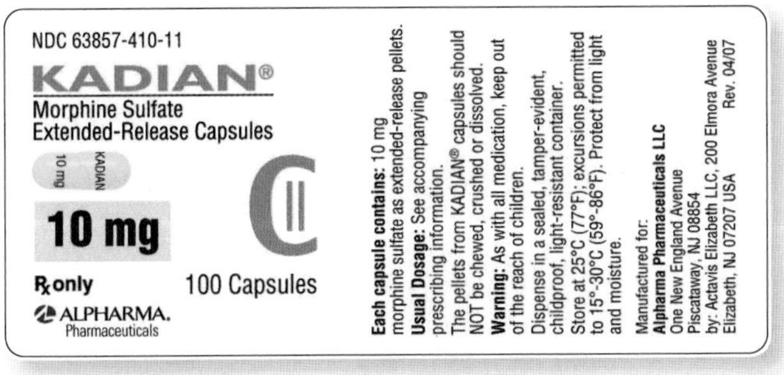

NDC 63857-410-11

KADIAN®

Morphine Sulfate
Extended-Release Capsules

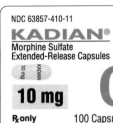

10 mg

Rx only   100 Capsules

ALPHARMA.
Pharmaceuticals

Each capsule contains: 10 mg morphine sulfate as extended-release pellets.
Usual Dosage: See accompanying prescribing information.
The pellets from KADIAN® capsules should NOT be chewed, crushed or dissolved.
Warning: As with all medication, keep out of the reach of children.
Dispense in a sealed, tamper-evident, childproof, light-resistant container.
Store at 25°C (77°F); excursions permitted to 15°-30°C (59°-86°F). Protect from light and moisture.
Manufactured for:
Alpharma Pharmaceuticals LLC
One New England Avenue
Piscataway, NJ 08854
by: Actavis Elizabeth LLC, 200 Elmora Avenue
Elizabeth, NJ 07207 USA   Rev. 04/07

NDC 0028-0051-10
6505-01-071-6557

Lopressor® 50 mg

metoprolol tartrate USP

1000 tablets

Rx only

ᘯ **NOVARTIS**

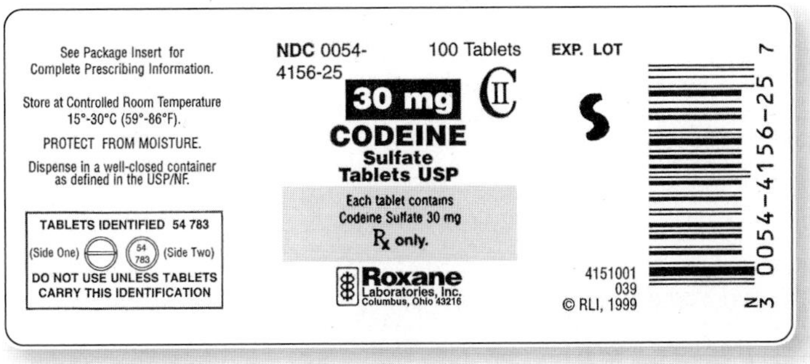

See Package Insert for Complete Prescribing Information.

Store at Controlled Room Temperature 15°-30°C (59°-86°F).

PROTECT FROM MOISTURE.

Dispense in a well-closed container as defined in the USP/NF.

TABLETS IDENTIFIED 54 783
(Side One) ⊖⊖ � 783 (Side Two)
DO NOT USE UNLESS TABLETS CARRY THIS IDENTIFICATION

NDC 0054-4156-25   100 Tablets   EXP. LOT

30 mg Ⅽ Ⅱ
CODEINE
Sulfate
Tablets USP

Each tablet contains
Codeine Sulfate 30 mg
℞ only.

Ⓡ **Roxane**
Laboratories, Inc.
Columbus, Ohio 43216

4151001
039
© RLI, 1999

3 0054-4156-25 7

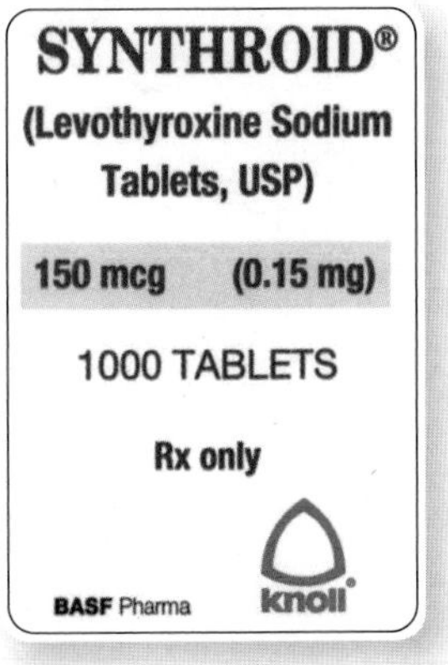

SYNTHROID®

(Levothyroxine Sodium Tablets, USP)

150 mcg   (0.15 mg)

1000 TABLETS

Rx only

BASF Pharma   △ **knoll**

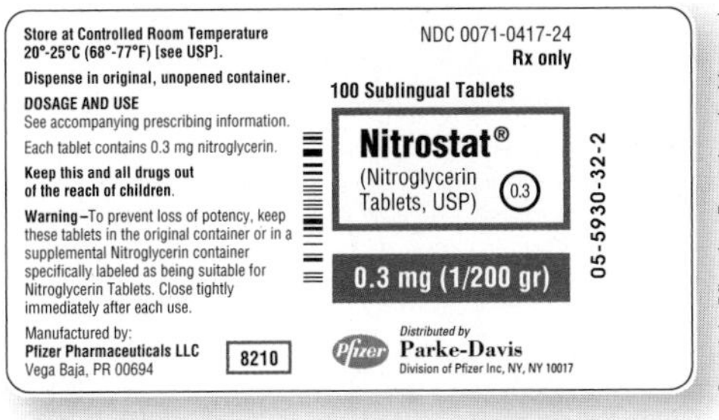

Store at Controlled Room Temperature
20°-25°C (68°-77°F) [see USP].

Dispense in original, unopened container.

DOSAGE AND USE
See accompanying prescribing information.

Each tablet contains 0.3 mg nitroglycerin.

Keep this and all drugs out of the reach of children.

Warning—To prevent loss of potency, keep these tablets in the original container or in a supplemental Nitroglycerin container specifically labeled as being suitable for Nitroglycerin Tablets. Close tightly immediately after each use.

Manufactured by:
Pfizer Pharmaceuticals LLC
Vega Baja, PR 00694   8210

NDC 0071-0417-24
Rx only

100 Sublingual Tablets

Nitrostat®
(Nitroglycerin Tablets, USP)   ⓪.3

0.3 mg (1/200 gr)

05-5930-32-2

Distributed by
Pfizer **Parke-Davis**
Division of Pfizer Inc, NY, NY 10017

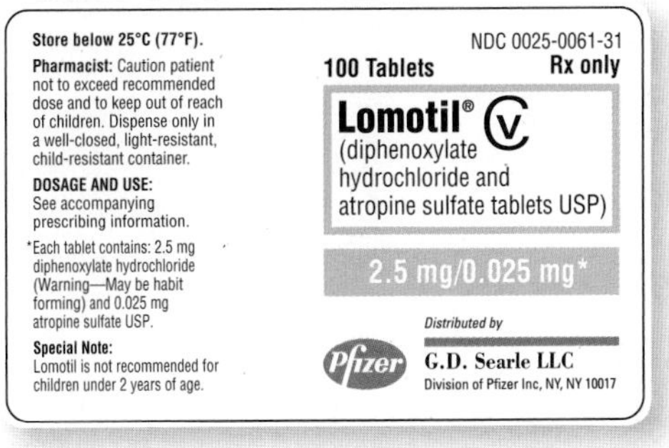

Store below 25°C (77°F).

Pharmacist: Caution patient not to exceed recommended dose and to keep out of reach of children. Dispense only in a well-closed, light-resistant, child-resistant container.

DOSAGE AND USE:
See accompanying prescribing information.

*Each tablet contains: 2.5 mg diphenoxylate hydrochloride (Warning—May be habit forming) and 0.025 mg atropine sulfate USP.

Special Note:
Lomotil is not recommended for children under 2 years of age.

NDC 0025-0061-31
Rx only

100 Tablets

Lomotil® Ⓒⓥ
(diphenoxylate hydrochloride and atropine sulfate tablets USP)

2.5 mg/0.025 mg*

Distributed by
Pfizer **G.D. Searle LLC**
Division of Pfizer Inc, NY, NY 10017

Batch:
Expires:

Store below 86°F (30°C).

RECOMMENDED STORAGE:
See accompanying literature for complete information on dosage and administration.

DOSAGE: See accompanying literature for complete information on dosage and administration.

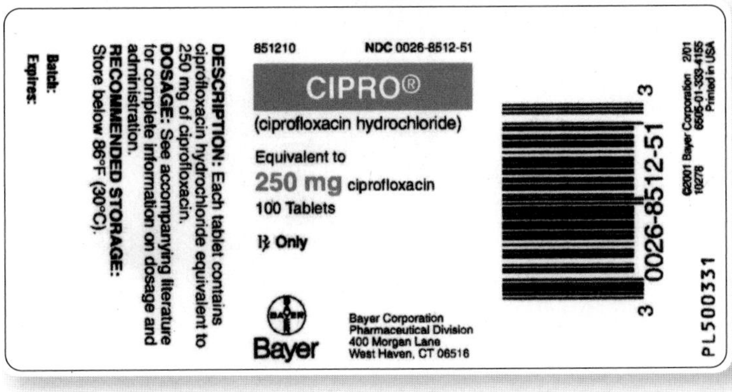

DESCRIPTION: Each tablet contains ciprofloxacin hydrochloride equivalent to 250 mg of ciprofloxacin.

851210   NDC 0026-8512-51

CIPRO®

(ciprofloxacin hydrochloride)

Equivalent to

250 mg ciprofloxacin
100 Tablets

℞ Only

Ⓑ **Bayer**

Bayer Corporation
Pharmaceutical Division
400 Morgan Lane
West Haven, CT 06516

©2001 Bayer Corporation
10278
6505-01-533-4155
Printed in USA

3 0026-8512-51 3

PL500331

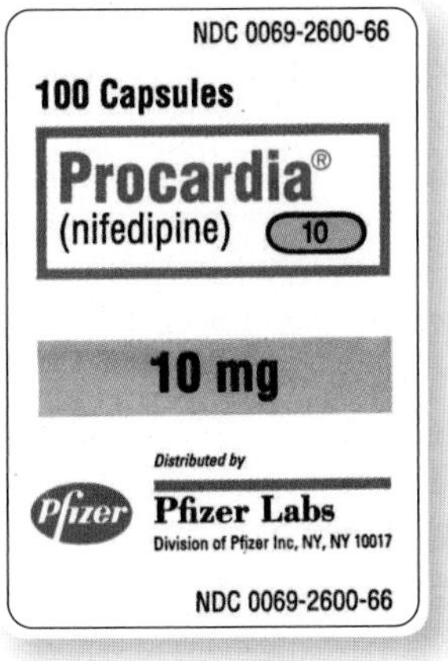

NDC 0069-2600-66

100 Capsules

Procardia®
(nifedipine)   ⟨ 10 ⟩

10 mg

Distributed by
Pfizer **Pfizer Labs**
Division of Pfizer Inc, NY, NY 10017

NDC 0069-2600-66

PART IV

30. cefaclor susp. 0.25 g _____

31. propanolol hydrocloride 120 mg _____

32. metronidazole 0.75 g _____

33. piroxicam 40 mg _____

34. Lopid® 300 mg _____

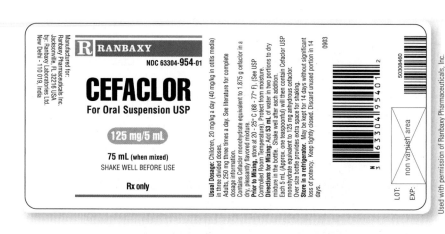

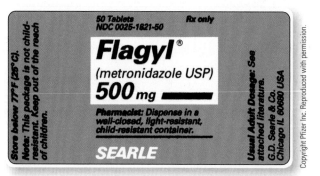

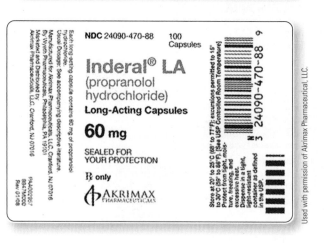

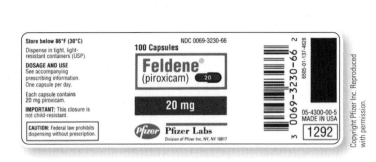

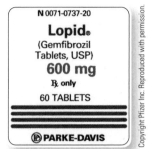

PART V

35. Vantin® 150 mg   _____

36. spironolactone 0.1 g   _____

37. cefpodoxime proxetil 0.2 g   _____

38. Azulfidine® 0.75 g   _____

39. potassium chloride 40 mEq   _____

40. Cipro® 250 mg   _____

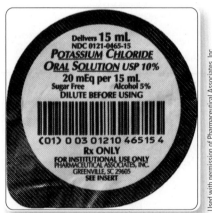

SECTION 3

Azulfidine®
sulfasalazine tablets, USP

500 mg

℞ only

MADE IN SWEDEN
Mfd. for: Pharmacia & Upjohn Co.
Kalamazoo, MI 49001, USA
by: Pharmacia & Upjohn AB
Stockholm, Sweden

300 Tablets

Pharmacia
&Upjohn

Copyright Pfizer Inc. Reproduced with permission.

NDC 0009-3615-03
50 mL (when mixed)

Vantin® *For Oral Suspension*
cefpodoxime proxetil
for oral suspension

100 mg per 5 mL

Equivalent to 100 mg per 5 mL
cefpodoxime when constituted

Pharmacia
&Upjohn

Copyright Pfizer Inc. Reproduced with permission.

Batch:
Expires:

DESCRIPTION: Each tablet contains
ciprofloxacin hydrochloride equivalent to
250 mg of ciprofloxacin.
DOSAGE: See accompanying literature
for complete information on dosage and
administration.
RECOMMENDED STORAGE:
Store below 86°F (30°C).

851210   NDC 0026-8512-51

CIPRO®
(ciprofloxacin hydrochloride)

Equivalent to
250 mg ciprofloxacin
100 Tablets

℞ Only

Bayer

Bayer Corporation
Pharmaceutical Division
400 Morgan Lane
West Haven, CT 06516

©2001 Bayer Corporation 2/01
10278   6505-01-333-4155
               Printed in USA

3 0026-8512-51 3

PL500331

Used with permission of Bayer Corporation.

Answers
1. 3 tab	**9.** 3 tab	**16.** 3 tab	**25.** 3 cap	**34.** ½ tab
2. 2 tab	**10.** 2 cap	**17.** 2 tab	**26.** 1½ tab	**35.** 7.5 mL
3. 2 cap	**11.** 2 tab (500 mg tablets)	**18.** 2 cap	**27.** 2 tab	**36.** 1 tab
4. 2 cap	**12.** 2 tab	**19.** 1½ tab	**28.** 1½ tab	**37.** 10 mL
5. 1 cap	**13.** 1 tab (500 mg tablets)	**20.** 3 tab	**29.** 2 tab	**38.** 1½ tab
6. 10 mL	**14.** 2 tab	**21.** 1 cap	**30.** 10 mL	**39.** 30 mL
7. 2 tab	**15.** 2 tab	**22.** 1 cap	**31.** 2 cap	**40.** 1 tab
8. 1 tab		**23.** 2 cap	**32.** 1½ tab	
		24. 1 tab	**33.** 2 cap	

CHAPTER 7

SAFE MEDICATION ADMINISTRATION

In this chapter you will be introduced to a sample **Medication Administration Record (MAR)** that may be used to prepare, administer, and chart medications. Additional instruction will include the **six rights of medication administration:** the basic guidelines for all medication administration; information on the most common sources of **medication errors;** and the **actions that you must take when errors occur**. You'll also be introduced to new transcription rules for medication dosages and abbreviations that have been addressed by the major watchdog organizations for medication safety: **The Joint Commission** and **The Institute for Safe Medication Practices (ISMP)**.

MEDICATION ADMINISTRATION RECORDS

The focus of this section is to familiarize you with a sample MAR so that you will understand the many columns and features it contains. Your instructors will orient you to the actual MARs you will use in your clinical experiences, and you will quickly discover that there is **no one universal form** in use. Each clinical facility using MARs makes its own determination on the particular format that suits its needs. What you will notice, however, is that **all MARs are more similar than different**. A MAR is, simply stated, **a paper record of all medications a patient is receiving and has received**.

The most prominent MAR feature is a **large column** where medications **given on a continuing basis** are listed. This column will contain a **drug name** (or names, if trade and generic listing is appropriate), **dosage, frequency, actual times of administration, and precautions related to administration, such as checking blood pressure, pulse, or body weight**. Other columns provide the following: an area that the person who transcribed the dosages initials; the start date of the medication; columns where dosages administered are recorded; an area for the initials of the nurse who gives the dosage; and an additional area where all staff initials are identified with a full name. A MAR may consist of a single sheet of paper printed on both sides, or two sheets, to allow separate space for p.r.n. (pro re nata or "as needed") medications (given on an as needed basis), for parenteral medications and site identification, and IV medications and/or fluids.

OBJECTIVES

The learner will:

1. read a MAR to identify medications to be administered.

2. record medications administered.

3. list and discuss the six rights of medication administration.

4. explain "partnering with the patient" in medication administration.

5. list common causes of dosage errors.

6. list the five steps to take when a dosage error occurs.

7. list the two major safety concerns addressed by The Joint Commission and ISMP.

Refer now to the sample MAR in Figure 7-1, and locate the following column headings and entries.

Column 1 Labeled "Start" and "Stop." The three drugs listed are being given on a continuing basis. They were started on "5–1." None has been discontinued.

Column 2 Labeled "Medication and Dose." The first drug listed is Lanoxin® including its generic name, digoxin. The dosage, "0.25 mg," and frequency, "daily," is next. There is a precautionary designation to "Check pulse" (ck pulse).

Column 3 Labeled "Schedule." Gives the actual times of each medication's administration. For Lanoxin, this is 8 am.

Column 4 This column has two designations: "Route," which is oral or "PO" for all three medications. The "Nurse" space, which "GJ" has initialed, identifies the transcriber of these medication orders.

Column 5 There are three designations here: "Time," the actual hour the drug is to be given (i.e., "8 am"); "Site" if the drug is parenteral; and "Initials," where the nurse who gave the drug, "BPP," verified administration. The pulse, "64," is recorded next to the 8 am dosage.

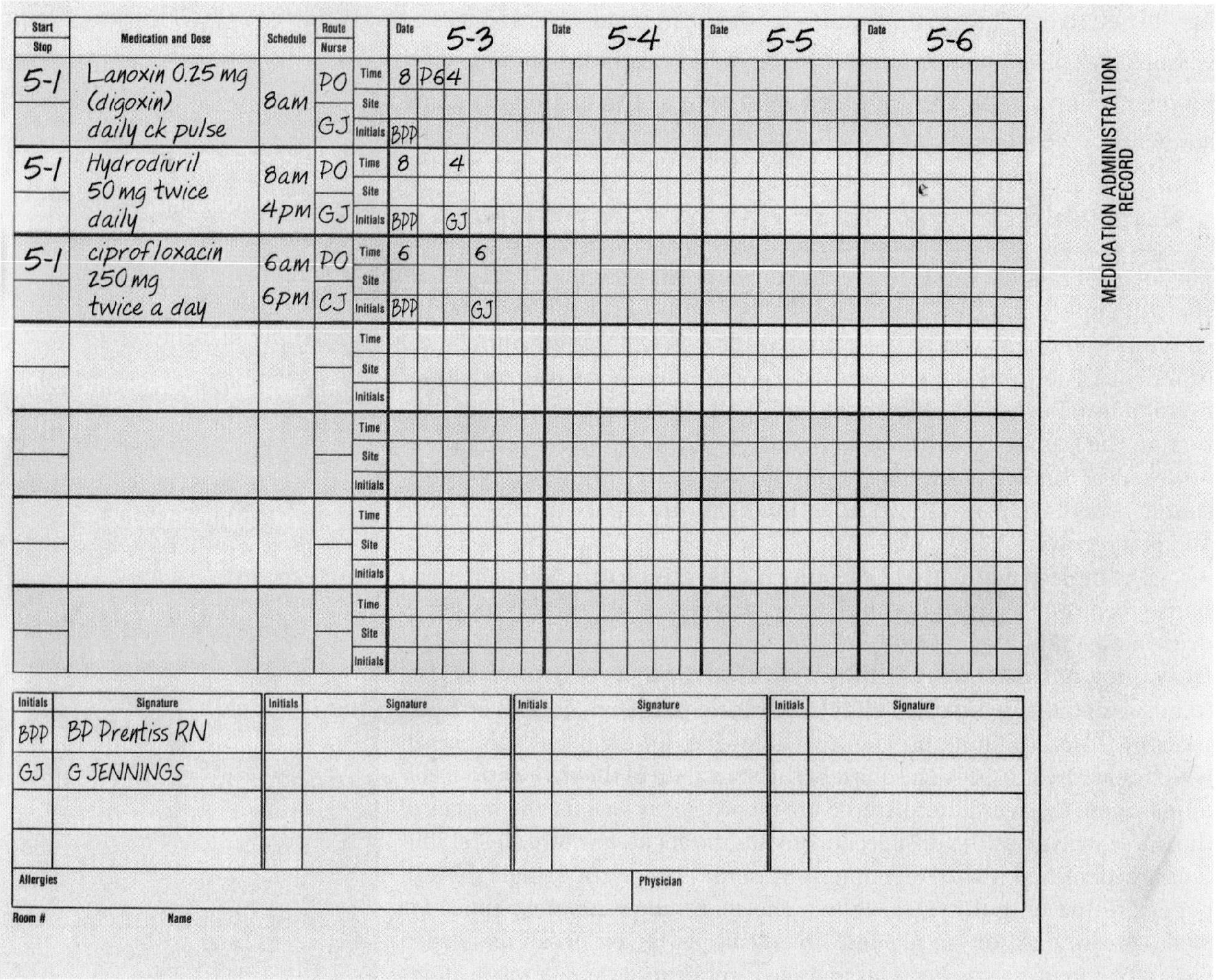

Start / Stop	Medication and Dose	Schedule	Route / Nurse		Date 5-3	Date 5-4	Date 5-5	Date 5-6
5-1	Lanoxin 0.25 mg (digoxin) daily ck pulse	8am	PO	Time	8 P64			
				Site				
			GJ	Initials	BPP			
5-1	Hydrodiuril 50 mg twice daily	8am 4pm	PO	Time	8 4			
				Site				
			GJ	Initials	BPP GJ			
5-1	ciprofloxacin 250 mg twice a day	6am 6pm	PO	Time	6 6			
				Site				
			CJ	Initials	BPP GJ			
				Time				
				Site				
				Initials				
				Time				
				Site				
				Initials				
				Time				
				Site				
				Initials				
				Time				
				Site				
				Initials				

Initials	Signature	Initials	Signature	Initials	Signature	Initials	Signature
BPP	BP Prentiss RN						
GJ	G JENNINGS						

Allergies

Physician

Room #

Name

MEDICATION ADMINISTRATION RECORD

FIGURE 7-1 Medication administration record.

This particular MAR covers only four days of medications, "5–3" through "5–6." However, most MARs provide for longer periods of up to a month. At the bottom of this MAR is an area for identification of staff initials, where "GJ" is clearly identified as "G Jennings" and "BPP" as "BP Prentiss."

▶▶▶ PROBLEMS 7.1

Refer to the MAR in Figure 7-1 to answer the following questions.

1. List the second and third listed drugs and dosages on this sample record.

   _____   _____

2. Who administered the 4 pm dosage for the second drug listed?

   _____   _____

3. Drug number 3 is administered twice a day. Identify the hours these dosages are to be given.

   _____   _____

Answers 1. Hydrodiuril 50 mg, ciprofloxacin 250 mg **2.** G. Jennings **3.** 6 am and 6 pm

▶▶▶ PROBLEMS 7.2

Use the drug entries on the MAR in Figure 7-1 as a guide to enter the following two additional drugs and dosages. Use today's date as the start date. Have your instructor or a fellow student check your entries.

1. Coumadin® (warfarin) 5 mg PO daily 6 pm.
2. Pronestyl® (procainamide) 1000 mg PO every 6 hours: 6 am, noon, 6 pm, and midnight.
3. Identify your initials as the transcriber of these dosages.
4. Sign for the initial 6 pm dosage administration for each drug.

Information needs to be filled in on the MAR.

Computer-controlled records, usually keyed to drug label bar codes, are making a strong appearance in the health care field. The Veterans Administration System in the United States is already completely computerized, and this has resulted in increased safety and lower costs in medication services. It is wise to remember, however, that errors can occur anywhere, and the newer systems of administration will have identified their own safety precautions for error-prone areas.

THE SIX RIGHTS OF MEDICATION ADMINISTRATION

The **six rights** of administration consist of the right **drug**, the right **dosage**, the right **route**, the right **time**, the right **person**, and the right **recording** of a dosage when it is administered. These rights will be covered in more detail in your fundamentals text, but it is appropriate to discuss them briefly here.

Right Drug

When preparing dosages, the **drug order and drug label are routinely checked against each other three times: when you locate the drug, just before you open or pour it, and immediately before you administer it**. There are three specific safety reminders related to reading labels that need to be revisited. The first is that **a drug may be ordered by trade name but available only in a generic** so make sure you have the drug ordered. The second concern is that **many drug names, particularly generic, are very similar** and must be identified carefully. And, finally, because it is easy to miss the **special initials that follow a drug name**—a familiar example is CR, for controlled release—look for and identify these. When doing the three required order and label cross checks, all these precautions to locate the correct drug apply.

Right Dosage

Dosage is **a particular concern in metric dosages containing a decimal**. Think back to your instruction in conversions between the different units of metric measure containing decimals. You know that in conversions in metric dosages, **the decimal point will always move three places**. If you are **converting from a greater to a lesser unit:** g to mg or mg to mcg, **the number will become larger**; if you are **converting from a lesser to a greater unit**: mcg to mg or mg to g, **the number will become smaller**. If you inadvertently **convert in the wrong direction, the numbers often don't make sense**: 0.25 mg **cannot** be 250 g; and 2 mg **cannot** be 0.002 mcg. Remember that medications are **prepared in average dosages** and usually consist of **one-half to three times the average dose (tablet or capsule) available**. Ask yourself if the conversion makes sense, and recognize when it doesn't.

Right Route

Oral medications are swallowed. This is not always easy for patients to do, and this is why many children's medications are prepared as liquids. This means you must **watch the patient actually take oral medications**. If you have any doubt that the medications have been swallowed, check the patient's mouth.

An additional oral route is the **sublingual: under the tongue**. There has been a considerable increase in the number of sublingual drugs in use, so this route designation is one to carefully identify. A sublingual drug swallowed will not have the desired effect, if it has any at all, because the acid of the stomach will destroy it.

Drops are another administration route, and eye, nose, and ear drops are quite common. Eye medications are also prepared as **ointments**, and, understandably, they are clearly labeled for their intended **ophthalmic** use. **Locating the ophthalmic designation** is mandatory before the use of any preparation on the eyes.

An increasing number of **topical** drugs is in use. These are **ointments** or, less commonly, **liquids** that are applied to the skin. The amount of ointment or liquid to be used is specific, as is the cleansing of a site for repeated ointment applications, and covering or not covering the site after application.

Now in very wide use are **transdermal patches**. The precautions in their use relate to where the patch must be applied, how long it is to stay on, and examination for local skin reaction to the adhesive that secures the patch. Unfortunately, many people are sensitive to transdermal patch adhesives. A rash may appear when a patch is used for the first time, or even after repeated use. Inflamed skin will not absorb well, and inflammation can cause acute discomfort.

A large number of **inhalation** medications is in common use. These medications are usually self-administered, and your responsibility will be to make sure that the patient understands how to use the inhalation device, how many activations each dosage requires, how many times a day to use the medication, and precautions in use, such as for temporary dizziness.

The **creams and suppositories** used for the genitorectal systems provide another method of direct medication application. These are very clearly labeled and recognizable.

Finally, there are the **parenterals: medications administered under the skin**. The **intravenous** is the primary parenteral route, with **intramuscular (IM)** and **subcutaneous** coming in second, and **intradermal** a distant third. Most injectable drugs are **site-specific**, and are labeled for either IV, IM, or subcutaneous use. You'll be reading many drug labels that identify specific parenteral site routes in the balance of this text.

Right Time

The time each drug is to be given is **often critical**, such as insulin immediately before a meal or, more correctly, a meal as soon as insulin is injected. Drugs may be ordered at **specific hours during the day or only at bedtime**. Some drugs must be given **before or after specific blood tests**. Pain medications are given **p.r.n.**, which means **as needed**. Pain medications are extremely **time sensitive**, and must be given before pain becomes severe in postoperative situations, and at least half an hour before a painful procedure, including postoperative ambulation.

Each clinical facility designates routine administration times; however, twice a day may mean 9 am and 5 pm or 9 am and 9 pm, depending on the action of the drug being given. Each MAR identifies **two time-related specifics: frequency**—for example, "twice a day"—then **specific hours**—for example, 9 (am) and 5 (pm) or, in international/military time, 09 and 17, representing 0900 and 1700.

A final consideration, just illustrated, is **standard versus international/military time**. A clinical facility will use **either one time or the other, but not both**. International/military time uses a 24-hour clock, starting with 0001 for one minute after midnight, to 2400 for midnight of the same (next date) day. To convert from standard to international/military time, add 12 hours to each hour beginning with 1 pm standard time. For example, 2 pm plus 12 hours is 1400; 4 pm plus 12 (hours) is 1600. Using international time, if you are unfamiliar with it, will initially require careful thought. Refer to Figure 7-2 for a complete time conversion chart.

Standard am	International/Military am	Standard pm	International/Military pm
1:00	0100	1:00	1300
2:00	0200	2:00	1400
3:00	0300	3:00	1500
4:00	0400	4:00	1600
5:00	0500	5:00	1700
6:00	0600	6:00	1800
7:00	0700	7:00	1900
8:00	0800	8:00	2000
9:00	0900	9:00	2100
10:00	1000	10:00	2200
11:00	1100	11:00	2300
12:00 noon	1200	12:00 midnight	2400

FIGURE 7-2 Comparison of standard and international/military time.

Right Person

Administering medications to the **right person** should be foolproof, but it isn't. All MARs identify patients by the **room number and bed** they occupy. But sometimes patients are moved, so room and bed number cannot be relied on for identification. The current identification procedure is to **ask an individual her or his name and birthdate**, then check the response against the wrist **Identa-Band**®. Obviously, some people will not be able to state their name. But if they can, they must be asked.

Of considerable concern is the possibility of having two people with the same surname on the same floor or even, though more rarely, in the same room. **Duplicate names** are a source of errors, so **read both surname, first name, and birthdate** on each Identa-Band®. **Do this every time you give a medication. No exceptions. Once a drug is administered, there is no way to get it back.**

Right Recording

If an administered drug **is not charted, it can be given again in error**. There is an **absolute rule that a drug given must be recorded immediately**. It is also necessary to **record and report unusual reactions to a medication**, such as nausea or dizziness, or a patient's **refusal to take a medication**. In such an occurrence, **record and report the incident immediately**.

If you give a **parenteral** medication other than by IV, **the injection site used is usually recorded,** so that a different site can be used next time. Diabetic or other patients receiving frequent injections may tell you which site they prefer, which they have a perfect right to do. Or, ask them if they have a preference. In actual practice, **sites are chosen by the condition of the tissues at acceptable sites,** because previous injection sites are generally easy to see and must be avoided.

THE SEVENTH RIGHT: PARTNERING WITH THE PATIENT

Partnering with the patient/recipient is so important a concern that it should be a seventh right. You are only half of a medication administration twosome. **The medication recipient is one of your best assists in preventing errors**. Consider the following, not uncommon, verbal reports: "I just had my medication." Or, "My doctor told me he was stopping this drug." Or, "The doctor said I needed a bigger dose." Or, "This pill doesn't look the same as the one I had before." Or, "Where is my . . . pill?" Or, "This pill made me sick the last time I took it." Learn to listen very carefully, and **consider the patient correct until proven otherwise**.

You will also be responsible for **helping the patient learn what drugs and dosages he or she is taking, what they are for, what time they must be taken, and how they must be taken**. Most individuals will be discharged with medications, so the sooner they—or, if they are not deemed responsible, their caretaker—can learn what they are taking, the better. They must also learn about common side effects and, if particularly relevant, what untoward effects they should watch for. Patients taking medications are essentially under chemical assistance, or assault, and they or their caretakers must be full partners in their medication administration.

 KEYpoint: An important safety precaution is recognition of the patient/recipient as a full partner in medication administration.

COMMON MEDICATION ERRORS

Prescription drugs are estimated to kill close to 100,000 people a year in the United States, although not all these deaths are hospital based. Medication errors happen, and they will continue to happen in **all three of the modalities** related to drug orders: the **prescribing** (done by a licensed practitioner), the **transcribing** (done by a person who specializes in this responsibility, frequently the pharmacy staff), or the **administering** (primarily a nursing responsibility). The vast majority of errors is in the prescribing and transcribing areas, but those attributable to administering still represent a very large number of incidents.

There has been a concerted **international** effort in recent years to identify the source of, and take active steps to reduce, the incidence of medication errors caused by the use of administration abbreviations. The primary and an ongoing leader in this project is **The Joint Commission**, formerly known as the **Joint Commission on Accreditation of Healthcare Organizations**.

Most safety recommendations fall into **two major categories: abbreviations for administration and drug names,** and **metric dosages containing decimals**.

Errors in Abbreviations and Drug Names

A number of abbreviations designating **the frequency and routes of medication administration** have been eliminated; for example, the abbreviations Q.D., QD, q.d., and qd used for a **single daily dose** and Q.O.D., QOD, q.o.d., and qod used for a dosage given **every other day**. These are no longer used but are now clearly written as **"daily"** or **"every other day."** Similarly, q.d. and QD for "every day" have been eliminated and are now designated "daily"; qhs, formerly used for "nightly" and misread as "every hour," is now written "nightly"; SC or sub q used for "subcutaneous" has been changed to "subcut" or "subcutaneous"; the use of "per os" for "by mouth" has been eliminated in favor of "PO," "by mouth," or "orally." An additional abbreviation, q2h or q2hr (or **any** specific hour) is now clearly written "every 2 hours." Another deletion is the use of a lowercase "u" or uppercase "U" or "IU" for "units." As you have already learned, units is not abbreviated, but is written as "units." A current list of acceptable administration abbreviations is available on the inside front cover of this text, but do keep in mind that there may be future changes in this evolving area of concern.

Common examples of confusing **drug name abbreviations** are MS for morphine sulfate and MSO_4 or $MgSO_4$ for magnesium sulfate. These drugs are now identified using their complete names. Figure 7-3, the Official "Do Not Use" List, identifies these changes.

Errors in Writing Metric Dosages

All the correct rules for writing metric dosages have been covered earlier in this text. But let's revisit the culprit areas, which are also identified in Figure 7-3. The first error is in **placing a decimal and a zero (0) following a whole number dosage** (called a **trailing zero**); for example, 4.0 g instead of 4 g. The decimal could easily be missed and 10 times the ordered dosage, 40 g, administered. The second error is **failing to place a zero in front of a decimal fraction** (referred to as lack of a **leading zero**); for example, .5 mg instead of **0**.5 mg. Once again, the decimal could be missed and 5 mg administered. Unfortunately, you may still see an occasional commercial drug label that has not yet been standardized to reflect the new recommended notation rules. But at least on a drug label you will not have the problem of trying to **interpret indecipherable handwriting**, which is often the direct cause of many of the errors just discussed. Commercial drug labels are being redesigned to reflect these new guidelines.

Additional changes have since been recommended by **ISMP**, the **Institute for Safe Medication Practices**. Those of you re-entering the health care field after a significant absence may want to review the ISMP lists in Appendix B. These tables are for reference only and need not be memorized.

Action Steps When Errors Occur

You will almost certainly meet with an error in one way or another during your career. So, let's look at the routine steps you must take when one occurs.

STEP 1   Errors must be reported as soon as they are discovered.

STEP 2   Necessary remedial measures must be instituted immediately.

STEP 3   The reason for the error must be determined.

STEP 4   An incident/accident report must be prepared.

STEP 5   Corrective policies/procedures must be instituted, if possible, to prevent the error from recurring.

Official "Do Not Use" List[1]

Do Not Use	Potential Problem	Use Instead
U, u (unit)	Mistaken for "0" (zero), the number "4" (four) or "cc"	Write "unit"
IU (International Unit)	Mistaken for IV (intravenous) or the number 10 (ten)	Write "International Unit"
Q.D., QD, q.d., qd (daily)	Mistaken for each other	Write "daily"
Q.O.D., QOD, q.o.d, qod (every other day)	Period after the Q mistaken for "I" and the "O" mistaken for "I"	Write "every other day"
Trailing zero (X.0 mg)* Lack of leading zero (.X mg)	Decimal point is missed	Write X mg Write 0.X mg
MS	Can mean morphine sulfate or magnesium sulfate	Write "morphine sulfate" Write "magnesium sulfate"
MSO$_4$ and MgSO$_4$	Confused for one another	

[1] Applies to all orders and all medication-related documentation that is handwritten (including free-text computer entry) or on pre-printed forms.

*Exception: A "trailing zero" may be used only where required to demonstrate the level of precision of the value being reported, such as for laboratory results, imaging studies that report size of lesions, or catheter/tube sizes. It may not be used in medication orders or other medication-related documentation.

▲ **FIGURE 7-3** Official "Do Not Use" list of medical abbreviations.

The most important step after ensuring the safety of the patient is reporting the error. If an error isn't reported, no action can be taken. Keep in mind that **an error is an accident, and it is not necessarily a reflection on competency, nor will reporting an error terminate your career. Distraction and fatigue play a significant role in medication errors**, and when in stressful situations, you must be particularly aware and vigilant that **you** do not become the person making an error.

KEY*point:* The major factors in nursing medication administration errors are distraction and fatigue, and particular vigilance is necessary in these stressful situations.

In time, and with repeat practice, administering medications will become familiar and comfortable. The irony is that when it does, you must **exercise more caution than ever. Routine medication administration must never be routine**.

 KEY*point:* Regardless of the source of an error, if you give a wrong drug or dosage, you are legally responsible for it.

Summary

This completes your introduction to safe medication administration. The important points to remember from this chapter are:

▼ When identifying a drug, pay particular attention to generic names and any initials that identify additional drug components or action.

▼ When identifying dosages, take special precautions with metric dosages containing a decimal.

▼ The route of administration is critical to medication safety and effectiveness.

▼ Parenteral medications are site specific: IV, IM, subcutaneous, and intradermal.

▼ Time of administration is especially important for p.r.n. medications for pain, and for drugs with a rapid action such as insulin.

▼ Identification of the right person begins with asking the patient his or her name, followed by checking the Identa-Band®.

▼ Making the patient or caretaker a full partner in medication administration is a major safety consideration.

▼ Recent changes in abbreviations for drug names and administration are creating increased safety in the clinical setting.

▼ Dosage errors must be reported as soon as discovered to set in motion the four additional steps you must take.

▼ Administering medications must never become routine.

▼ Fatigue and/or clinical distractions are major factors in medication errors.

▼ MARs are the immediate reference for medication administration, and keeping them up-to-the-minute is of prime importance.

Summary Self-Test

Answer the questions as succinctly as possible.

1. List the six rights of medication administration. _____
    _____

2. What consideration was stressed regarding reading generic names? _____
    _____

3. What might extra initials following a drug name identify? _____
    _____
    _____

4. List the two major transcribing considerations for metric dosages containing
    a decimal. _____
    _____
    _____

5. What use will you make of the fact that medications are prepared in average dosages?
    _____
    _____

6. Name and discuss the two time-sensitive medications that were identified in this chapter.
    _____
    _____
    _____

7. What two patient identification steps follow arrival at the room and bed number
    indicated on a MAR? _____
    _____

8. What will you do if a patient refuses a medication? _____
    _____

9. List the steps you must take when a medication error occurs. _____
    _____
    _____
    _____

10. List your medication responsibilities in preparing a patient for discharge.
    _____
    _____
    _____

Answers 1. Drug, dosage, route, person, time, and recording **2.** Read carefully; they are often similar
3. Additional medications in a preparation or special action **4.** Use a zero in front of a decimal to draw
attention to it; no decimal or zero following a whole-number dosage **5.** An unusual number of oral tablets
or capsules or excessively large mL volumes must be questioned **6.** Pain medications—give before pain becomes severe or half an hour before a painful procedure; insulin—make sure a meal is available shortly after
administration **7.** Ask the patient for his or her name and birthdate; check response against the Identa-Band®
8. Ask why, record it, report it **9.** Report the error, take remedial measures as necessary, determine the
cause, complete an incident report, and institute a policy to prevent a repeat **10.** Review all the discharge
drugs by asking the patient to explain the dosage, frequency, time, and route of administration for each.
Review these again as necessary, including side effects and precautions

CHAPTER 8

HYPODERMIC SYRINGE MEASUREMENT

A variety of hypodermic syringes is in clinical use. This chapter focuses most heavily on the frequently used 3 mL syringe. However, larger volume syringes are used on occasion, so it is necessary that you learn the **differences** as well as the **similarities** of all syringes in use.

Regardless of a syringe's volume or capacity–0.5, 1, 3, 5, 10, or 20 mL–all except specialized insulin syringes **are calibrated in mL**. Because some syringe manufacturers have not yet replaced the labeling on their syringes with the official mL volume measurement, you may still see cc on syringes. Keep in mind, however, that these two measures, mL and cc, are essentially identical. They will be correctly referred to throughout this text as mL. The various capacity syringes contain **calibrations that differ from each other**. Recognizing the difference in syringe calibrations is the chief safety concern of this chapter.

KEYpoint: The calibrations on different volume syringes differ from each other, requiring particular care in dosage measurement.

STANDARD 3 mL SYRINGE

The most commonly used hypodermic syringe is the 3 mL size illustrated in Figure 8-1. Notice the calibrations for the metric mL scale, and that **longer calibrations** identify zero (0) and each ½ and full mL measure. These longer calibrations are numbered: ½, 1, 1½, 2, 2½, and 3.

Next, notice the **number of calibrations in each mL**, which is **10**, indicating that, on this syringe, each mL is **calibrated in tenths**. Tenths of a mL are written as **decimal fractions**; for example 1.2 mL, 2.5 mL, or 0.4 mL. Also, notice the arrow on this syringe, which identifies a 0.8 mL dosage.

OBJECTIVES

The learner will measure parenteral solutions using:

1. a standard 3 mL syringe.
2. a tuberculin syringe.
3. 5 and 10 mL syringes.
4. a 20 mL syringe.

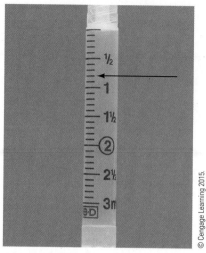

▲ **FIGURE 8-1** A 3 mL syringe.

▶▶▶ PROBLEMS 8.1

Use decimal numbers—for example, 2.2 mL—to identify the measurements indicated by the arrows on the standard 3 mL syringes that follow.

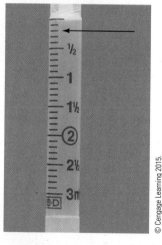

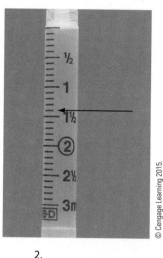

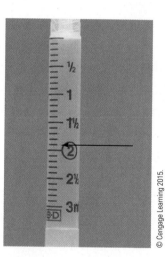

1. _____

2. _____

3. _____

Answers **1.** 0.2 mL **2.** 1.4 mL **3.** 1.9 mL

Did you have difficulty with the 0.2 mL calibration in Problem 1? Remember that **the first long calibration on all syringes is zero**. It is slightly longer than the 0.1 mL and subsequent one-tenth calibrations. Be careful not to mistakenly count it as 0.1 mL.

You have just been looking at photos of syringe barrels only. In assembled syringes, the colored suction tip of the plunger has two widened areas in contact with the barrel that look like two distinct rings. **Calibrations are read from the front, or top, ring.** Do not become confused by the second, or bottom, ring or by the raised middle section of the suction tip.

▶▶▶ PROBLEMS 8.2

What dosages are measured by the following three assembled syringes?

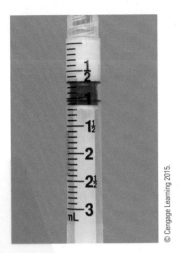

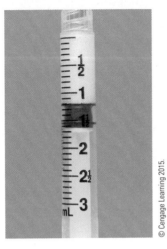

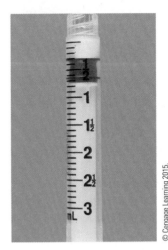

1. _____   2. _____   3. _____

Answers **1.** 0.7 mL **2.** 1.2 mL **3.** 0.3 mL

▶▶▶ PROBLEMS 8.3

Draw an arrow or shade in the following syringe barrels to indicate the required dosages. Have your instructor check your accuracy.

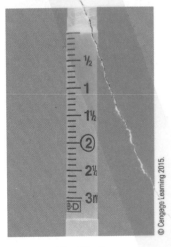

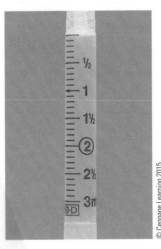

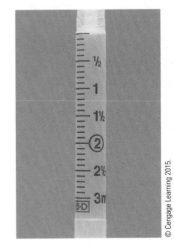

1. 1.3 mL   2. 2.4 mL   3. 0.9 mL

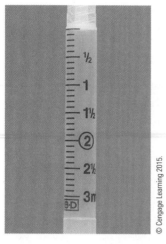

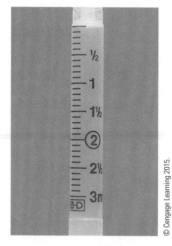

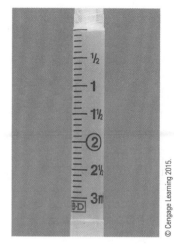

4. 2.5 mL   5. 1.7 mL   6. 2.1 mL

Verify your answers with your instructor.

▶▶▶ PROBLEMS 8.4

Identify the dosages measured on the following 3 mL syringes.

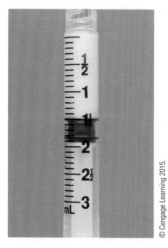

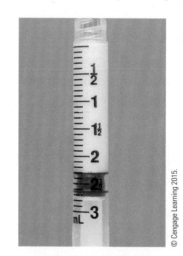

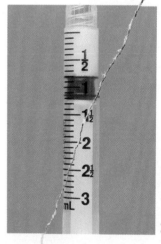

1. _____   2. _____   3. _____

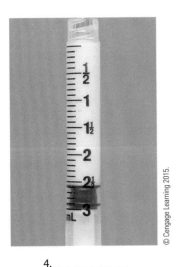

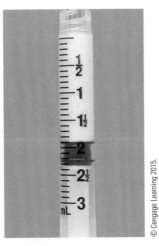

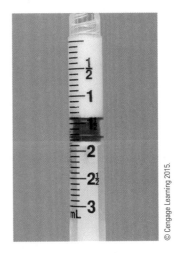

4. _____

5. _____

6. _____

Answers **1.** 1.5 mL **2.** 2.3 mL **3.** 0.8 mL **4.** 2.6 mL **5.** 1.9 mL **6.** 1.4 mL

SAFETY SYRINGES

A number of safety syringes has been developed in recent years to reduce the danger of accidental contaminated needle sticks. Several of these syringes are illustrated in the following photos. Take a few minutes to become familiar with them, because you will in all probability be using them in the clinical setting.

Refer first to the photos in Figure 8-2, which show two BD SafetyGlide™ syringes. Each of these syringes contains a protective needle guard that can be activated by a single finger to cover and seal the needle after injection.

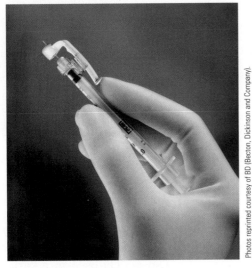

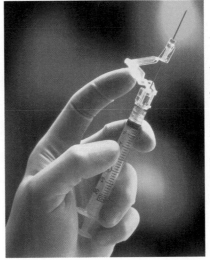

▲ **FIGURE 8-2** SafetyGlide™ syringes.

The syringe shown in Figure 8-3, the VanishPoint®, has a needle that automatically retracts into the barrel after injection.

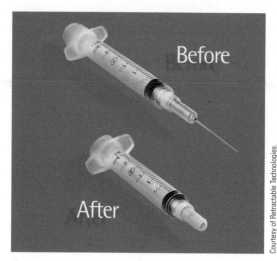

▲ **FIGURE 8-3** VanishPoint®.

A third type of safety needle commonly used is the Magellan Safety Needle by Covidien™, as shown in Figure 8-4. This design also offers one-handed activation. It can be activated one of three ways: by thumb, forefinger, or on a flat surface. As with the other safety syringes, once activated, its safety shield covers the entire needle, providing protection during and after disposal.

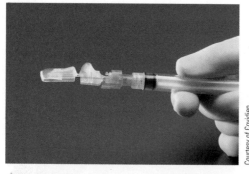
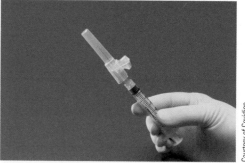

▲ **FIGURE 8-4** Magellan Safety Needle.

TUBERCULIN (TB) SYRINGE

When very small dosages are required, they are measured in special tuberculin (TB) **0.5 or 1 mL syringes calibrated in hundredths**. Originally designed for the small dosages required for tuberculin skin testing, these syringes are also widely used in a variety of sensitivity and allergy tests. Pediatric dosages frequently require measurement in hundredths, as does heparin, an anticoagulant drug.

Refer to the 0.5 mL TB syringe in Figure 8-5, and take a careful look at its metric calibrated hundredth scale. Notice that slightly longer calibrations identify zero, 0.05, 0.1, 0.15, 0.2, and so on, through the 0.5 mL measure. Shorter calibrations lie between these to measure the hundredths. Each tenth mL, .1, .2, .3, .4, and .5, is numbered on this particular TB syringe. Take a moment to study the dosage measured by the arrow in Figure 8-5, which is 0.43 mL.

The closeness and small size of TB syringe calibrations mandate particular care and an unhurried approach in TB syringe dosage measurement.

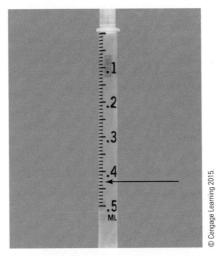

▲ **FIGURE 8-5** A tuberculin (TB) syringe.

▶▶▶ PROBLEMS 8.5

Identify the measurements on the six TB syringes provided.

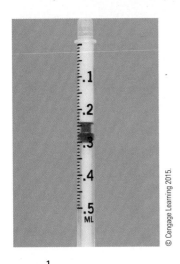

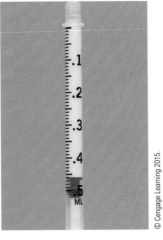

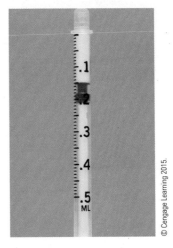

1. _____   2. _____   3. _____

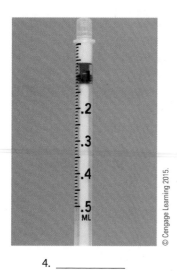

© Cengage Learning 2015.

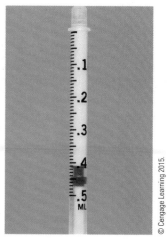

© Cengage Learning 2015.

© Cengage Learning 2015.

4. _____   5. _____   6. _____

Answers   **1.** 0.24 mL   **2.** 0.46 mL   **3.** 0.15 mL   **4.** 0.06 mL   **5.** 0.27 mL   **6.** 0.41 mL

▶▶▶ PROBLEMS 8.6

Draw an arrow on the barrel to identify the dosages indicated on these TB syringes. Have your instructor check your answers.

© Cengage Learning 2015.

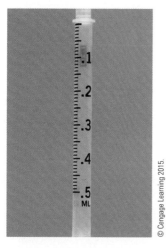

© Cengage Learning 2015.

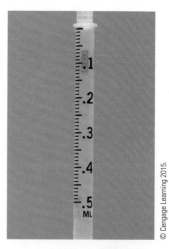

© Cengage Learning 2015.

1. 0.28 mL   2. 0.32 mL   3. 0.45 mL

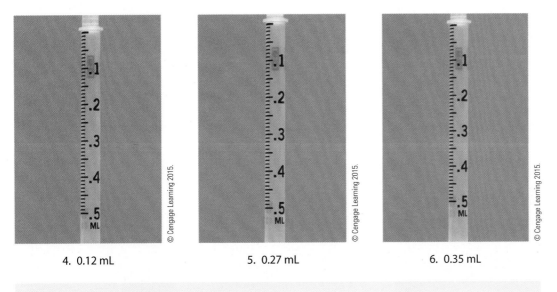

4. 0.12 mL   5. 0.27 mL   6. 0.35 mL

Verify your answers with your instructor.

5 AND 10 mL SYRINGES

When volumes larger than 3 mL are required, a 5 or 10 mL syringe is typically used. Refer to Figure 8-6, and examine the calibrations between the numbered mLs to determine how these syringes are calibrated.

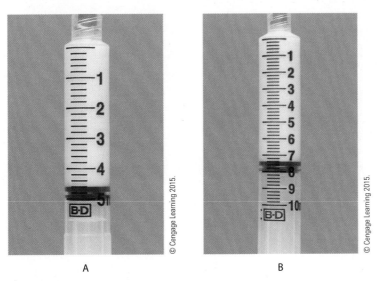

A   B

△ **FIGURE 8-6** A 5 mL (A) and a 10 mL (B) syringe.

As you may have discovered, the calibrations divide each mL of these syringes into **five** so that **each shorter calibration actually measures 0.2 mL**. The 5 mL syringe on the left measures 4.6 mL, and the 10 mL syringe on the right measures 7.4 mL. These syringes are most often used to measure whole rather than fractional dosages, but in your practice readings, we will include a full range of measurements.

SECTION 3

▶▶▶ PROBLEMS 8.7

What dosages are measured on the following syringes?

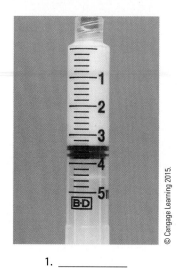

© Cengage Learning 2015.

1. _____

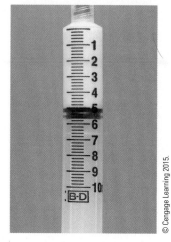

© Cengage Learning 2015.

2. _____

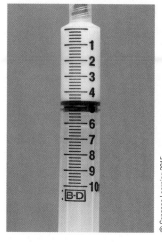

© Cengage Learning 2015.

3. _____

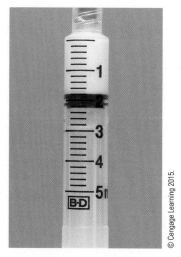

© Cengage Learning 2015.

4. _____

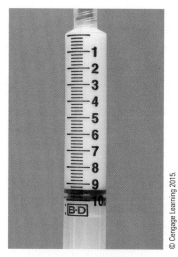

© Cengage Learning 2015.

5. _____

Answers   1. 3.4 mL   **2.** 5 mL   **3.** 4.6 mL   **4.** 1.8 mL   **5.** 9.4 mL

▶▶▶ PROBLEMS 8.8

Measure the dosages indicated on the syringes provided. Have an instructor check your accuracy.

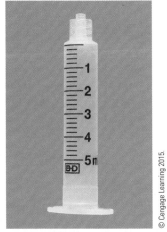

1. 1.4 mL

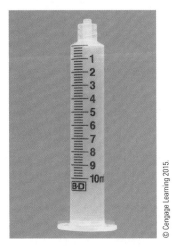

2. 3.2 mL

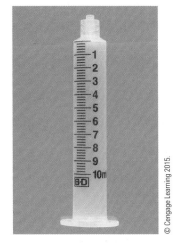

3. 6.8 mL

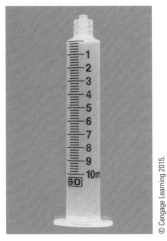

4. 9.4 mL

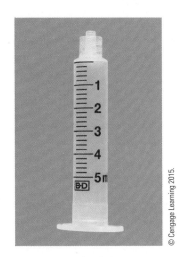

5. 3 mL

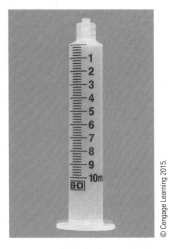

6. 5.6 mL

Verity your answers with your instructor.

20 mL AND LARGER SYRINGES

Examine the 20 mL syringe in Figure 8-7, and determine how it is calibrated.

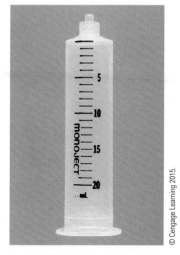

△ **FIGURE 8-7** A 20 mL syringe.

As you can see, this syringe is calibrated in **1 mL increments,** with longer calibrations identifying the 0, 5, 10, 15, and 20 mL volumes. Syringes with a capacity larger than 20 mL are also calibrated in full mL measures. These syringes are used only for measurement of very large volumes.

▶▶▶ PROBLEMS 8.9

What dosages are measured on these syringes?

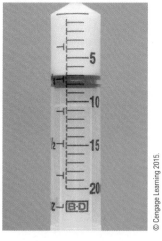

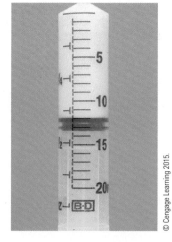

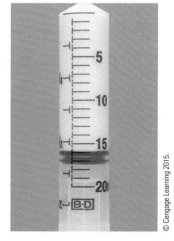

1. _____

2. _____

3. _____

Answers   **1.** 7 mL   **2.** 12 mL   **3.** 16 mL

PROBLEMS 8.10

Shade in or draw arrows on the three syringe barrels provided to identify the volumes listed. Have your answers checked by your instructor.

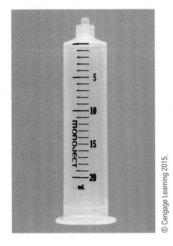

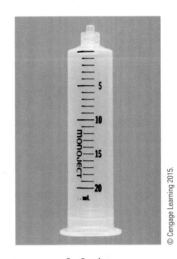

1. 11 mL   2. 18 mL   3. 9 mL

Verify your answers with your instructor.

Summary

This concludes your introduction to syringe calibrations. The important points to remember from this chapter are:

▽ 3 mL syringes are calibrated in tenths.

▽ TB syringes are calibrated in hundredths.

▽ 5 and 10 mL syringes are calibrated in fifths (two-tenths).

▽ Syringes larger than 10 mL are calibrated in full mL measures.

▽ The first long calibration on all syringes indicates zero.

▽ All syringe calibrations must be read from the top, or front, ring of the plunger's suction tip.

Summary Self-Test

Identify the dosages measured on the following syringes.

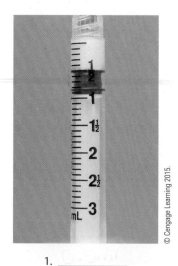

1. _____

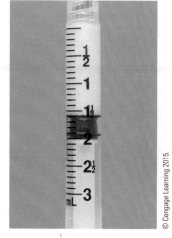

2. _____

3. _____

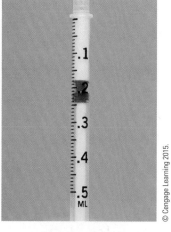

4. _____

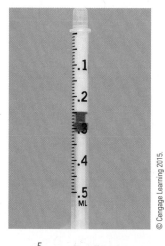

5. _____

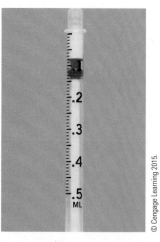

6. _____

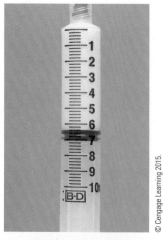

7. _____

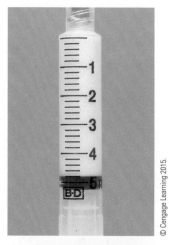

8. _____

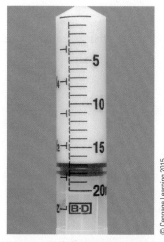

9. _____

Draw arrows or shade the barrels on the following syringes/cartridges to measure the indicated dosages. Have your answers checked by your instructor.

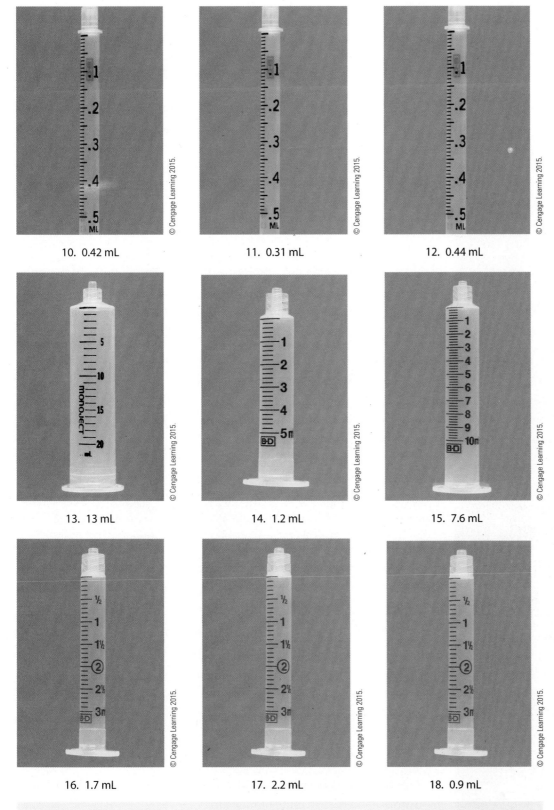

10. 0.42 mL   11. 0.31 mL   12. 0.44 mL

13. 13 mL   14. 1.2 mL   15. 7.6 mL

16. 1.7 mL   17. 2.2 mL   18. 0.9 mL

Answers **1.** 0.5 mL **2.** 2.5 mL **3.** 1.6 mL **4.** 0.18 mL **5.** 0.25 mL **6.** 0.08 mL **7.** 6.4 mL **8.** 4.8 mL **9.** 17 mL **10–18.** Verify your answers with your instructor.

CHAPTER 8

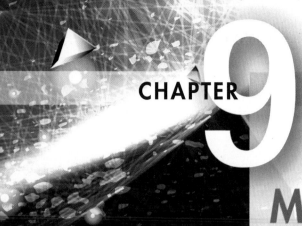

CHAPTER 9

PARENTERAL MEDICATION LABELS AND DOSAGE CALCULATION

OBJECTIVES

The learner will:

1. read parenteral solution labels and identify dosage strengths.

2. calculate average parenteral dosages from the labels provided.

3. measure parenteral dosages in metric, milliequivalent, unit, percentage, and ratio strengths using 3 mL, TB, 5, 10, and 20 mL syringes.

Parenteral medications are administered by injection, with intravenous (IV), intramuscular (IM), and subcutaneous (subcut) being the most frequently used routes. The labels of oral and parenteral solutions are very similar, but the size of the average parenteral dosage label is much smaller. Intramuscular solutions are manufactured so that the **average adult dosage will be contained in a volume of between 0.5 mL and 3 mL**, with subcutaneous injections being smaller, and seldom exceeding 1 mL. Excessively larger or smaller volumes would need to be questioned and calculations rechecked.

 KEY*point:* Volumes larger than 3 mL are difficult for a single IM injection site to absorb, and the 0.5 to 3 mL volume can be used as a guideline for accuracy of calculations in IM and subcutaneous dosages.

Intravenous medication administration is usually a two-step procedure. The dosage is prepared first, then may be further diluted in IV fluids before administration. In this chapter, we will be concerned only with the **first step of IV drug preparation, which is accurate measurement of the prescribed dosage.**

Parenteral medications are packaged in a variety of single-use glass ampules, single- and multiple-use rubber-stoppered vials, and premeasured syringes and cartridges. See Figure 9-1.

READING METRIC/SI SOLUTION LABELS

Let's begin by looking at parenteral solution labels on which the dosages are expressed in metric units of measure.

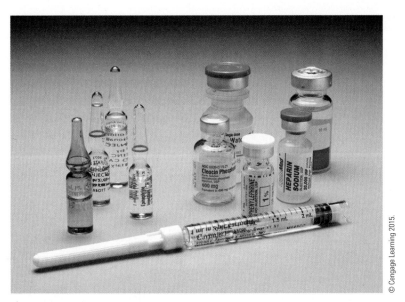

▲ **FIGURE 9-1** Ampules, vials, and a prefilled cartridge.

EXAMPLE 1

Refer to the Vistaril® label in Figure 9-2. The immediate difference you will notice between this and oral solution labels is the **size**. Ampules and vials are small and their labels are small, which requires that they be **read with particular care**. The information, however, is similar to oral labels. Vistaril is the trade name of the drug; hydroxyzine hydrochloride is the generic name. The dosage strength is 50 mg per mL (in the red rectangular area). The total vial contents are 10 mL (in black, center). Keep in mind that average intramuscular and subcutaneous dosages usually consist of one-half to double the average dosage strength, which for this IM Vistaril is 50 mg per mL.

> For 50 mg, you would give 1 mL
> For 25 mg, you would give 0.5 mL
> For 100 mg, you would give 2 mL
> For 75 mg, you would give 1.5 mL

These average dosages are within the usual 0.5 to 3 mL IM volume.

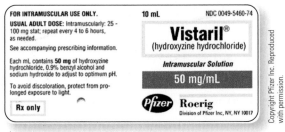

▲ **FIGURE 9-2**

EXAMPLE 2

The Robinul® (glycopyrrolate) medication in Figure 9-3 has a dosage strength of 0.2 mg/mL.

For a 0.2 mg dosage, you would give 1 mL

For a 0.1 mg dosage, you would give 0.5 mL

For a 200 mcg dosage, you would give 1 mL

For a 100 mcg dosage, you would give 0.5 mL

For a 0.4 mg dosage, you would give 2 mL

For a 400 mcg dosage, you would give 2 mL

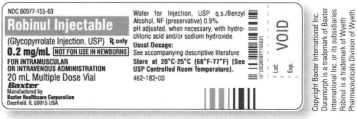

▲ **FIGURE 9-3**

▶▶▶ PROBLEMS 9.1

Refer to the antibiotic solution label in Figure 9-4 to answer the following questions.

1. What is the dosage strength of this solution? _____

2. How many mL are required for a dosage of 3 mg? _____

3. How many mL for a 6 mg dosage? _____

4. How many mL for a 9 mg dosage? _____

5. How many mL for a 12 mg dosage? _____

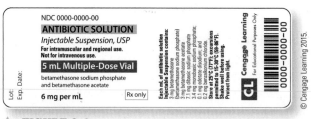

▲ **FIGURE 9-4**

Answers **1.** 6 mg/mL **2.** 0.5 mL **3.** 1 mL **4.** 1.5 mL **5.** 2 mL

▶▶▶ PROBLEMS 9.2

Refer to the Ativan label in Figure 9-5 to answer the following questions.

1. What is the total volume of this vial? _____

2. What is the dosage strength? _____

3. If 8 mg were ordered, how many mL would this be? _____

4. If 6 mg were ordered, how many mL would this be? _____

5. How many mL would you need to prepare a 20 mg dosage? _____

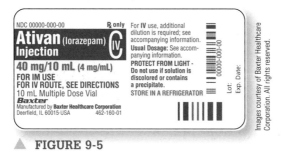

▲ **FIGURE 9-5**

Answers   1. 10 mL **2.** 40 mg/10 mL or 4 mg/mL **3.** 20 mL **4.** 15 mL **5.** 5 mL

PERCENT (%) AND RATIO SOLUTION LABELS

Drugs labeled as **percentage solutions** often express the dosage strength in **metric measures in addition to percentage strength**. The lidocaine label in Figure 9-6, a 2% solution, is an example.

But directly underneath this is a "20 mg/mL" designation. Lidocaine HCl is most often ordered in mg, but it is also used as a local anesthetic, and when it is, a physician may ask you to prepare a volume dosage specifying % strength.

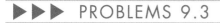 PROBLEMS 9.3

Refer to the lidocaine label in Figure 9-6 to answer the following questions.

1. How many mL are needed for a 10 mg dosage? _____

2. How many mL for a 20 mg dosage? _____

3. If you are asked to prepare 5 mL of a 2% solution, how many mL would you draw up? _____

4. If you are asked to prepare 15 mg? _____

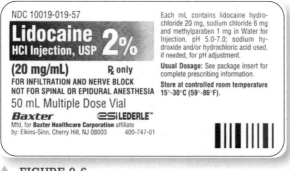

▲ **FIGURE 9-6**

Answers   1. 0.5 mL **2.** 1 mL **3.** 5 mL **4.** 0.75 mL

▶▶▶ PROBLEMS 9.4

Refer to the lidocaine label in Figure 9-7 to answer the following questions.

1. What is the percentage strength of this lidocaine solution?   _____

2. How many mL does the vial contain?   _____

3. If you are asked to prepare 20 mL of a 1% lidocaine solution, how many mL will you draw up in the syringe?   _____

4. What is the metric dosage strength of this solution?   _____

5. If you are asked to prepare 25 mg from this vial, what volume will you draw up?   _____

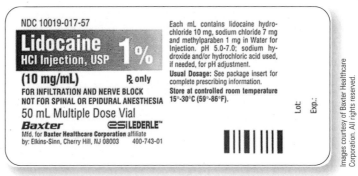

NDC 10019-017-57

Lidocaine 1%
HCl Injection, USP

(10 mg/mL)   ℞ only
FOR INFILTRATION AND NERVE BLOCK
NOT FOR SPINAL OR EPIDURAL ANESTHESIA
50 mL Multiple Dose Vial
Baxter   ℮SILEDERLE™
Mfd. for **Baxter Healthcare Corporation** affiliate
by: Elkins-Sinn, Cherry Hill, NJ 08003   400-743-01

Each mL contains lidocaine hydrochloride 10 mg, sodium chloride 7 mg and methylparaben 1 mg in Water for Injection. pH 5.0-7.0; sodium hydroxide and/or hydrochloric acid used, if needed, for pH adjustment.
Usual Dosage: See package insert for complete prescribing information.
Store at controlled room temperature 15°-30°C (59°-86°F).

Lot:
Exp.:

▲ FIGURE 9-7

Refer to the calcium gluconate label in Figure 9-8 to answer the following questions.

6. What is the percentage strength of this solution?   _____

7. How many mL does this preparation contain?   _____

8. What is the per mL mEq dosage strength of this solution?   _____

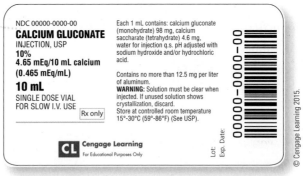

NDC 00000-0000-00

CALCIUM GLUCONATE
INJECTION, USP
10%
4.65 mEq/10 mL calcium
(0.465 mEq/mL)

10 mL
SINGLE DOSE VIAL
FOR SLOW I.V. USE   Rx only

CL **Cengage Learning**
For Educational Purposes Only

Each 1 mL contains: calcium gluconate (monohydrate) 98 mg, calcium saccharate (tetrahydrate) 4.6 mg, water for injection q.s. pH adjusted with sodium hydroxide and/or hydrochloric acid.

Contains no more than 12.5 mg per liter of aluminum.
WARNING: Solution must be clear when injected. If unused solution shows crystallization, discard.
Store at controlled room temperature 15°-30°C (59°-86°F) (See USP).

Lot:
Exp. Date:

© Cengage Learning 2015.

▲ FIGURE 9-8

Answers 1. 1% **2.** 50 mL **3.** 20 mL **4.** 10 mg/mL **5.** 2.5 mL **6.** 10% **7.** 10 mL **8.** 0.465 mEq/mL

Parenteral medications expressed in **ratio strengths** are not common, and **when they are ordered, it will be by number of mL**. Ratio labels may also contain dosages in metric weights.

PROBLEMS 9.5

Refer to the epinephrine label in Figure 9-9 to answer the following questions.

1. What is the ratio strength of this solution?   _____

2. What volume is this contained in?   _____

3. What is the metric dosage strength of this solution?   _____

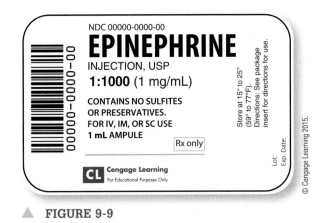

NDC 00000-0000-00

EPINEPHRINE

INJECTION, USP

1:1000 (1 mg/mL)

CONTAINS NO SULFITES
OR PRESERVATIVES.
FOR IV, IM, OR SC USE
1 mL AMPULE

Rx only

Store at 15° to 25°
(59° to 77°F).
Directions: See package
insert for directions for use.

Lot:
Exp. Date:

© Cengage Learning 2015.

CL **Cengage Learning**
For Educational Purposes Only

▲ **FIGURE 9-9**

Answers   1. 1 : 1000   **2.** 1 mL   **3.** 1 mg/mL

SOLUTIONS MEASURED IN INTERNATIONAL UNITS

A number of drugs are measured in **International Units**. The following labels will introduce you to several examples.

 PROBLEMS 9.6

Refer to the heparin label in Figure 9-10 to answer the following questions.

1. What is the total volume of this vial?   _____

2. What is the dosage strength?   _____

3. If a volume of 1.5 mL is prepared, how many units
   will this be?   _____

4. How many mL will you need to prepare a dosage of
   5500 units?   _____

5. If 0.25 mL of this medication is prepared, what dosage
   will this be?   _____

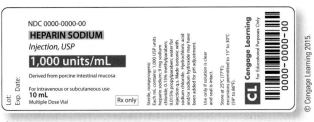

NDC 0000-0000-00

HEPARIN SODIUM

Injection, USP

1,000 units/mL

Derived from porcine intestinal mucosa

For intravenous or subcutaneous use
10 mL
Multiple Dose Vial

Rx only

Sterile, nonpyrogenic.
Each mL contains: 1,000 USP units
heparin sodium; 9 mg sodium
chloride; 0.15% methylparaben;
0.015% propylparaben; water for
injection q.s. Made isotonic with
sodium chloride. Hydrochloric acid
and/or sodium hydroxide may have
been added for pH adjustment.

Store at 25°C (77°F);
excursions permitted to 15° to 30°C
(59° to 86°F).

Use only if solution is clear
and seal is intact.

Cengage Learning
For Educational Purposes Only

CL

0000-0000-00

© Cengage Learning 2015.

Lot:
Exp. Date:

▲ **FIGURE 9-10**

Refer to the penicillin G procaine label in Figure 9-11 to answer the following questions.

6. What is the dosage strength of this medication? _____

7. If 600,000 units are ordered, how many mL would this require? _____

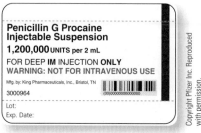

FIGURE 9-11

Answers 1. 10 mL **2.** 1000 units/mL **3.** 1500 units **4.** 5.5 mL **5.** 250 units **6.** 1,200,000 units/2 mL
7. 1 mL

SOLUTIONS MEASURED AS MILLIEQUIVALENTS (mEq)

The next four labels will introduce you to milliequivalent (mEq) dosages. Refer to the calcium gluconate label in Figure 9-12 and notice that in addition to its 10% strength, this vial has a dosage of 0.465 mEq/mL. If a dosage of 0.465 mEq were ordered, you would draw up 1 mL in the syringe.

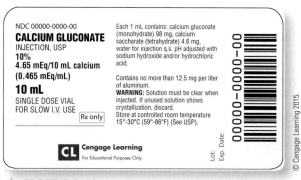

FIGURE 9-12

▶▶▶ PROBLEMS 9.7

Refer to the potassium chloride label in Figure 9-13 to answer the following questions.

1. What are the total dosage and volume of this vial? _____

2. What is the dosage in mEq per mL? _____

3. If you were asked to prepare 15 mEq for addition to an IV, what volume would you draw up? _____

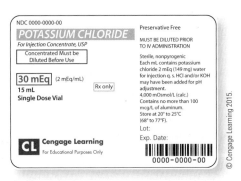

▲ **FIGURE 9-13**

Refer to the potassium acetate label in Figure 9-14 to answer the following dosage questions.

4. What is the strength of this solution in mEq per mL?   _____

5. If you were asked to prepare 40 mEq for addition to an IV solution, what volume would you draw up in the syringe?   _____

6. What volume would you need for a dosage of 20 mEq?   _____

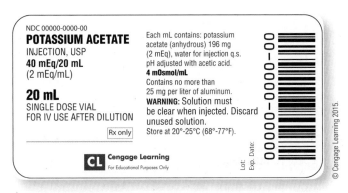

▲ **FIGURE 9-14**

Refer to the sodium bicarbonate label in Figure 9-15. Notice that this solution lists the drug strength in mEq, percentage, and g. Read the label very carefully to answer the following questions.

7. What is the dosage strength expressed in mEq/mL?   _____

8. What is the total volume of the vial, and how many mEq does this volume contain?   _____

9. What is the strength per mL expressed as g?   _____

10. If you were asked to prepare 10 mL of an 8.4% sodium bicarbonate solution, what volume would you draw up in a syringe?   _____

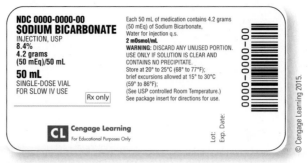

FIGURE 9-15

Answers   1. 30 mEq; 15 mL   **2.** 2 mEq/mL   **3.** 7.5 mL   **4.** 2 mEq/mL   **5.** 20 mL   **6.** 10 mL   **7.** 1 mEq/mL   **8.** 50 mL; 50 mEq   **9.** 0.084 g/mL   **10.** 10 mL

Summary

This concludes the introduction to parenteral solution labels. The important points to remember from this chapter are:

▽ The most commonly used parenteral administration routes are IV, IM, and subcutaneous.

▽ The labels of most parenteral solutions are quite small and must be read with particular care.

▽ The average IM dosage will be contained in a volume of between 0.5 mL and 3 mL.

▽ These 0.5 to 3 mL volumes can be used as a guideline to accuracy of calculations.

▽ The average subcutaneous dosage volume is between 0.5 and 1 mL.

▽ IV medication preparation is usually a two-step procedure: measurement of the dosage, then dilution according to manufacturer's recommendations or a physician's or prescriber's order.

▽ Parenteral drugs may be measured in metric, ratio, percentage, unit, or mEq dosages.

▽ If dosages are ordered by percentage or ratio strength, they are usually specified in mL to be administered.

▽ Most IM dosages are prepared using a 3 mL syringe.

▽ Most subcutaneous dosages are prepared using a 3 mL or tuberculin syringe.

Summary Self-Test

Read the parenteral drug labels provided to measure the following dosages. Then, indicate on the syringe provided exactly how much solution you will draw up to obtain these dosages. Have your answers checked by your instructor to be sure you have measured the dosages correctly.

Dosage Ordered   **mL Needed**

1. terbutaline sulfate 500 mcg   _____

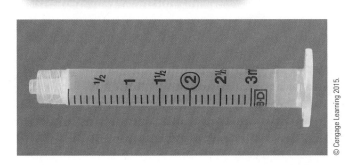

TERBUTALINE SULFATE INJECTION USP	NDC 55390-101-10
FOR SC INJECTION ONLY.	Sterile Vial
1 mg/mL	Protect from light.
Rx ONLY	Manufactured for: Bedford Laboratories™ Bedford, OH 44146
	TBT-V00

Used with permission of Bedford Laboratories, a division of Ben Venue Laboratories, Inc. A Boehringer-Ingelheim Company.

© Cengage Learning 2015.

2. furosemide 10 mg   _____

NDC 0000-0000-00

FUROSEMIDE
INJECTION, USP

20 mg/2 mL
(10 mg/mL)

2 mL
SINGLE DOSE VIAL
FOR IV OR IM USE

Rx only

CL Cengage Learning
For Educational Purposes Only

WARNING: Use only if solution is clear and colorless.
Protect from light.
Store at controlled room temperature between 15°-30°C (59°-86°F).

0000-0000-00

Lot:
Exp. Date:

© Cengage Learning 2015.

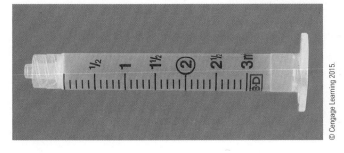

© Cengage Learning 2015.

CHAPTER 9

1, 4, 6, 8, 12, 13, 14, 16, 21, 22, 28
38, 40

Dosage Ordered	**mL Needed**
3. heparin 2500 units	_____

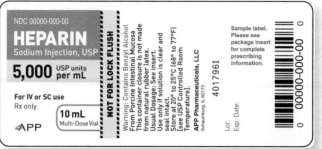

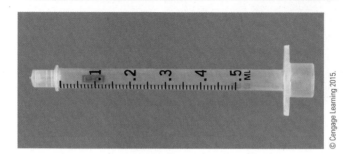

4. acyclovir Na 100 mg _____

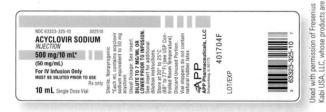

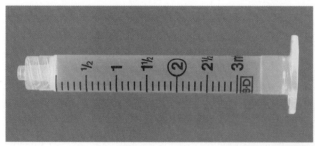

Dosage Ordered   **mL Needed**

5. atropine 0.2 mg   _____

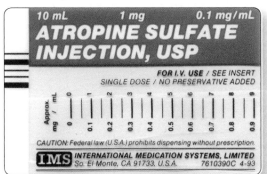

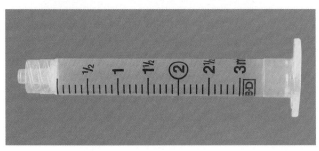

6. hydroxyzine HCl 25 mg   _____

FOR INTRAMUSCULAR USE ONLY
USUAL ADULT DOSE: Intramuscularly: 25 - 100 mg stat; repeat every 4 to 6 hours, as needed. See accompanying prescribing information.

Each mL contains **25 mg** of hydroxyzine hydrochloride, 0.9% benzyl alcohol and sodium hydroxide to adjust to optimum pH.

To avoid discoloration, protect from prolonged exposure to light.

CAUTION: Federal law prohibits dispensing without prescription.

10 mL   NDC 0049-5450-74

Vistaril®
(hydroxyzine hydrochloride)

Intramuscular Solution

25 mg/mL

Pfizer **Roerig**
Division of Pfizer Inc, NY, NY 10017

Copyright Pfizer Inc. Reproduced with permission.

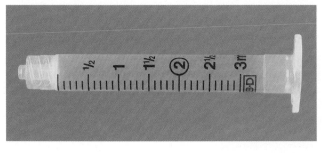

© Cengage Learning 2015.

Dosage Ordered   **mL Needed**

7. Robinul® 100 mcg   _____

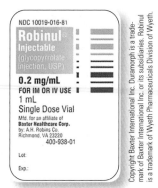
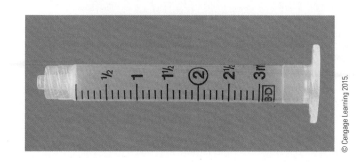

8. diltiazem 25 mg   _____

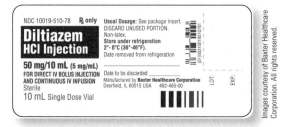

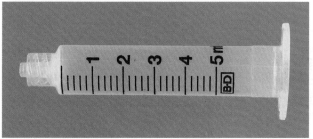

9. methotrexate 0.25 g   _____

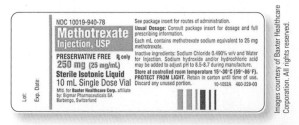

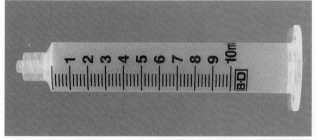

Dosage Ordered	**mL Needed**
10. cyanocobalamin 1 mg	_____

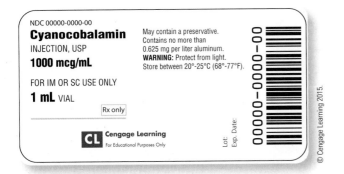

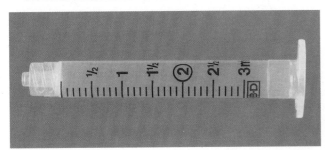

---

11. nubain 10 mg	_____

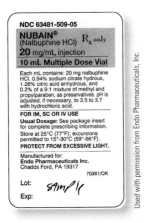

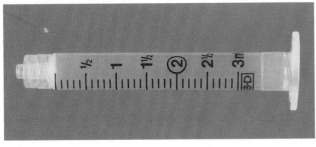

Dosage Ordered   **mL Needed**

12. epinephrine 2 mg   _____

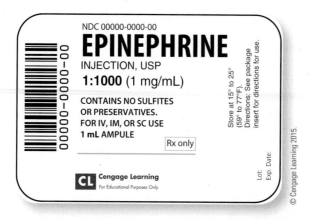

NDC 00000-0000-00

EPINEPHRINE

INJECTION, USP

1:1000 (1 mg/mL)

CONTAINS NO SULFITES
OR PRESERVATIVES.
FOR IV, IM, OR SC USE
1 mL AMPULE

Rx only

Store at 15° to 25°
(59° to 77°F).
Directions: See package
insert for directions for use.

Lot:
Exp. Date:

CL Cengage Learning
For Educational Purposes Only

© Cengage Learning 2015.

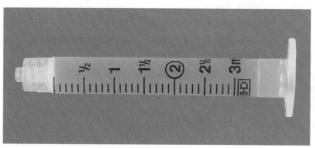

© Cengage Learning 2015.

13. Fentanyl® 125 mcg   _____

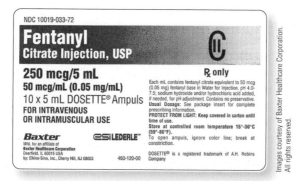

NDC 10019-033-72

Fentanyl
Citrate Injection, USP

C II

R only

250 mcg/5 mL
50 mcg/mL (0.05 mg/mL)
10 x 5 mL DOSETTE® Ampuls
FOR INTRAVENOUS
OR INTRAMUSCULAR USE

Baxter
Mfd. for an affiliate of
Baxter Healthcare Corporation
Deerfield, IL 60015 USA
by: Elkins-Sinn, Inc., Cherry Hill, NJ 08003

©Si LEDERLE™

460-120-00

Each mL contains fentanyl citrate equivalent to 50 mcg
(0.05 mg) fentanyl base in Water for Injection. pH 4.0–
7.5; sodium hydroxide and/or hydrochloric acid added,
if needed, for pH adjustment. Contains no preservative.
Usual Dosage: See package insert for complete
prescribing information.
**PROTECT FROM LIGHT: Keep covered in carton until
time of use.**
**Store at controlled room temperature 15°–30°C
(59°–86°F).**
To open ampuls, ignore color line; break at
constriction.

DOSETTE® is a registered trademark of A.H. Robins
Company

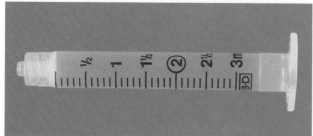

© Cengage Learning 2015.

Dosage Ordered   **mL Needed**

14. calcium gluconate 0.93 mEq   _____

NDC 00000-0000-00

CALCIUM GLUCONATE
INJECTION, USP
10%
4.65 mEq/10 mL calcium
(0.465 mEq/mL)

10 mL
SINGLE DOSE VIAL
FOR SLOW I.V. USE   Rx only

Each 1 mL contains: calcium gluconate (monohydrate) 98 mg, calcium saccharate (tetrahydrate) 4.6 mg, water for injection q.s. pH adjusted with sodium hydroxide and/or hydrochloric acid.

Contains no more than 12.5 mg per liter of aluminum.
WARNING: Solution must be clear when injected. If unused solution shows crystallization, discard.
Store at controlled room temperature 15°-30°C (59°-86°F) (See USP).

CL Cengage Learning
For Educational Purposes Only

Lot:
Exp. Date:

00000-0000-00

© Cengage Learning 2015.

© Cengage Learning 2015.

15. ceftriaxone 0.7 g I.M.   _____

NDC 0000-0000-00   Rx only

Ceftriaxone
for Injection, USP

1 gram

For I.M. or I.V. Use
Single Use Vial

TEVA

Each vial contains: ceftriaxone sodium powder equivalent to 1 gram ceftriaxone.
For I.M. Administration : Reconstitute with 2.1 mL 1% Lidocaine Hydrochloride Injection (USP) or Sterile Water for Injection (USP). Each 1 mL of solution contains approximately 350 mg equivalent of ceftriaxone.
For I.V. Administration : See Package Insert
Usual Dosage: See Package Insert
Iss. 9/2009
39C1701450909

Storage Prior to Reconstitution:
Store powder at 20° to 25°C (68° to 77°F) [See USP Controlled Room Temperature].
Protect from Light.
Storage After Reconstitution: See Package Insert
Mfd for: Teva Parenteral Medicines Irvine, CA 92618

Used with permission of Teva Pharmaceuticals, USA.

© Cengage Learning 2015.

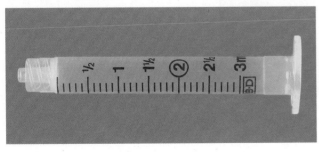

Dosage Ordered   **mL Needed**

16. heparin 500 units   _____

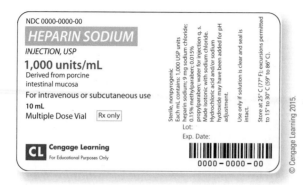

NDC 0000-0000-00

HEPARIN SODIUM

INJECTION, USP

1,000 units/mL
Derived from porcine
intestinal mucosa

For intravenous or subcutaneous use

10 mL
Multiple Dose Vial   Rx only

Sterile, nonpyrogenic.
Each mL contains: 1,000 USP units
heparin sodium; 9 mg sodium chloride;
0.15% methylparaben; 0.015%
propylparaben; water for injection q. s.
Made isotonic with sodium chloride.
Hydrochloric acid and/or sodium
hydroxide may have been added for pH
adjustment.

Use only if solution is clear and seal is
intact.

Store at 25° C (77° F); excursions permitted
to 15° to 30° C (59° to 86° C).

Lot:
Exp. Date:

CL Cengage Learning
For Educational Purposes Only

0000-0000-00

© Cengage Learning 2015.

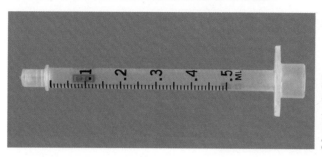

© Cengage Learning 2015.

17. ondansetron 3 mg   _____

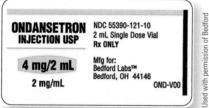

ONDANSETRON
INJECTION USP

4 mg/2 mL

2 mg/mL

NDC 55390-121-10
2 mL Single Dose Vial
Rx ONLY

Mfg for:
Bedford Labs™
Bedford, OH 44146

OND-V00

Used with permission of Bedford
Laboratories, a division of Ben
Venue Laboratories, Inc. A
Boehringer-Ingelheim Company.

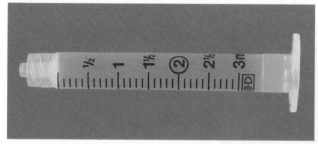

© Cengage Learning 2015.

Dosage Ordered   **mL Needed**

18. epinephrine 0.5 mg   _____

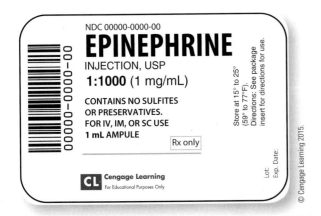

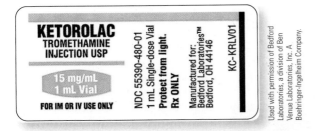

19. ketorolac tromethamine 30 mg   _____

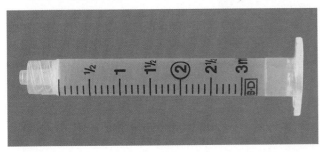

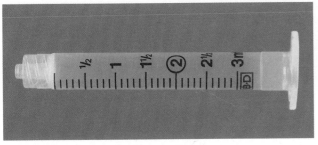

Dosage Ordered   **mL Needed**

20. Ativan 6 mg   _____

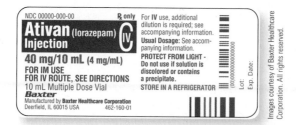

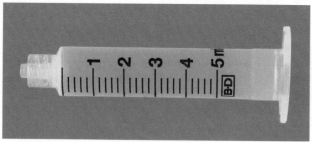

21. lidocaine HCl 50 mg   _____

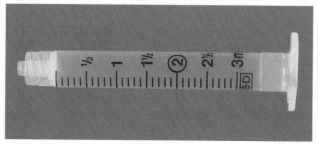

Dosage Ordered

mL Needed

22. sodium chloride 40 mEq

_____

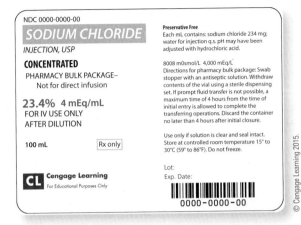

NDC 0000-0000-00

SODIUM CHLORIDE

INJECTION, USP

CONCENTRATED

PHARMACY BULK PACKAGE–
Not for direct infusion

23.4% 4 mEq/mL
FOR IV USE ONLY
AFTER DILUTION

100 mL   Rx only

CL **Cengage Learning**
For Educational Purposes Only

0000-0000-00

Preservative Free
Each mL contains: sodium chloride 234 mg;
water for injection q.s. pH may have been
adjusted with hydrochloric acid.

8008 mOsmol/L 4,000 mEq/L
Directions for pharmacy bulk package: Swab
stopper with an antiseptic solution. Withdraw
contents of the vial using a sterile dispensing
set. If prompt fluid transfer is not possible, a
maximum time of 4 hours from the time of
initial entry is allowed to complete the
transferring operations. Discard the container
no later than 4 hours after initial closure.

Use only if solution is clear and seal intact.
Store at controlled room temperature 15° to
30°C (59° to 86°F). Do not freeze.

Lot:
Exp. Date:

© Cengage Learning 2015.

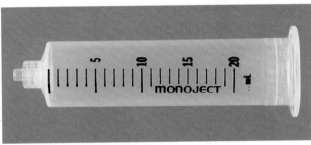

© Cengage Learning 2015.

23. atropine 200 mcg

_____

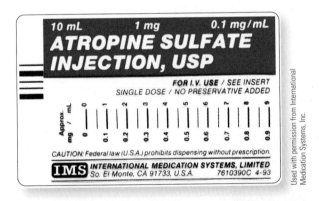

10 mL   1 mg   0.1 mg/mL

**ATROPINE SULFATE
INJECTION, USP**

FOR I.V. USE / SEE INSERT
SINGLE DOSE / NO PRESERVATIVE ADDED

CAUTION: Federal law (U.S.A.) prohibits dispensing without prescription.

IMS **INTERNATIONAL MEDICATION SYSTEMS, LIMITED**
So. El Monte, CA 91733, U.S.A.   7610390C 4-93

Used with permission from International
Medication Systems, Inc.

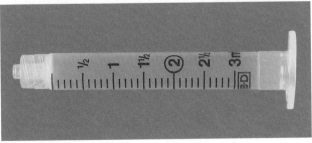

© Cengage Learning 2015.

Dosage Ordered   **mL Needed**

24. meperidine 50 mg

_____

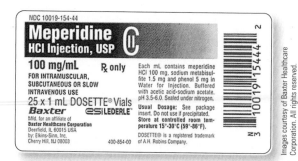

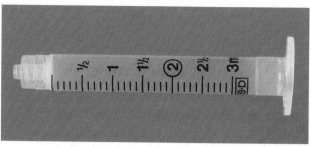

25. clindamycin 0.3 g

_____

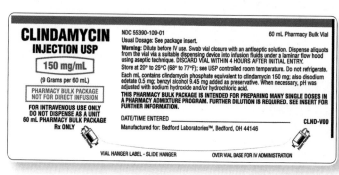

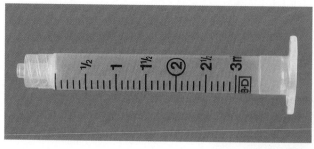

Dosage Ordered   **mL Needed**

26. morphine sulfate 15 mg   _____

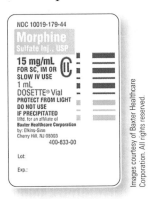

NDC 10019-179-44

Morphine
Sulfate Inj., USP

15 mg/mL
FOR SC, IM OR
SLOW IV USE
1 mL
DOSETTE® Vial
PROTECT FROM LIGHT
DO NOT USE
IF PRECIPITATED
Mfd. for an affiliate of
Baxter Healthcare Corporation
by: Elkins-Sinn
Cherry Hill, NJ 08003
400-833-00

Lot:

Exp.:

27. acyclovir Na 150 mg   _____

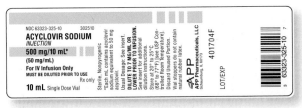

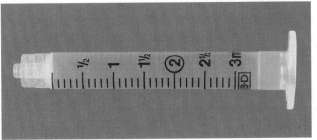

NDC 63323-325-10   302510

ACYCLOVIR SODIUM
INJECTION

500 mg/10 mL*

(50 mg/mL)

For IV Infusion Only
MUST BE DILUTED PRIOR TO USE
Rx only

10 mL Single Dose Vial

APP
APP Pharmaceuticals, LLC
Schaumburg, IL 60173

401704F

LOT/EXP

28. cisplatin 20 mg   _____

CISplatin doses greater than 100 mg/m² once every 3 to 4 weeks are rarely used. See package insert.

CISplatin
Injection

50 mg/50 mL

FOR IV USE ONLY   1 mg/mL Aqueous

NDC 55390-112-50   50 mL MULTIPLE DOSE VIAL
USUAL DOSAGE: See package insert.
Each mL contains 1 mg cisplatin and 9 mg sodium chloride in water for injection. HCl and/or sodium hydroxide added to adjust pH to 3.5 to 4.5.
Store at 15° to 25°C (59° to 77°F).
Protect from light. DO NOT REFRIGERATE. STERILE SOLUTIONS FOR INTRAVENOUS USE. Rx ONLY
Manufactured for:
Bedford Laboratories™ BEDFORD
Bedford, OH 44146
Manufactured by:
Ben Venue Labs, Inc.
Bedford, OH 44146
CIS-AQ-VA01

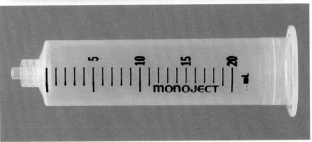

SECTION 3

Dosage Ordered   **mL Needed**

29. sodium chloride 20 mEq   _____

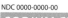

NDC 0000-0000-00

SODIUM CHLORIDE

INJECTION, USP

CONCENTRATED

PHARMACY BULK PACKAGE–
    Not for direct infusion

23.4% 4 mEq/mL
FOR IV USE ONLY
AFTER DILUTION

100 mL   Rx only

CL **Cengage Learning**
For Educational Purposes Only

Preservative Free
Each mL contains: sodium chloride 234 mg;
water for injection q.s. pH may have been
adjusted with hydrochloric acid.

8008 mOsmol/L 4,000 mEq/L
Directions for pharmacy bulk package: Swab
stopper with an antiseptic solution. Withdraw
contents of the vial using a sterile dispensing
set. If prompt fluid transfer is not possible, a
maximum time of 4 hours from the time of
initial entry is allowed to complete the
transferring operations. Discard the container
no later than 4 hours after initial closure.

Use only if solution is clear and seal intact.
Store at controlled room temperature 15° to
30°C (59° to 86°F). Do not freeze.

Lot:
Exp. Date:

0000-0000-00

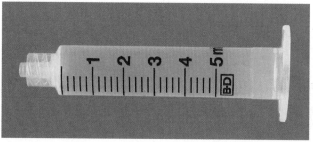

30. meperidine 50 mg   _____

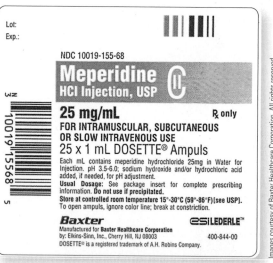

Lot:
Exp.:

NDC 10019-155-68

Meperidine
HCI Injection, USP

25 mg/mL   R͟x only
FOR INTRAMUSCULAR, SUBCUTANEOUS
OR SLOW INTRAVENOUS USE
25 x 1 mL DOSETTE® Ampuls

Each mL contains meperidine hydrochloride 25mg in Water for
Injection. pH 3.5-6.0; sodium hydroxide and/or hydrochloric acid
added, if needed, for pH adjustment.
Usual Dosage: See package insert for complete prescribing
information. Do not use if precipitated.
Store at controlled room temperature 15°-30°C (59°-86°F) [see USP].
To open ampuls, ignore color line; break at constriction.

Baxter
Manufactured for **Baxter Healthcare Corporation**
by: Elkins-Sinn, Inc., Cherry Hill, NJ 08003
DOSETTE® is a registered trademark of A.H. Robins Company.   400-844-00

⊘SILEDERLE™

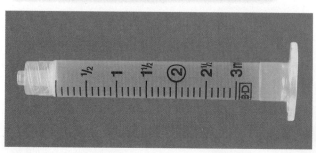

Dosage Ordered   **mL Needed**

31. furosemide 30 mg   _____

NDC 0000-0000-00
FUROSEMIDE
INJECTION, USP
40 mg/4 mL
(10 mg/mL)

4 mL
SINGLE DOSE VIAL
FOR IV OR IM USE

Rx only

Each mL contains furosemide 10 mg, water for injections q.s., sodium chloride, hydrochlonic acid to adjust pH between 8.0 and 9.3.
WARNING: Use only if solution is clear and Colorless. Protect from light. Discard unused portion. Store at controlled room temperature between 15°-30°C (59°-86°F).

CL Cengage Learning
For Educational Purposes Only

Lot:
Exp. Date:

0000-0000-00

© Cengage Learning 2015.

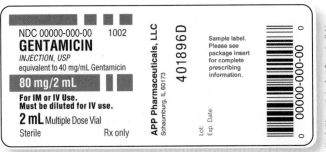

© Cengage Learning 2015.

32. gentamicin 60 mg   _____

NDC 00000-000-00   1002
GENTAMICIN
INJECTION, USP
equivalent to 40 mg/mL Gentamicin

80 mg/2 mL

For IM or IV Use.
Must be diluted for IV use.

2 mL Multiple Dose Vial
Sterile   Rx only

APP Pharmaceuticals, LLC
Schaumburg, IL 60173

401896D

Sample label. Please see package insert for complete prescribing information.

Lot:
Exp. Date:

00000-000-00

Used with permission from Fresenius Kabi, USA, LLC, whose products are available only in the United States.

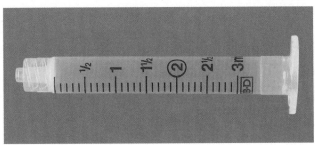

© Cengage Learning 2015.

Dosage Ordered   **mL Needed**

33. meperidine 50 mg   _____

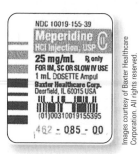

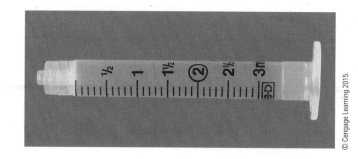

34. dexamethasone 2 mg   _____

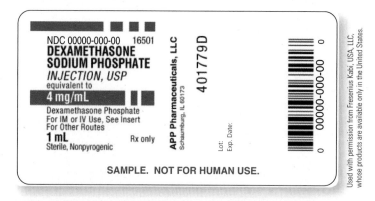

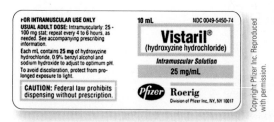

35. Vistaril® 50 mg   _____

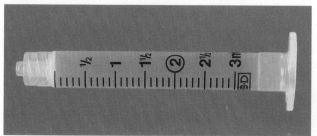

CHAPTER 9

Dosage Ordered	**mL Needed**

36. fentanyl 0.05 mg _____

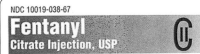

NDC 10019-038-67

Fentanyl
Citrate Injection, USP

100 mcg/2 mL
50 mcg/ mL (0.05 mg/mL) R̥ only
FOR INTRAVENOUS OR INTRAMUSCULAR USE
10 x 2 mL DOSETTE® Ampuls

Each mL contains fentanyl citrate equivalent to 50 mcg (0.05 mg) fentanyl base in Water for Injection. pH 4.0-7.5; sodium hydroxide and/or hydrochloric acid added, if needed, for pH adjustment. CONTAINS NO PRESERVATIVE.
Usual Dosage: See package insert for complete prescribing information.
PROTECT FROM LIGHT: Keep covered in carton until time of use.
Store at controlled room temperature 15°-30°C (59°-86°F).
To open ampuls, ignore color line; break at constriction.

Baxter
Mfd. for an affiliate of **Baxter Healthcare Corporation**
by: Elkins-Sinn, Cherry Hill, NJ 08003
DOSETTE® is a registered trademark of A.H. Robins Company   400-762-01

⊖SILEDERLE

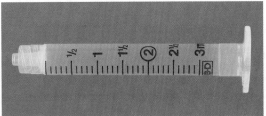

37. morphine 15 mg _____

NDC 10019-178-44

Morphine
Sulfate Inj., USP

10 mg/mL
FOR SC, IM OR
SLOW IV USE
1 mL DOSETTE® Vial
PROTECT FROM LIGHT
DO NOT USE
IF PRECIPITATED

Mfd. for an affiliate of
Baxter Healthcare Corporation
by: Elkins-Sinn,
Cherry Hill, NJ 08003
400-829-01

Lot.:

Exp.:

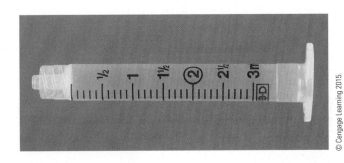

38. cyanocobalamin 1 mg _____

NDC 00000-0000-00
Cyanocobalamin
INJECTION, USP
1000 mcg/mL

FOR IM OR SC USE ONLY
1 mL VIAL

Rx only

May contain a preservative.
Contains no more than
0.625 mg per liter aluminum.
WARNING: Protect from light.
Store between 20°-25°C (68°-77°F).

CL Cengage Learning
For Educational Purposes Only

Lot: Exp. Date:

00000-0000-00

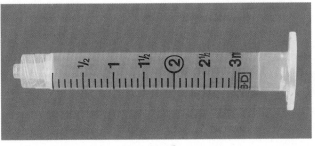

Dosage Ordered

mL Needed

39. ketorolac tromethamine 15 mg

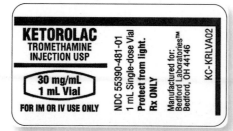

KETOROLAC
TROMETHAMINE
INJECTION USP

30 mg/mL
1 mL Vial

FOR IM OR IV USE ONLY

NDC 55390-481-01
1 mL Single-dose Vial
Protect from light.
Rx ONLY

Manufactured for:
Bedford Laboratories™
Bedford, OH 44146

KC-KRLVA02

Used with permission of Bedford Laboratories, a division of Ben Venue Laboratories, Inc. A Boehringer-Ingelheim Company.

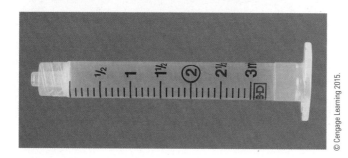

© Cengage Learning 2015.

40. Robinul® 200 mcg

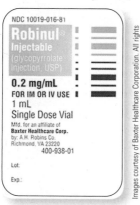

NDC 10019-016-81

Robinul®
Injectable
(glycopyrrolate
injection, USP)

0.2 mg/mL
FOR IM OR IV USE
1 mL
Single Dose Vial

Mfd. for an affiliate of
Baxter Healthcare Corp.
by: A.H. Robins Co.
Richmond, VA 23220
400-938-01

Lot:

Exp.:

Images courtesy of Baxter Healthcare Corporation. All rights reserved.

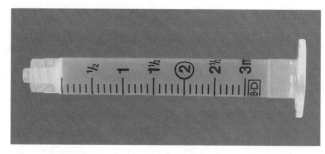

© Cengage Learning 2015.

Answers				
1. 0.5 mL	**9.** 10 mL	**18.** 0.5 mL	**27.** 3 mL	**36.** 1 mL
2. 1 mL	**10.** 1 mL	**19.** 2 mL	**28.** 20 mL	**37.** 1.5 mL
3. 0.5 mL	**11.** 0.5 mL	**20.** 1.5 mL	**29.** 5 mL	**38.** 1 mL
4. 2 mL	**12.** 2 mL	**21.** 5 mL	**30.** 2 mL	**39.** 0.5 mL
5. 2 mL	**13.** 2.5 mL	**22.** 10 mL	**31.** 3 mL	**40.** 1 mL
6. 1 mL	**14.** 2 mL	**23.** 2 mL	**32.** 1.5 mL	
7. 0.5 mL	**15.** 2 mL	**24.** 0.5 mL	**33.** 2 mL	
8. 5 mL	**16.** 0.5 mL	**25.** 2 mL	**34.** 0.5 mL	
	17. 1.5 mL	**26.** 1 mL	**35.** 2 mL	

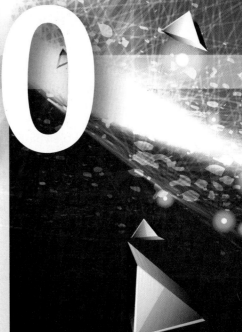

CHAPTER

10

RECONSTITUTION OF POWDERED DRUGS

Many drugs are shipped in powdered form because they **retain their potency only a short time in solution**. Reconstitution of these drugs is often the responsibility of clinical pharmacies, but you will need to know how to read and follow reconstitution directions and how to label drugs with an expiration date and time once they have been reconstituted. The drug label, or instructional package insert, will give specific directions for reconstitution of the drug. Reading these requires care, and this chapter will take you step by step through the entire process.

RECONSTITUTION OF A SINGLE-STRENGTH SOLUTION

Let's start with the simplest type of reconstitution instructions, for a single strength solution. Examine the label for the Solu-Medrol® 500 mg vial in Figure 10-1.

℞ only 81 2365909 See package insert for complete product information. Store at controlled room temperature 20° to 25°C (68° to 77°F) [see USP]. Protect from light. Reconstitute with 8 mL Bacteriostatic Water for Injection with Benzyl Alcohol. **When reconstituted as directed each 8 mL contains:** *Methylprednisolone sodium succinate equivalent to 500 mg methylprednisolone (62.5 mg per mL). Store solution at controlled room temperature 20° to 25°C (68° to 77°F) [see USP] and use within 48 hours after mixing. Lyophilized in container. Protect from light. Reconstituted: _____ Pharmacia & Upjohn Co., Kalamazoo, MI 49001, USA	NDC 0009-0758-01 4—125 mg doses **Solu-Medrol®** methylprednisolone sodium succinate for injection, USP **500 mg*** For intramuscular or intravenous use Diluent Contains Benzyl Alcohol as a Preservative

Copyright Pfizer Inc. Reproduced with permission.

▲ FIGURE 10-1

 KEY*point:* Reconstitution directions on vial labels may be small and difficult to read, and extreme care in reading them is essential.

The first step in reconstitution is to locate the directions. They are on the left side of this label.

OBJECTIVES

The learner will:

1. prepare solutions from powdered drugs using directions printed on vial labels.

2. prepare solutions from powdered drugs using drug literature or inserts.

3. determine the expiration date and time for reconstituted drugs.

4. calculate dosages for reconstituted drugs.

Locate the **Reconstitute with 8 mL Bacteriostatic Water for injection with Benzyl Alcohol** instructions. Water, or any other solution specified for reconstitution, is called the **diluent**. The **type of diluent** specified will be **different for different drugs**. The **volume of diluent will also vary**. Therefore, reading the label carefully to identify both the type and the volume of diluent to be used is mandatory.

Once the type of diluent is identified, the next step is to use a **sterile syringe and aseptic technique** to draw up the 8 mL volume required. Inject it slowly into the vial **above the medication level, because air bubbles can distort drug dosages**. If the diluent volume is large, as in this case, be aware that **the syringe plunger will be forced out to expel air to reequalize the internal vial pressure as you inject**. Very large volumes of diluent will have to be injected in divided amounts to keep the internal vial pressure equalized. When all the diluent has been injected, the vial is rotated and upended until all the medication has been dissolved. **Do not shake** unless directed to do so, because this also can add air bubbles to some medications and distort dosages.

After reconstitution locate the information that relates to the **length of time the reconstituted solution may be stored**, and **how it must be stored**. Look again at the Solu-Medrol directions and locate this information. You will find that this solution can be stored at room temperature and that it must be used within 48 hours of reconstitution.

The next step is to **print your initials on the label as the person who reconstituted the drug**, in case any questions subsequently arise concerning the preparation. Next, **add the expiration date and time to the label**. Let's assume you reconstituted this Solu-Medrol solution at **2 pm on January 3**. What expiration (EXP) date and time will you print on the label? The reconstituted drug lasts only 48 hours at room temperature, so you would print **Exp. Jan. 5, 2 pm**, which is 48 hours (2 days) from the time you reconstituted it.

KEY*point:* The person who reconstitutes a drug is responsible for labeling it with the date and time of expiration, and with his or her initials.

Next, identify the total dosage strength of this vial, which is **500 mg**. Near the top of the label, you can locate the individual dosage strength: **4–125 mg doses**. Because you have injected 8 mL of diluent, this will be approximately **2 mL for each 125 mg** dose, but if you read the small print on the label, you will see that the individual dosage is clearly identified as **62.5 mg per mL**.

Reconstituted volumes do not always exactly equal the amount of diluent added; in fact, most do not. This is because the medication itself has a volume, and it usually makes the total volume somewhat larger than the amount of diluent injected. Our next examples of a single-strength reconstitution will illustrate this increased volume concept.

If a 62.5 mg dosage is ordered, you will need 1 mL.

If a 125 mg dosage is needed, you will need 2 mL (125 mg = 62.5 mg × 2).

If a 250 mg dosage is needed, you will need 4 mL; and if 500 mg is ordered, the total is 8 mL.

KEY*point:* Reconstituted volumes may exceed the volume of the diluent added, because the drug itself has a volume.

▶▶▶ PROBLEMS 10.1

Other drugs shipped in powdered form are antibiotics. Read the label in Figure 10-2 to answer the following questions about reconstituting this drug. All the information you need is printed sideways on the right of the label.

1. How should this drug be stored before reconstitution? _____

2. How is this drug administered? _____

3. How long will this solution retain its potency at room temperature after reconstitution? _____

4. How long if refrigerated? _____

5. If you reconstitute this drug at 10:10 am on October 3 and it is refrigerated, what expiration time will you print on the label? _____

6. What else will you print on the label? _____

7. What is the total dosage of this reconstituted IV solution? _____

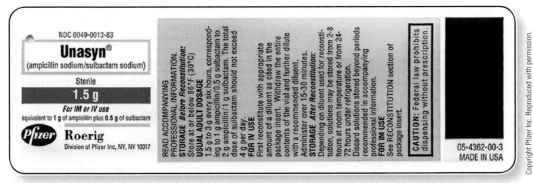

▲ **FIGURE 10-2**

Answers **1.** at or below 86°F (30°C) **2.** IM or IV **3.** 2–8 hours **4.** 24–72 hours **5.** Exp. Oct. 4 10:10 am to Oct. 6 10:10 am (your answer must include "Exp." to be correct) **6.** your initials **7.** 1.5 g

▶▶▶ PROBLEMS 10.2

Refer to the penicillin V potassium oral suspension label in Figure 10-3 to answer the following questions.

1. How much diluent is needed to reconstitute this large-volume oral suspension preparation? _____

2. What kind of diluent will you use? _____

3. The label is specific about how to add this diluent. What does it tell you? _____

4. This is an oral suspension. Does the diluent need to be sterile? _____

5. What is the mg dosage strength of the prepared solution? _____

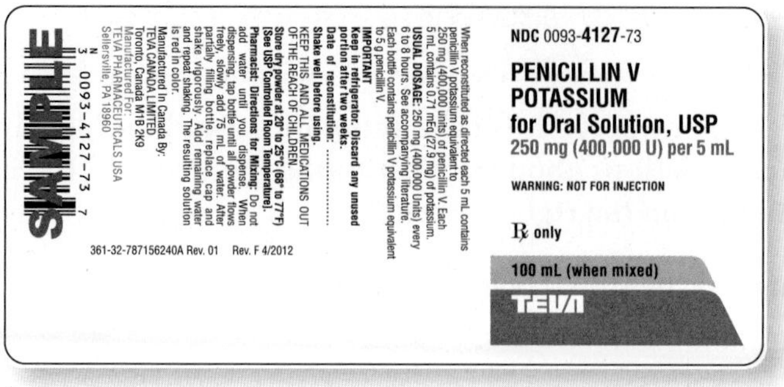

FIGURE 10-3

6. Determine the expiration date if you reconstitute this drug on March 15 at 4:40 pm.   _____

7. How must the reconstituted solution be stored?   _____

8. If the dosage ordered is 125 mg, how many mL are needed?   _____

9. For a 500 mg dosage, how many mL are needed?   _____

10. How many units of medication will there be in a 5 mL dose?   _____

11. What should you do to this medication before administering it?   _____

12. What must the person who reconstitutes the medication print on the label?   _____

Answers   1. 75 mL **2.** water **3.** Slowly add water, partially fill bottle, and shake vigorously. Add remaining water and shake. **4.** No, this is an oral medication. **5.** 250 mg/5 mL **6.** Exp. March 29 4:40 pm **7.** in a refrigerator **8.** 2.5 mL **9.** 10 mL **10.** 400,000 units **11.** shake well **12.** his or her initials

▶▶▶ PROBLEMS 10.3

Refer to the ceftriaxone label in Figure 10-4 to answer the following questions.

1. What is the total dosage of this vial?   _____

2. How much diluent is used for IM reconstitution?   _____

3. What kind of diluent is specified for IM reconstitution?   _____

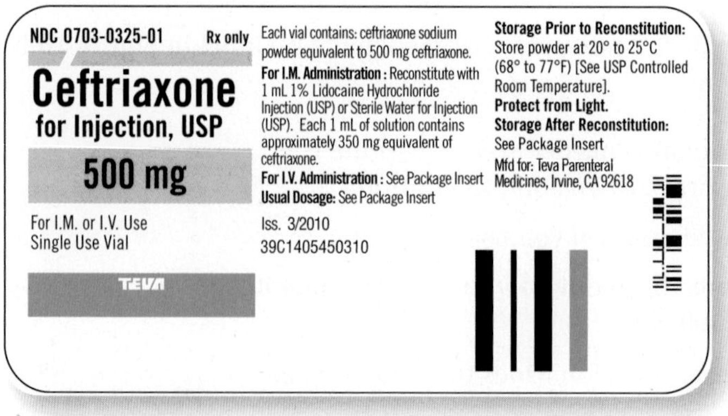

FIGURE 10-4

4. What dosage will 1 mL of IM reconstituted solution contain?   _____

5. Where does it tell you to look for information on the
kind of diluent to use for IV reconstitution?   _____

6. Where will you find storage and expiration details?   _____

7. What will you print on the label in addition to the expiration date?   _____

Answers 1. 500 mg **2.** 1 mL **3.** 1% lidocaine hydrochloride injection or sterile water for injection **4.** 350 mg
5. package insert **6.** package insert **7.** your initials

▶▶▶ PROBLEMS 10.4

Refer to the clindamycin label provided in Figure 10-5 to answer the following questions.

1. What is the total dosage in this vial?   _____

2. Where will you locate reconstitution instructions?   _____

3. How long may the reconstituted solution be used?   _____

4. How much clindamycin will a 6 mL IV volume contain?   _____

5. How many mL will be needed for a 1500 mg IV dosage?   _____

6. What is the mL strength of the reconstituted solution?   _____

7. How is this drug administered?   _____

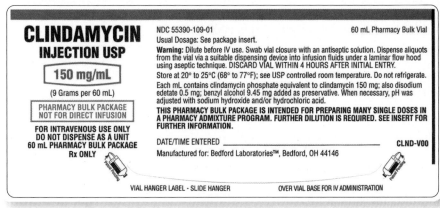

▲ **FIGURE 10-5**

Answers 1. 9 grams **2.** on the package insert directions **3.** 4 hours **4.** 900 mg/6 mL **5.** 10 mL
6. 150 mg/mL **7.** IV

▶▶▶ PROBLEMS 10.5

Refer to the cytarabine label in Figure 10-6 to answer the following questions.

1. What is the total dosage strength of this vial?   _____

2. How much diluent is required for reconstitution?   _____

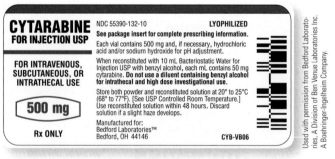

FIGURE 10-6

3. What will be the dosage strength per mL of the reconstituted solution? _____

4. What type of diluent is to be used? _____

5. How long can the reconstituted solution be retained? _____

6. How is this medication administered? _____

Answers **1.** 1 g **2.** 10 mL **3.** 100 mg per mL **4.** bacteriostatic water **5.** 48 hours **6.** intravenously, subcutaneously, or intrathecally

▶▶▶ PROBLEMS 10.6

Refer to the cytarabine label in Figure 10-7 to answer the following questions.

1. What is the total dosage strength of this vial? _____

2. How much diluent is required for reconstitution? _____

3. What will be the dosage per mL of the reconstituted solution? _____

4. What is the expiration time of the reconstituted solution? _____

5. What diluent must be used for subcutaneous injection?

FIGURE 10-7

Answers **1.** 500 mg **2.** 10 mL **3.** 50 mg per mL **4.** 48 hours **5.** bacteriostatic water for injection USP with benzyl alcohol

RECONSTITUTION FROM PACKAGE INSERT DIRECTIONS

The package insert directions provided represent just a small portion of the information that drug package inserts contain. Additional information includes specific use of the drug for diagnosed conditions, such as bacterial meningitis, infections of the gastrointestinal or genitourinary tracts, and so forth; dosage recommendations if the vial label does not contain them; and untoward or adverse reactions, to name just a sample of the topics covered.

▶▶▶ PROBLEMS 10.7

Refer to the selected package insert information in Figure 10-8 to answer the following questions.

1. Identify the types of diluent that may be used for reconstitution under the section labeled **For Intramuscular Use**.   _____

2. Look next at the four-column table for reconstitution, and notice that information is provided for the four different strengths of vials available: 250 mg, 500 mg, 1 g, and 2 g. What volume of diluent is specified for a 250 mg vial?   _____

3. How much diluent is required for a 500 mg vial?   _____

4. How much diluent is required for a 1 g vial?   _____

5. How much diluent is required for a 2 g vial?   _____

6. The mL dosage strength of all four reconstituted solutions is the same. What is it?   _____

7. Refer to the information under **For Direct Intravenous Use**. How much diluent must be added to the 250 mg or 500 mg vials?   _____

8. What stipulation is made for direct IV administration of the 250 mg and 500 mg reconstituted solution?   _____

9. What is the caution pertaining to rapid IV administration?   _____

NDC 0000-0000-00

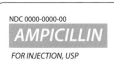

FOR INJECTION, USP

Use ampicillin for injection to treat and/or prevent infections that are known to be caused by bacteria.

DIRECTIONS:
Use only freshly prepared solutions. Use intramuscular and intravenous injections within one hour of preparation.

For Intramuscular Use
Dissolve contents of a vial with the amount of sterile water for injection or bacteriostatic water for injection as outlined in the following table.

Vial Amount	Amount of Diluent to Be Added (mL)	Approximate Available Volume (mL)	Approximate Concentration (in mg/mL)
250 mg	0.9	1	250
500 mg	1.7	2	250
1 g	3.4	4	250
2 g	6.8	8	250

Ampicillin for injection 1 g and 2 g vials are intended for intravenous use; however, intramuscular administration is permissible when 250 mg or 500 mg vials are unavailable. In these instances, dissolve in 3.4 or 6.8 mL sterile water for injection or bacteriostatic water for injection, respectively. The resulting solution will provide a concentration of 250 mg per mL.

For Direct Intravenous Use
Add 5 mL sterile water for injection or bacteriostatic water for injection to the 250 and 500 mg vials. Administer slowly over 3 to 5 minutes. Ampicillin for injection 1 g or 2 g, may also be given by direct intravenous administration. Dissolve in 7.4 or 14.8 mL sterile water for injection or bacteriostatic water for injection, respectively.

Administer slowly over at least 10 to 15 minutes.

CAUTION: More rapid administration may result in convulsive seizures.

Lot:
Exp. Date:

© Cengage Learning 2015.

CL Cengage Learning
For Educational Purposes Only

▲ **FIGURE 10-8**

Answers   1. sterile water for injection or bacteriostatic water for injection   **2.** 0.9 mL   **3.** 1.7 mL   **4.** 3.4 mL   **5.** 6.8 mL   **6.** 250 mg per 1 mL   **7.** 5 mL   **8.** Inject slowly over 3 to 5 minutes.   **9.** Rapid administration may result in seizures.

In this section, you were concentrating specifically on locating vial label and package insert directions for reconstitution of a single-strength solution. And you quickly discovered that there is no standard way that this information is presented. But the information is all there somewhere; you must persist until you locate it.

The next section will introduce you to labels and package inserts that contain directions for preparation of multiple-strength solutions.

RECONSTITUTION OF MULTIPLE-STRENGTH SOLUTIONS

Some powdered drugs offer a choice of dosage strengths. When this is the case, you must choose the strength most appropriate for the dosage ordered. For example, refer to the penicillin label in Figure 10-9. The dosage strengths that can be obtained are listed on the right.

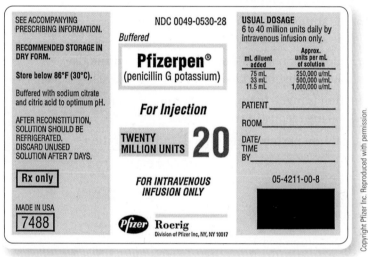

▲ **FIGURE 10-9**

Notice that three dosage strengths are listed: 250,000 units, 500,000 units, and 1,000,000 units/mL. If the dosage ordered is 500,000 units, the most appropriate strength to mix would be 500,000 units/mL. Read across from this strength, and determine how much diluent must be added to obtain it. The answer is 33 mL. If the dosage ordered is 1,000,000 units, what would be the most appropriate strength to prepare, and how much diluent would this require? The answers are 1,000,000 units/mL and 11.5 mL.

KEY*point:* A multiple-strength solution requires that you add one additional piece of information to the label after reconstitution: the dosage strength just mixed.

▶▶▶ PROBLEMS 10.8

Refer to the Pfizerpen® label in Figure 10-9 to answer these additional questions.

1. If you add 75 mL of diluent to prepare a solution of penicillin, what dosage strength will you print on the label? _____

2. Does this prepared solution require refrigeration? _____

3. If you reconstitute it on June 1 at 2 pm, what expiration time and date will you print on the label? _____

4. What is the total dosage strength of this vial? _____

5. What else do you print on the label besides the dosage strength just reconstituted? _____

6. Where will you locate information on the diluent to be used? _____

Answers 1. 250,000 units per mL **2.** yes **3.** Exp. June 8 2 pm **4.** 20 million units **5.** your initials **6.** package insert

The next problems consist of two simulated vial labels with solution strengths of 500 mg and 1 g and a package insert that gives the directions for their reconstitution.

▶▶▶ PROBLEMS 10.9

Refer to the Antibiotic for Intravenous Use labels and insert in Figure 10-10, Figure 10-11, and Figure 10-12. Use both the insert and label information to answer the following questions.

1. How much diluent must be used to reconstitute a 500 mg vial? _____

2. How much diluent will be needed for a 1 g vial? _____

3. What kind of diluent is specified? _____

4. What is the reconstituted dosage per mL of both of these solutions? _____

5. How long can the solution be used if stored in a refrigerator? _____

6. If the drug is reconstituted on May 4 at 1350, what expiration date and time will you print on the label? _____

7. What else must you print on the label? _____

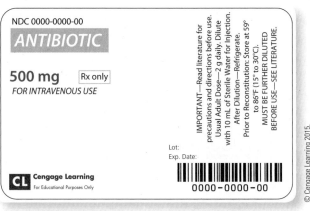

▲ **FIGURE 10-10**

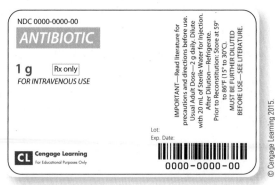

IMPORTANT—Read literature for precautions and directions before use. Usual Adult Dose—2 g daily. Dilute with 20 mL of Sterile Water for Injection. After Dilution—Refrigerate. Prior to Reconstitution: Store at 59° to 86°F (15° to 30°C). MUST BE FURTHER DILUTED BEFORE USE—SEE LITERATURE.

NDC 0000-0000-00
ANTIBIOTIC
1 g   Rx only
FOR INTRAVENOUS USE
Lot:
Exp. Date:
CL Cengage Learning
For Educational Purposes Only
0000-0000-00
© Cengage Learning 2015.

PREPARATION AND STABILITY
At the time of use, reconstitute by adding either 10 mL of Sterile Water for Injection to the 500-mg vial or 20 mL of Sterile Water for Injection to the 1-g vial of dry, sterile powder. Vials reconstituted in this manner will give a solution of 50 mg/mL. FURTHER DILUTION IS REQUIRED.
After reconstitution, the vials may be stored in a refrigerator for 14 days without significant loss of potency. Reconstituted solutions containing 500 mg must be diluted with at least 100 mL of diluent. Reconstituted solutions containing 1 g must be diluted with at least 200 mL of diluent. The desired dose, diluted in this manner, should be administered by intermittent intravenous infusion over a period of at least 60 minutes.
© Cengage Learning 2015.

▲ **FIGURE 10-11**   ▲ **FIGURE 10-12**

Answers 1. 10 mL **2.** 20 mL **3.** sterile water for injection **4.** 50 mg per mL **5.** 14 days
6. Exp. May 18 1350 **7.** your initials

Summary

This concludes the chapter on the reconstitution of powdered drugs. The important points to remember from this chapter are:

▽ If the medication label does not contain reconstitution directions, these may be located on the medication package insert.

▽ The type and amount of diluent to be used for reconstitution must be exactly as specified in the reconstitution instructions.

▽ If directions are given for both IM and IV reconstitution, be careful to read the correct set for the solution you are preparing.

▽ The person who reconstitutes a drug must initial the vial and print the expiration time and date on the label, unless all the drug is used immediately.

▽ If a solution is prepared using multiple-strength medication directions, the strength reconstituted must also be printed on the label.

Summary Self-Test

Refer to the ceftriaxone label in Figure 10-13 to answer the following questions about reconstitution.

1. What is the total dosage of this vial? _____

2. What volume of diluent must be used for I.M. reconstitution? _____

3. What will be the dosage strength of 1 mL of reconstituted I.M. solution?_____

NDC 0703-0335-01   Rx only Each vial contains: ceftriaxone sodium powder equivalent to 1 gram ceftriaxone.
Ceftriaxone
for Injection, USP
1 gram
For I.M. or I.V. Use
Single Use Vial
TEVA

For I.M. Administration : Reconstitute with 2.1 mL 1% Lidocaine Hydrochloride Injection (USP) or Sterile Water for Injection (USP). Each 1 mL of solution contains approximately 350 mg equivalent of ceftriaxone.
For I.V. Administration : See Package Insert
Usual Dosage: See Package Insert
Iss. 9/2009
39C1701450909

Storage Prior to Reconstitution: Store powder at 20° to 25°C (68° to 77°F) [See USP Controlled Room Temperature].
Protect from Light.
Storage After Reconstitution: See Package Insert
Mfd for: Teva Parenteral Medicines Irvine, CA 92618

Used with permission from Teva Pharmaceuticals USA.

▲ **FIGURE 10-13**

Refer to the levothyroxine sodium label in Figure 10-14 to answer the following questions.

4. What is the dosage strength of this vial in mcg? In mg?   _____ _____

5. What volume of diluent must you add to prepare the solution for use?   _____

6. What kind of diluent must be used?   _____

7. How long will this reconstituted solution retain its potency?   _____

8. What is the per mL strength of the reconstituted solution?   _____

9. Where will you find average dosage instructions?   _____

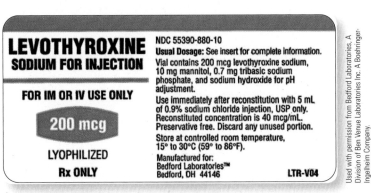

▲ FIGURE 10-14

Refer to the cytarabine label in Figure 10-15 to answer the following questions.

10. How much diluent is used to reconstitute this solution?   _____

11. What type of diluent?   _____

12. What is the total vial dosage?   _____

13. At what temperature should this medication be stored?   _____

14. What dosage will each 1 mL contain?   _____

15. What is the expiration time of the reconstituted solution?   _____

16. If the solution is reconstituted on Feb 14 at 0840,
    what expiration date must be printed on the label?   _____

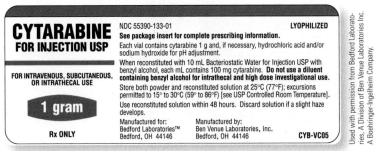

▲ FIGURE 10-15

Refer to the Vfend® I.V. label in Figure 10-16 to answer the following questions.

17. How much diluent is required to reconstitute this Vfend I.V. solution?   _____

18. What diluent is specified for use?   _____

19. What is the strength of each 1 mL of the reconstituted solution?   _____

20. What is the total dosage of this vial?   _____

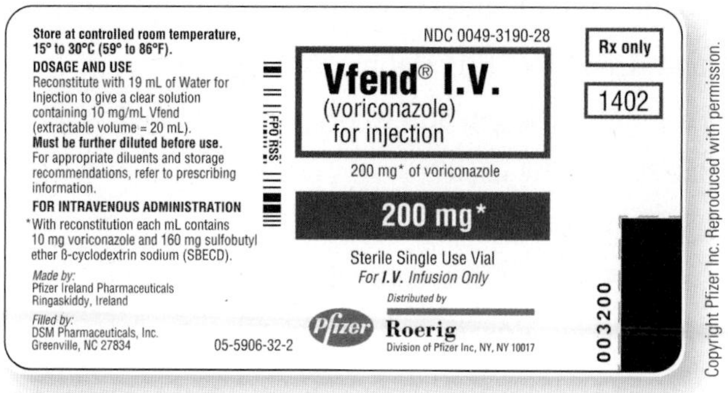

▲ FIGURE 10-16

Refer to the Vantin® Oral Suspension label in Figure 10-17 to answer the following questions.

21. How much diluent will be required to reconstitute this medication? _____

22. What type of diluent is listed for reconstitution? _____

23. How is this diluent to be added? _____

24. What is the reconstituted dosage strength? _____

25. How long will the reconstituted Vantin solution retain its potency? _____

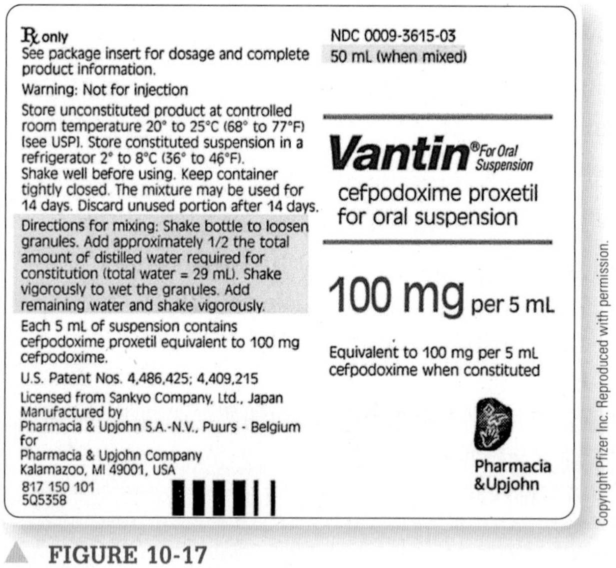

▲ FIGURE 10-17

Refer to the cytarabine label in Figure 10-18 to answer the following questions.

26. What is the total strength of this medication? _____

27. What diluent must be used for reconstitution? _____

28. How much? _____

29. What is the dosage per reconstituted mL? _____

30. How long does the reconstituted cytarabine solution retain its potency at room temperature? _____

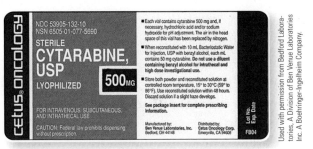

▲ **FIGURE 10-18**

Refer to the acyclovir label in Figure 10-19 to answer the following questions for reconstitution.

31. What type of diluent is recommended for reconstitution? _____

32. How much diluent must be added? _____

33. What is the total dosage strength of this vial? _____

34. How soon must this solution be used? _____

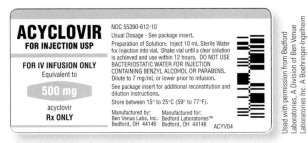

▲ **FIGURE 10-19**

Refer to the cytarabine label in Figure 10-20 and answer the following questions.

35. What is the total dosage strength of this vial? _____

36. What volume of diluent must be added? _____

37. What kind of diluent must be used? _____

38. What is the reconstituted dosage strength per mL? _____

39. How long will this medication retain its potency? _____

CYTARABINE
FOR INJECTION USP

NDC 55390-134-01   LYOPHILIZED

See package insert for complete prescribing information.

Each vial contains cytarabine 2 g and, if necessary, hydrochloric acid and/or sodium hydroxide for pH adjustment.

When reconstituted with 20 mL Bacteriostatic Water for Injection USP with benzyl alcohol, each mL contains 100 mg cytarabine. **Do not use a diluent containing benzyl alcohol for intrathecal and high dose investigational use.**

Store both powder and reconstituted solution at 25°C (77°F); excursions permitted to 15° to 30°C (59° to 86°F) [see USP Controlled Room Temperature]. Use reconstituted solution within 48 hours. Discard solution if a slight haze develops.

Manufactured for: Bedford Laboratories™
Bedford, OH 44146   **CYB-VD05**

FOR INTRAVENOUS, SUBCUTANEOUS, OR INTRATHECAL USE

2 gram

Rx ONLY

▲ **FIGURE 10-20**

Refer to the Pfizerpen® label in Figure 10-21 to answer the following questions.

40. What is the total dosage strength of this vial? _____

41. How much diluent must be added to prepare a
    100,000 units/mL strength? _____

42. How much diluent must be added to prepare a
    500,000 units/mL strength? _____

43. How much diluent must be added to prepare a
    50,000 units/mL strength? _____

44. This label has no information on the type of diluent to use.
    Where will you find this? _____

45. How must this solution be stored? _____

46. If reconstituted at 1:10 am on December 18, what must
    you print on the label? _____

47. What else must you print on the label? _____

48. Why should you print? _____

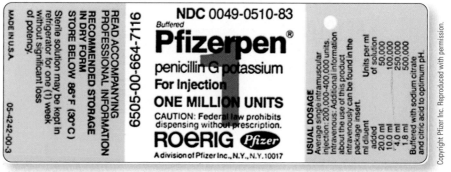

▲ FIGURE 10-21

Refer to the Zithromax® label in Figure 10-22 to answer the following questions.

49. What is the generic name for Zithromax? _____

50. What is the dosage strength of this vial? _____

51. What diluent is specified for reconstitution? _____

52. How much diluent is required? _____

53. What is the reconstituted dosage strength? _____

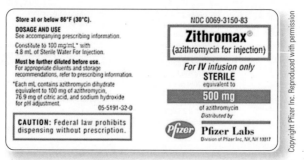

▲ FIGURE 10-22

Answers

1. 1 g
2. 2.1 mL
3. 350 mg/mL
4. 200 mcg; 0.2 mg
5. 5 mL
6. 0.9% sodium chloride
7. must be used immediately
8. 40 mcg/mL
9. package insert
10. 10 mL
11. bacteriostatic water for injection USP with benzyl alcohol
12. 1 gram
13. 25°C (77°F)
14. 100 mg/mL
15. 48 hours
16. Exp. Feb. 16 0840
17. 19 mL
18. water for injection
19. 10 mg/mL
20. 200 mg
21. 29 mL
22. distilled water
23. Shake the bottle to loosen granules, add half (15 mL) of the distilled water, and shake vigorously to dissolve granules; add balance of water and shake vigorously.
24. 100 mg/5 mL
25. 14 days
26. 500 mg
27. bacteriostatic water for injection USP with benzyl alcohol
28. 10 mL
29. 50 mg/mL
30. 48 hours
31. sterile water for injection
32. 10 mL
33. 500 mg
34. within 12 hours
35. 2 g
36. 20 mL
37. bacteriostatic water for injection USP with benzyl alcohol
38. 100 mg/mL
39. 48 hours
40. one million units
41. 10 mL
42. 1.8 mL
43. 20 mL
44. package insert
45. refrigerate
46. Exp. Dec. 25 1:10 am
47. your initials
48. Space considerations; handwriting is difficult to read.
49. azithromycin
50. 500 mg
51. sterile water for injection
52. 4.8 mL
53. 100 mg/mL

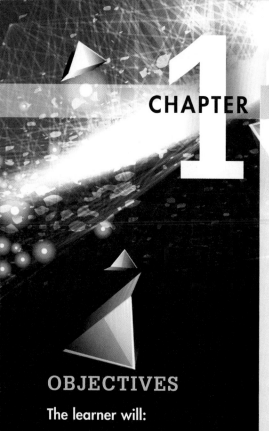

MEASURING INSULIN DOSAGES

OBJECTIVES

The learner will:

1. identify insulins in current use.

2. read insulin labels to identify type.

3. read calibrations on 100 units/mL insulin syringes.

4. measure single insulin dosages.

5. measure combined insulin dosages.

6. discuss the difference between rapid-, short-, intermediate-, and long-acting insulins.

7. discuss insulin injection sites and techniques.

Diabetes is one of the fastest-growing health problems in both the United States and Canada. Since the advent of DNA technology in the 1980s, the number of insulin products has almost quadrupled in an effort to keep pace with treatment needs.

This chapter will introduce you to the current insulin preparations available; provide real insulin vial labels to familiarize you with the different insulins; describe the physical appearance of insulins; instruct you in the use of specialized insulin syringes; and provide a step-by-step procedure for the combination of two different insulins in a single syringe, a skill you may use on an ongoing basis throughout your career.

We will briefly introduce you to insulin action times and injection techniques, which will be covered in detail in your pharmacology text.

TYPES OF INSULIN

Prior to the 1980s, all insulin was produced from animal sources. Today, **all are products of DNA**. The two earliest DNA insulins, **R (Regular)** and **N (NPH)***, are made from **recombinant DNA** (cut and spliced DNA fragments). Both of these insulins incorporate the **"lin"** of the word insu**lin** in their trade names: Humu**lin**® R and Humu**lin**® N manufactured by the Eli Lilly Co., and Novo**lin**® R and Novo**lin**® N from Novo Nordisk. **Regular** insulin is a **clear** solution, and it is **fast acting**, while **N** is **cloudy**, classified as **intermediate acting**, and has a **slower start but longer action**. Regular and N insulin are often **combined in a single syringe** to reduce the number of injections an individual must have. They may be combined at first to determine an individual's R and NPH insulin requirements, then ordered in **commercially combined insulin preparations**, such as **70/30** and **50/50** mixes, to provide both a fast and more prolonged action.

Another type of DNA preparation is the **analogs**, which are **chemically altered DNA**. Depending on their structure, the analogs offer an extremely rapid action, or a longer and more balanced control of blood

---

***NOTE:** The N intermediate action insulin takes its "N" designation from NPH, the first intermediate action insulin developed in the mid 1930s. The NPH initials represent neutral protamine Hagedorn, the chemical structure and name of the developer of NPH, Hans Hagedorn.*

glucose levels. Once again, some of the trade names of these products reflect their origin: the **"log"** of ana**log** is incorporated in two of the frequently used trade-named insulins: Huma**log**® and Novo**log**®. Among the analogs whose trade names do not identify their analog structure are Apidra® (glulisine), Lantis® (glargine), and Levemir® (detemir).

KEY_point:_ The -lin ending of regular and N insulin trade names can be used as an additional safeguard in distinguishing them from several of the analogs, which incorporate -log at the end of their trade names.

Unfortunately, most insulin **vials, solutions, and labels look very much alike**, and it is here where the first precaution in insulin preparation must be stressed.

INSULIN VIAL AND INSULIN INJECTION PEN LABEL IDENTIFICATION

Like other medications, insulin preparations have both trade and generic names. Eli Lilly and Novo Nordisk are the major insulin manufacturers; however, there are now other manufacturers producing and marketing insulin. In the insulin label identification problems that follow, you will be asked to identify insulin manufacturers, as well as insulin types and dosages. Some of the labels included are from **insulin pen** preparations: **prefilled, self-injection syringes** that contain **multiple doses** of insulin (Figure 11-1). To see an excellent demonstration of insulin pen use, go to http://www.levemir-us.com. All insulin is prepared in units per mL doses.

It would be hard to watch television today and not see advertisements for **prefilled insulin injection pens**, which are also called simply **insulin pens**. Many prefilled pens contain two insulins, one rapid acting and the other intermediate or long acting, which are combined to **establish maintenance doses for each individual patient**. All have a mechanism to set the dosage to be injected and each contains multiple doses that require multiple injections. Most contain a single needle, which is reused several times by the individual until a new insulin pen dosage is ordered. **Pen insulins do not require refrigeration**.

Pens are beginning to be used in the clinical setting, either for initial patient instruction in use, or ongoing therapy. The same label identity checks that are required for other meds are critical prior to administration. Ongoing supervision is essential to determine if a patient, who is being instructed in self-injection, is correctly administering the ordered dosage independently.

As with all medications, errors in insulin pen use have begun to creep in, and the pens are now a source of concern for in-hospital use. **Under no circumstances are insulin pens to be used for anyone other than the patient they are ordered for**.

KEY_point:_ Pens are prescribed for exclusive use with a single patient.

SECTION 3

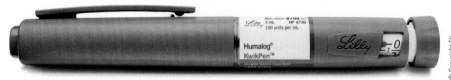

A. Humalog KwikPen 100 units/mL

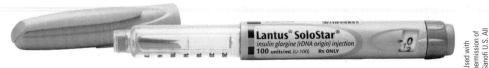

B. Lantus SoloStar 100 units/mL

▲ **FIGURE 11-1** Prefilled insulin pens.

Insulin pens are ordered for exclusive use for a single patient. This applies even if the pen needles are removable, which in most cases they are not.

▶▶▶ PROBLEMS 11.1

1. What does the 70 on the label in Figure 11-2 represent? _____

2. What does the 30 identify? _____

3. What company manufactured this insulin? _____

4. What is the dosage strength of this insulin? _____

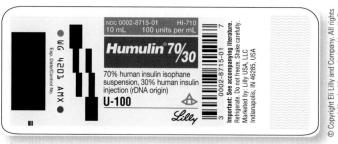

▲ **FIGURE 11-2**

5. What is the generic name of the insulin preparation in Figure 11-3? _____

6. What is the dosage strength? _____

7. What volume of insulin does this pen contain? _____

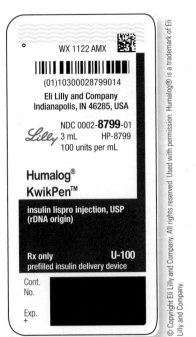

▲ FIGURE 11-3

8. What is the generic name of the insulin in Figure 11-4? _____

9. What exactly does the 50/50 identify? _____

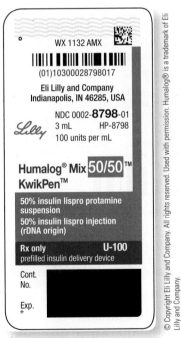

▲ FIGURE 11-4

10. What is the generic name of the insulin in Figure 11-5?

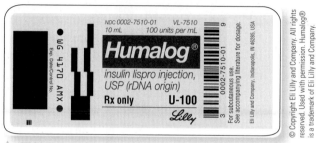

▲ **FIGURE 11-5**

11. What is the generic name of the insulin in Figure 11-6?

12. What is the trade name of this insulin?

13. What is the dosage strength of this preparation?

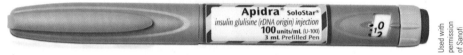

▲ **FIGURE 11-6**

14. What is the trade name of the insulin in Figure 11-7?

15. What is the generic name?

16. Who manufactures this insulin?

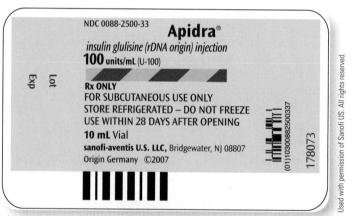

▲ **FIGURE 11-7**

17. What does the R on the label in Figure 11-8 identify?

18. Identify the precaution for using this particular insulin.

19. What is the total volume of this vial?

20. What is the dosage strength of this insulin?

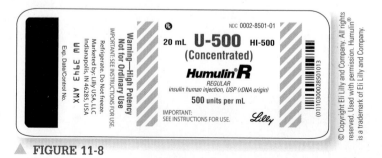

▲ **FIGURE 11-8**

21. What is the generic name of the insulin in the combination preparation in Figure 11-9? _____

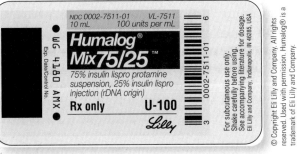

▲ **FIGURE 11-9**

22. What is the trade name of the insulin label in Figure 11-10? _____

23. What is its generic name? _____

24. What is its dosage strength? _____

25. Who manufactures this insulin? _____

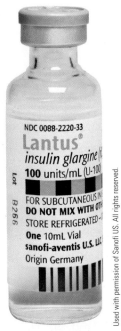

▲ **FIGURE 11-10**

Answers **1.** 70% isophane suspension **2.** 30% human insulin **3.** Lilly USA **4.** 100 units/mL
5. insulin lispro injection (rDNA origin) **6.** 100 units/mL **7.** 3 mL **8.** lispro
9. 50% insulin lispro protamine suspension; 50% insulin lispro injection **10.** lispro **11.** glulisine
12. Apidra® **13.** 100 units/mL **14.** Apidra® **15.** glulisine **16.** sanofi-aventis **17.** regular insulin
18. high potency; not for ordinary use **19.** 20 mL **20.** 500 units/mL **21.** lispro **22.** Lantus®
23. glargine **24.** 100 units/mL **25.** sanofi-aventis

 KEY_point:_ Diligence in the identification of insulin preparations is critical, because many vials, solutions, and labels are strikingly similar.

INSULIN SYRINGES

Think back for a moment to the insulin labels you have just read, and you will recall that all, except one high-potency vial, have a dosage strength of **100 units per mL**. You may have also noticed that these vials are additionally labeled **U-100**, which similarly identifies the 100 units per mL strength.

Insulin is administered using special **insulin syringes calibrated in units**. In diameter, these are quite like the smaller TB syringes, but the calibrations are totally different. **Insulin syringes are used only for insulin administration**, and they are available in the **100 unit, 50 unit, and 30 unit sizes** in Figure 11-11. The smaller 30 and 50 unit syringe calibrations are larger, and they provide an added degree of safety in measurement of small dosages.

Because of their small diameter, insulin syringe calibrations and numbering wrap around the small syringe barrel. Refer to the insulin syringes in Figure 11-11 again, and notice the calibrations there. For accurate measurement, you will learn **to rotate insulin syringes side to side to locate the calibration you need and to draw up the insulin dosage ordered**. To make your instruction in measuring insulin dosages easier, sample flattened out versions of calibrated syringes are provided. You will be using these flattened out syringes for your initial instruction in preparing insulin dosages.

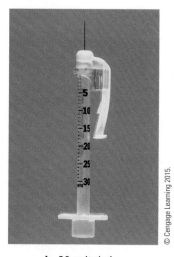
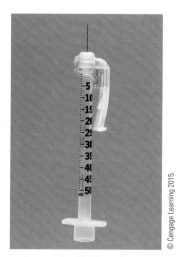
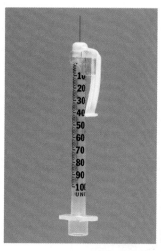

A. 30 units/mL   B. 50 units/mL   C. 100 units/mL

© Cengage Learning 2015.

▲ **FIGURE 11-11**

The calibrations for the 50 unit dosage syringes are used in the first problems that follow. Notice that the **first long calibration**, as on all other syringes, identifies **zero** and that **each subsequent calibration measures 1 unit. Each 5 unit calibration is numbered: 5, 10, 15, 20, and so forth**.

▶▶▶ PROBLEMS 11.2

Refer to the syringe calibrations for the 50 unit calibrated syringes provided to identify the dosages indicated by the shaded areas and arrows.

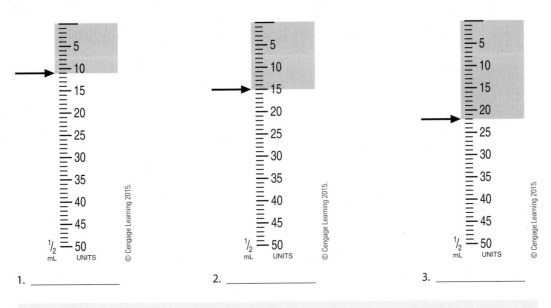

1. _____   2. _____   3. _____

Answers   1. 11 units   **2.** 15 units   **3.** 22 units

▶▶▶ PROBLEMS 11.3

Use the 50 unit calibrations provided to shade in the following dosages.

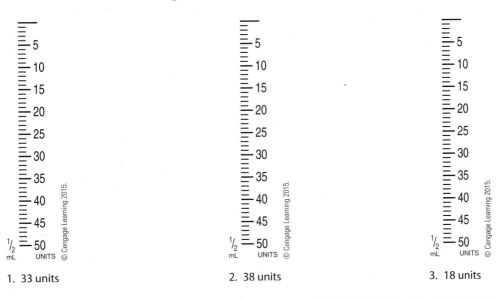

1. 33 units   2. 38 units   3. 18 units

Answers Have your instructor check your accuracy.

There are two 100 unit insulin syringes in common use. Refer to the first of these syringe calibrations in Problems 11.4. First, notice the 100 unit capacity and that, in contrast to the smaller dose syringes, only **each 10 unit increment is numbered: 10, 20, 30, and so forth**. Next, notice the number of calibrations in each 10 unit increment, which is 5, indicating that **this syringe is calibrated in 2 unit increments. Odd-numbered units cannot be measured accurately using this syringe**.

▶▶▶ PROBLEMS 11.4

Identify the dosages indicated by the shading and arrows on the 100 unit syringes provided.

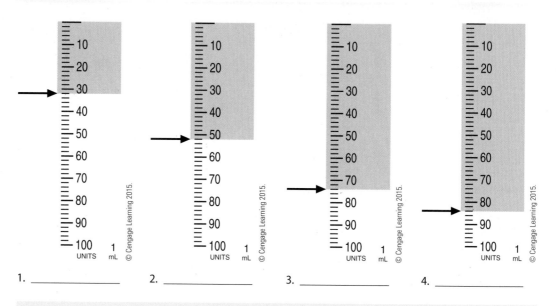

1. _____ 2. _____ 3. _____ 4. _____

Answers **1.** 32 units **2.** 52 units **3.** 74 units **4.** 84 units

▶▶▶ PROBLEMS 11.5

Shade in the syringe calibrations provided to measure the dosages indicated.

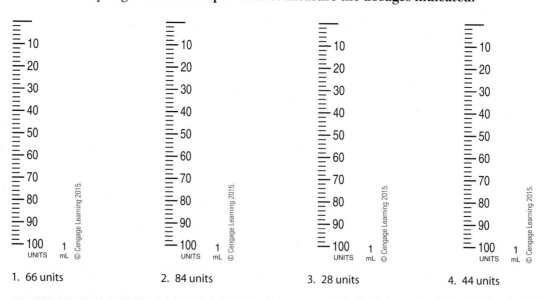

1. 66 units   2. 84 units   3. 28 units   4. 44 units

Answers Have your instructor check your accuracy.

The second type of 100 unit syringe calibration is illustrated in Figure 11-12. Notice that this syringe has a **double scale: the odd numbers are on the left, and the even are on the right**. Each 5 unit increment is numbered, but on **opposite sides** of the syringe. This syringe does have a calibration for each 1 unit increment, but in order to count every calibration to measure a dosage, the syringe would have to be rotated back and forth. This could cause confusion. There is a safer way to read the calibrations. **To measure uneven numbered dosages**—for example, 7, 13, and 27—**use the uneven (left) scale only; for even-numbered dosages**—such as 6, 10, and 56—**use the even (right) scale only. Count each calibration (on one side only) as 2 units, because that is what it is measuring**.

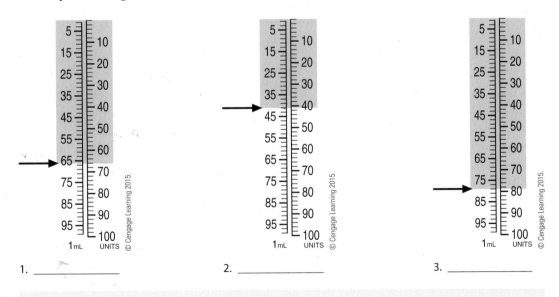

▲ **FIGURE 11-12**

EXAMPLE 1

To prepare an 89 unit dosage, start at 85 units on the uneven left scale, count the first calibration beyond this as 87 units and the next as 89 units (**each calibration on the same side measures 2 units**).

EXAMPLE 2

To measure a 26 unit dosage, use the even-numbered right side calibrations. Start at 20 units, move up one calibration to 22 units, another to 24 units, and one more to 26 units (**each calibration is 2 units**).

▶▶▶ PROBLEMS 11.6

Identify the dosages measured on the 100 unit syringe calibrations provided.

1. _____   2. _____   3. _____

Answers   1. 66 units **2.** 41 units **3.** 79 units

PROBLEMS 11.7

Shade in the syringe calibrations provided to identify the following dosages.

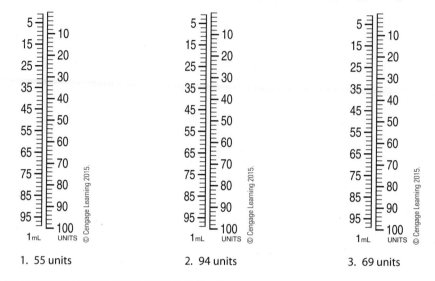

1. 55 units   2. 94 units   3. 69 units

Answers   Have your instructor check your accuracy.

COMBINING INSULIN DOSAGES

Insulin-dependent individuals may have one or even several subcutaneous injections of insulin per day. In order to reduce the number of injections as much as possible, it is common to combine two insulins in a single syringe: a short-acting Regular with an intermediate-acting NPH insulin.

 KEY*point:* When two insulins are combined in the same syringe, the clear Regular (shortest-acting) insulin is drawn up first.

Both insulins will be withdrawn from sealed 10 mL vials. This requires that an amount of air equal to the insulin to be withdrawn be injected into each vial as a preliminary step, to **keep the pressure inside the vials equalized after the insulin is withdrawn.** An additional step concerns preparation of the insulin itself. Regular clear insulin does not need to be mixed, but **N (NPH) is cloudy and precipitates out**. It must be **gently rotated to mix immediately before withdrawal**.

The smallest volume insulin syringe available is used to measure the dosages you need, because their larger calibrations provide additional ease and safety in reading. Examples of the actual step-by-step combination procedure follow.

EXAMPLE 1

The order is for a dosage of 10 units of Regular and 48 units of NPH.

STEP   1   Locate the correct R and NPH insulin and use an alcohol wipe to cleanse both vial tops.

STEP   2   The combined dosage, 10 units of Regular and 48 units of NPH, is 58 units. This requires the use of a 100 unit syringe.

STEP 3 Draw up 48 units of replacement air for the NPH in the syringe, and insert the needle tip into the NPH vial. Keep the needle tip above the insulin level so as to not inject air into the insulin and possibly distort the dosage. Inject the air and remove the needle.

STEP 4 Draw up 10 units of replacement air for the Regular insulin vial. Insert the needle into the vial, again above the insulin level, and inject the air. Draw up the 10 units of Regular insulin.

STEP 5 Pick up and gently rotate the NPH vial until the insulin is mixed. Insert the needle back into the vial and draw up the 48 units of NPH.

STEP 6 Administer the insulin dosage at once so that the NPH has no chance to precipitate out. Chart the administration.

EXAMPLE 2

A dosage of 16 units Regular and 22 units of NPH has been ordered.

STEP 1 Locate the correct Regular and NPH insulin and use an alcohol wipe to cleanse both vial tops.

STEP 2 The combined dosage, 16 units of Regular and 22 units of NPH, totals 38 units. For this administration, you can use a 50 unit volume syringe.

STEP 3 Draw up 22 units of replacement air for the NPH in the syringe. Insert the needle tip into the NPH vial. Keep the needle tip above the insulin level so as to not inject air into the insulin and possibly distort the dosage. Inject the air and remove the needle.

STEP 4 Draw up 16 units of replacement air for the Regular insulin vial. Insert the needle into the vial, again above the insulin level, and inject the air. Draw up the 16 units of Regular insulin.

STEP 5 Pick up and gently rotate the NPH vial until the insulin is mixed. Insert the needle and draw up the 22 units of NPH.

STEP 6 Administer the insulin at once so that the NPH has no chance to precipitate out. Chart the administration.

INSULIN ACTION TIMES

As equally important as insulin type and dosage is **the timing of insulin administration,** based on **onset of action, peak and duration, and relationship to dietary intake**.

Insulin is classified by action as **rapid, short, intermediate, or long acting**. The **rapid-acting** insulins aspart, glulisine, and lispro, whose onset of action varies from 10 to 30 minutes, **must be followed immediately by a meal**. Failure to immediately ingest food would result in a rapidly lowered blood glucose level and **insulin reaction from hypoglycemia**. Also note that these rapid-acting insulins have a peak and duration of from 0.5 to 5 hours. Their action is relatively short.

Next, compare the **short-acting, regular** insulins which have an onset of 30 minutes, a peak of 1–5 hours, and a duration of 8 hours. These also require that the individual **eat shortly after administration**.

KEY_point:_ Rapid- and short-acting insulin must be followed immediately by a meal.

The **intermediate-acting** insulins are moving into the longer action range, with an onset of 1–4 hours, a peak of 4–12 hours, and duration of 14–26 hours. And, finally, the **long-acting** detemir and glargine insulins have an onset of 1–2 hours but a sustained minimal peak of up to 24 hours. Their administration is not related to dietary intake. Insulin detemir may be administered once or twice a day, while glargine is administered at night.

 KEY_point:_ Long-acting insulins are not administered in relation to immediate food ingestion.

The number of diabetic products will continue to increase because of the rapidly rising incidence of Type 2 diabetes. An inhalation insulin, Exubera®, is now available, and two additional new drugs are now in increasing use: Byetta® and Symlin®. Both of the latter act to change the body's response to food, either by promoting insulin secretion, delaying gastric emptying, and/or altering glucose metabolism.

INSULIN INJECTION SITES AND TECHNIQUES

Insulin is injected subcutaneously. As with other parenteral medications, the **injection sites must be rotated,** keeping **at least an inch away from each previously used site**. The abdomen has the most rapid absorption, followed by the upper arm. The outer thigh, a full hand's breadth above the knee and below the hip, may be used, but absorption is somewhat slower at this site. Your responsibility is, and will continue to be, to give the correct insulin and dosage at the correct time, taking special care to ensure that a meal immediately follows rapid- and short-acting insulin injection.

▶▶▶ PROBLEMS 11.8

For each of the following combined Regular and NPH insulin dosages, indicate the total volume of the combined dosage and the smallest capacity syringe you can use to prepare it; 30, 50, and 100 unit capacity syringes are available.

	Total Volume	Syringe Size
1. 28 units Regular, 64 units NPH	_____	_____
2. 16 units NPH, 6 units Regular	_____	_____
3. 33 units Regular, 41 units NPH	_____	_____
4. 21 units Regular, 52 units NPH	_____	_____
5. 13 units Regular, 27 units NPH	_____	_____

Answers   1. 92 units; 100 unit **2.** 22 units; 30 unit **3.** 74 units; 100 unit **4.** 73 units; 100 unit **5.** 40 units; 50 unit

Summary

This concludes the chapter on insulin dosages. The important points to remember from this chapter are:

▼ Insulin labels must be read with extreme care because they look very similar.

▼ Insulin is measured using specially calibrated insulin syringes.

▼ Insulin syringes are available in 100, 50, and 30 unit capacities.

▼ The smaller 30 or 50 unit capacity syringes provide a greater degree of safety because of their larger calibrations.

▼ Each calibration on 30 and 50 unit volume syringes measures 1 unit.

▼ Calibrations on 100 unit capacity insulin syringes may measure 1 or 2 unit increments, depending on their design.

▼ The "lin" in the trade names of Regular and N (NPH) insulin identifies their recombinant DNA origin.

▼ The "log" in several of the analog insulins identifies their chemically altered DNA structure.

▼ Regular (R) and N (NPH) insulin can be mixed in a single syringe.

▼ Regular insulin is drawn up first in combination R and N dosages.

▼ N insulins are cloudy because they contain insoluble particles.

▼ Because N insulins precipitate out, they must be gently and thoroughly mixed before withdrawal, and injected immediately after preparation.

▼ Insulin is administered subcutaneously.

▼ The abdomen and upper arm provide the most rapid subcutaneous absorption sites.

▼ Insulin injection sites are routinely rotated.

Summary Self-Test

Use the syringe calibrations provided to measure the following dosages. For combined insulin dosages, use arrows to indicate the exact calibration to be used for each insulin ordered. Have your instructor check your answers.

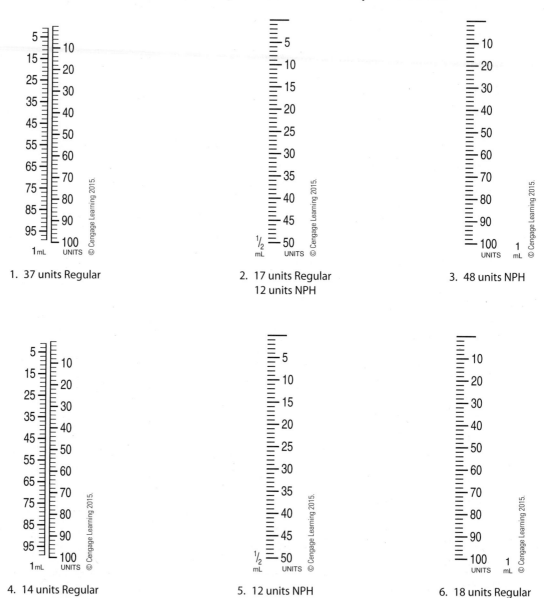

1. 37 units Regular

2. 17 units Regular
   12 units NPH

3. 48 units NPH

4. 14 units Regular
   58 units NPH

5. 12 units NPH

6. 18 units Regular
   8 units NPH

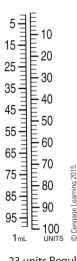
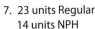

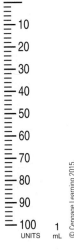

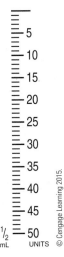

7. 23 units Regular
   14 units NPH

8. 8 units Regular
   20 units NPH

9. 24 units Regular

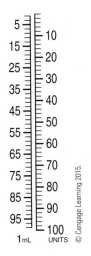

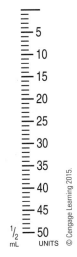

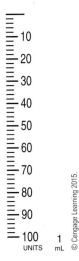

10. 57 units NPH

11. 22 units Regular

12. 14 units Regular
    44 units NPH

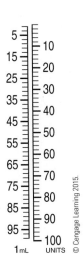

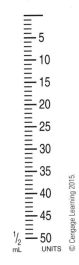

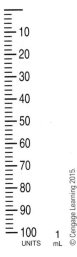

13. 24 units Regular
    27 units NPH

14. 33 units Regular
    10 units NPH

15. 56 units Regular

Identify the dosages measured on the following syringes.

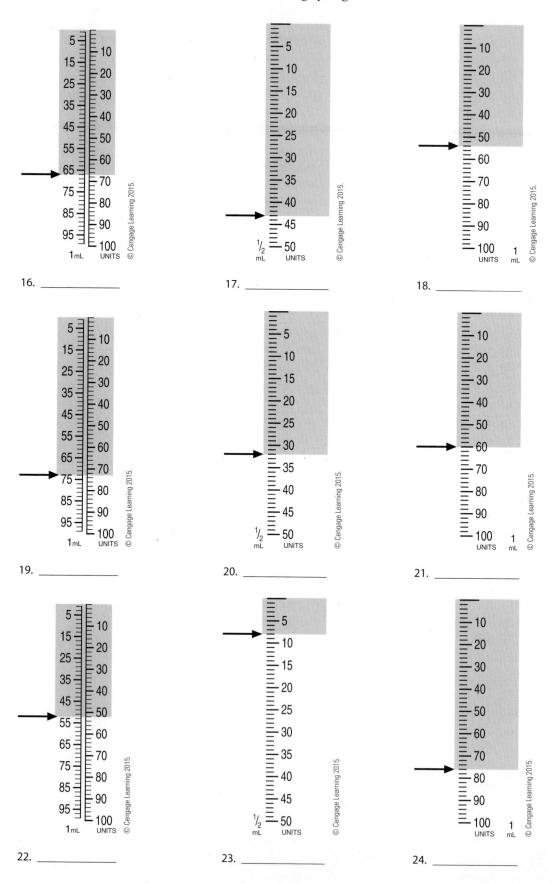

16. _____

17. _____

18. _____

19. _____

20. _____

21. _____

22. _____

23. _____

24. _____

CHAPTER 11

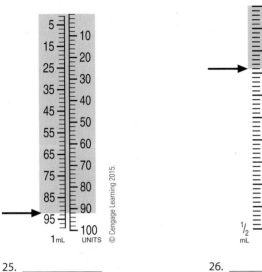

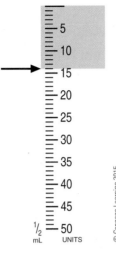

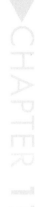

25. _____

26. _____

27. _____

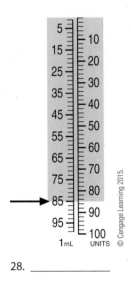

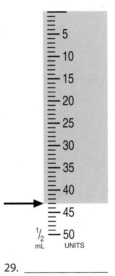 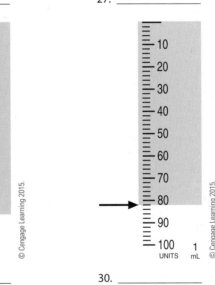

28. _____

29. _____

30. _____

Answers			
1-15. See instructor	**19.** 73 units	**24.** 76 units	**29.** 43 units
16. 67 units	**20.** 32 units	**25.** 92 units	**30.** 82 units
17. 43 units	**21.** 60 units	**26.** 14 units	
18. 54 units	**22.** 52 units	**27.** 58 units	
	23. 8 units	**28.** 85 units	

SECTION

Dosage Calculations

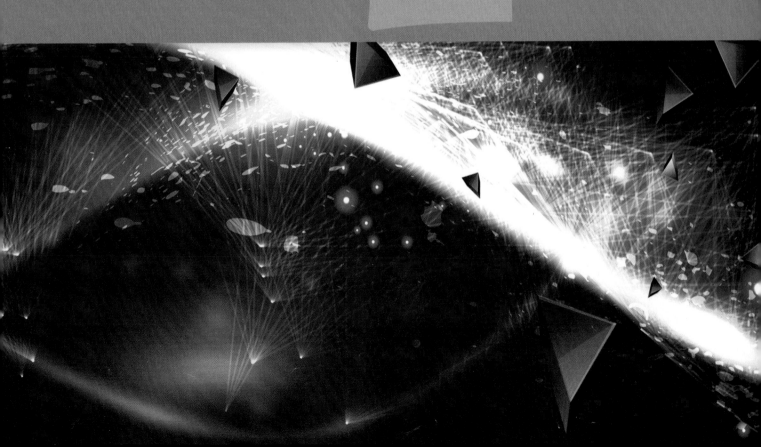

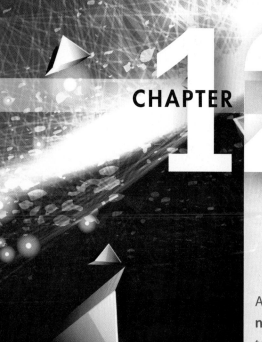

12 RATIO AND PROPORTION

OBJECTIVES

The learner will:

1. define ratio.
2. define proportion.
3. solve dosage problems using ratio and proportion.
4. assess answers obtained to determine if they are logical.

PREREQUISITES

Chapters 1–8

A **ratio** consists of **two different numbers or quantities that have a significant relationship to each other.** Earlier in the text, you learned how to read the dosage on drug labels. Each of these dosages was expressed as a ratio: a certain weight (strength) of drug in a tablet (tab), capsule (cap), or a certain volume of solution, most commonly mL; for example, 50 mg per mL, 100 mcg per tab, 1000 units per mL.

RATIOS

There are **two ways to express (write)** a ratio. The numbers can be written as a **common fraction**, or **separated by a colon**.

As a common fraction		Separated by a colon
$\dfrac{50 \text{ mg}}{1 \text{ mL}}$	or	50 mg : 1 mL
$\dfrac{100 \text{ mcg}}{1 \text{ tab}}$	or	100 mcg : 1 tab
$\dfrac{1000 \text{ units}}{1 \text{ mL}}$	or	1000 units : 1 mL

KEYpoint: A ratio consists of two numbers that have a significant relationship to each other. It can be expressed as a common fraction or with the numbers separated by a colon.

▶▶▶ PROBLEMS 12.1

Express dosages using the ratio format you prefer.

1. An injectable solution that contains 100 mg
   in each 1.5 mL   _____

2. An injectable solution that contains 250 mg
   in each 0.7 mL   _____

3. A tablet that contains 0.4 mg of drug   _____

4. Two tablets that contain 450 mg of drug   _____

Answers **1.** $\dfrac{100 \text{ mg}}{1.5 \text{ mL}}$; 100 mg : 1.5 mL **2.** $\dfrac{250 \text{ mg}}{0.7 \text{ mL}}$; 250 mg : 0.7 mL; **3.** $\dfrac{0.4 \text{ mg}}{1 \text{ tab}}$; 0.4 mg : 1 tab

4. $\dfrac{450 \text{ mg}}{2 \text{ tab}}$; 450 mg : 2 tab

Note: If you did not include the units of measure, your answers are incorrect.

 To complete the chapter, choose the ratio format you prefer. If you choose the
common fraction format, continue on this page. If you prefer ratios using
the colon format, turn now to page 171 to "Ratio and Proportion Expressed
Using Colons."

RATIO AND PROPORTION EXPRESSED USING COMMON FRACTIONS

Whereas a ratio is an expression of a significant relationship between two numbers, **a proportion** is used **to show the relationship between two ratios**. In a proportion, the ratios are separated by an **equal (=) sign**.

$$\frac{50}{1} = \frac{100}{2}$$

 KEY*point:* A true proportion contains two ratios that are equal.

The previous example is a true proportion. This is a simple comparison, and by using drug strength examples, we can verify that the ratios are equal and that the proportion is true.

EXAMPLE 1 $\dfrac{50 \text{ mg}}{\textbf{1 tab}} = \dfrac{100 \text{ mg}}{\textbf{2 tab}}$

If 1 tablet contains 50 mg, 2 tablets will contain 100 mg.

EXAMPLE 2
$$\frac{50 \text{ mg}}{1 \text{ mL}} = \frac{100 \text{ mg}}{2 \text{ mL}}$$

If 1 mL contains 50 mg, 2 mL will contain 100 mg.

You can also prove mathematically that these ratios are equal and that the proportion is true. Look again at Example 1.

$$\frac{50 \text{ mg}}{1 \text{ tab}} = \frac{100 \text{ mg}}{2 \text{ tab}}$$

 KEYpoint: In a true proportion, the cross-multiplied products will be identical.

To prove that a proportion is true, cross multiply. The products (answers) you obtain will be identical.

EXAMPLE 1
$$\frac{50 \text{ mg}}{1 \text{ tab}} = \frac{100 \text{ mg}}{2 \text{ tab}}$$

$$\frac{50}{1} \diagdown\!\!\!\!\diagup \frac{100}{2} \qquad \text{Drop the measurement units}$$

$$50 \times 2 = 100 \times 1 \qquad \text{Cross multiply}$$

$$100 = 100$$

The products of cross multiplying in this proportion, 100, are the same. We have now proved mathematically what we previously proved mentally: The ratios are equal and the proportion is true.

EXAMPLE 2
$$\frac{500 \text{ mg}}{2 \text{ mL}} \diagdown\!\!\!\!\diagup \frac{250 \text{ mg}}{1 \text{ mL}}$$

$$250 \times 2 = 500 \times 1 \qquad \text{Drop the measurement units, then cross multiply}$$

$$500 = 500$$

The products of cross multiplying, 500, are identical. This is a true proportion; the ratios are equal.

EXAMPLE 3
$$\frac{10 \text{ units}}{1 \text{ mL}} = \frac{20 \text{ units}}{2 \text{ mL}}$$

$$10 \times 2 = 20 \times 1$$

$$20 = 20$$

This is a true proportion. The products of cross multiplying, 20, are equal.

▶▶▶ PROBLEMS 12.2

Determine mathematically if these proportions are true.

1. $\dfrac{34 \text{ mg}}{2 \text{ mL}} = \dfrac{51 \text{ mg}}{3 \text{ mL}}$ _____

2. $\dfrac{15 \text{ mg}}{4 \text{ mL}} = \dfrac{45 \text{ mg}}{12 \text{ mL}}$ _____

3. $\dfrac{46 \text{ mg}}{1.3 \text{ mL}} = \dfrac{23 \text{ mg}}{0.65 \text{ mL}}$ _____

4. $\dfrac{150 \text{ units}}{2.3 \text{ mL}} = \dfrac{130 \text{ units}}{1.9 \text{ mL}}$ _____

5. $\dfrac{40 \text{ mg}}{1.1 \text{ mL}} = \dfrac{80 \text{ mg}}{2.2 \text{ mL}}$ _____

Answers **1.** true $(2 \times 51 = 102$ and $34 \times 3 = 102)$ **2.** true $(4 \times 45 = 180$ and $15 \times 12 = 180)$
3. true $(46 \times 0.65 = 29.9$ and $23 \times 1.3 = 29.9)$ **4.** not true $(150 \times 1.9 = 285$ and $130 \times 2.3 = 299)$
5. true $(40 \times 2.2 = 88$ and $1.1 \times 80 = 88)$

DOSAGE CALCULATION USING RATIO AND PROPORTION EXPRESSED AS COMMON FRACTIONS

Ratio and proportion are important in dosage calculations because they can be used when only **one ratio is known**, or **complete**, and **the second is incomplete**. Look carefully at the following examples for mL parenteral dosages, which is where calculations are most often required.

EXAMPLE 1 A solution strength of **8 mg per mL** will be used to prepare a dosage of **10 mg**.

The **known ratio** is provided by the **solution strength available**, 8 mg per mL. The **incomplete ratio** is the **dosage to be given**, 10 mg, and X is used to represent the mL which will contain 10 mg.

$$\frac{8 \text{ mg}}{1 \text{ mL}} = \frac{10 \text{ mg}}{X \text{ mL}}$$

$\left(\begin{array}{c}\text{complete ratio}\\ \text{drug strength}\end{array}\right)$ $\left(\begin{array}{c}\text{incomplete ratio}\\ \text{dosage to give}\end{array}\right)$

KEY*point:* The ratios in a proportion are written in the same sequence of measurement units.

In the previous example, they are:

$$\frac{mg}{mL} = \frac{mg}{mL}$$

Both **numerators** are **mg**; both **denominators** are **mL**.

Next, let's look at the math steps used to determine the value of the unknown, X mL. The math will be familiar because it was covered earlier in the refresher math section.

$$\frac{8\ mg}{1\ mL} = \frac{10\ mg}{X\ mL}$$	Set up the proportion to include the measurement units; make sure they are in the same sequence
$$\frac{8\ mg}{1\ mL} \underset{}{\overset{}{\times}} \frac{10\ mg}{X\ mL}$$	Drop the measurement units as you cross multiply
$$8X = 10$$	Keep X on the left of the equation
$$X = \frac{\overset{5}{\cancel{10}}}{\underset{4}{\cancel{8}}}$$	Divide 10 by the number in front of X; reduce by the highest common denominator (2)
$$= \frac{5}{4}$$	Divide the final fraction to obtain a decimal fraction
$$= \textbf{1.25 mL}$$	The X in the original proportion was **mL**, so the answer is 1.25 **mL**

The ordered dosage of 10 mg is contained in 1.25 mL.

It is routine to check your math twice in dosage calculations. However, it is also necessary to **assess each answer to determine if it is logical**, and here is where the review of the relative value of numbers is put to use. Consider the answer just obtained in Example 1.

$$\frac{8\ mg}{1\ mL} = \frac{10\ mg}{X\ mL}$$

$$X = \textbf{1.25 mL}$$

If **1 mL** contains **8 mg**, you will need a **larger** volume than 1 mL to obtain **10 mg**. The answer obtained, **1.25 mL**, is larger; therefore, it is logical. This routine check does not guarantee that your math is correct, but it does indicate that you did not mix up the units of measure when you set up the proportion and cross multiplied.

 KEY*point:* Assess each answer obtained to determine if it is logical.

EXAMPLE 2 The strength available is **25 mg in 1.5 mL**. A dosage of **20 mg** has been ordered.

$$\frac{25 \text{ mg}}{1.5 \text{ mL}} = \frac{20 \text{ mg}}{X \text{ mL}}$$ Make sure the units are in the same sequence

$$25X = 1.5 \times 20$$ Cross multiply; keep X on the left

$$X = \frac{\cancel{30}^{6}}{\cancel{25}_{5}}$$ Reduce by 5, then divide the final fraction

$$= \textbf{1.2 mL}$$ Include the measurement unit in your answer

The dosage ordered, 20 mg, is smaller than the strength available, 25 mg in 1.5 mL. So, the answer should be smaller than 1.5 mL, and it is. The answer is logical.

EXAMPLE 3 A dosage of **200 mg** must be prepared from a solution strength of **80 mg per mL**.

$$\frac{80 \text{ mg}}{1 \text{ mL}} = \frac{200 \text{ mg}}{X \text{ mL}}$$

$$80X = 200$$

$$\frac{\cancel{200}^{5}}{\cancel{80}_{2}} = \textbf{2.5 mL}$$

The unknown, X, was mL, so the answer must be mL. The dosage ordered, 200 mg, is larger than the 80 mg per mL strength being used, so it must be contained in more than 1 mL. The answer, 2.5 mL, is larger. Therefore, it is logical.

As soon as you are comfortable with the math for ratio and proportion, you can combine several steps and work even more efficiently. You may already have been doing this, but here are a few examples to demonstrate the shortcuts.

EXAMPLE 4 A **300 mg in 1.2 mL** solution will be used to prepare a dosage of **120 mg**.

$$\frac{300 \text{ mg}}{1.2 \text{ mL}} = \frac{120 \text{ mg}}{X \text{ mL}}$$ Set up the proportion, with the known ratio written first

$$X = \frac{1.2 \times 120}{300}$$ Cross multiply, and **immediately** divide by the number in front of X

$$\frac{1.2 \times \cancel{120}^{2}}{\cancel{300}_{5}} = \frac{2.4}{5} = 0.48 = \textbf{0.5 mL}$$ Reduce (by 60); do final division; round to nearest tenth

A dosage of 120 mg will require fewer mL than the 300 mg per 1.2 mL strength available. The smaller 0.5 mL answer is logical.

EXAMPLE 5   Prepare a **2 mg** dosage using a **1.5 mg in 0.5 mL** solution.

$$\frac{1.5 \text{ mg}}{0.5 \text{ mL}} = \frac{2 \text{ mg}}{X \text{ mL}}$$

$$X = \frac{\cancel{0.5}^{1} \times 2}{\cancel{1.5}_{3}} = 0.66 = \textbf{0.7 mL}$$

The 0.7 mL answer is a larger volume than the 1.5 mg in 0.5 mL dosage strength available; therefore, it is logical for this 2 mg dosage.

EXAMPLE 6   A **120 mg** dosage is ordered. The solution available is labeled **80 mg per mL**.

$$\frac{80 \text{ mg}}{1 \text{ mL}} = \frac{120 \text{ mg}}{X \text{ mL}}$$

$$X = \frac{\cancel{120}^{3}}{\cancel{80}_{2}} = \textbf{1.5 mL}$$

The 120 mg dosage ordered will require a volume larger than the 80 mg per mL available dosage strength. The answer, 1.5 mL, is larger; therefore, it is logical.

▶▶▶ PROBLEMS 12.3

Calculate these dosages. Express answers to the nearest tenth. Assess answers to determine if they are logical.

1. A dosage of 24 mg has been ordered. The solution strength available is 12.5 mg in 1.5 mL.   _____

2. A 40 mg in 2.5 mL solution will be used to prepare a 30 mg dosage.   _____

3. Prepare 0.3 mg from a solution strength of 0.6 mg in 0.8 mL.   _____

4. A 36 mg per 2 mL strength solution is used to prepare 24 mg.   _____

5. A dosage of 52 mg is to be prepared from a 78 mg in 0.9 mL solution.   _____

6. A dosage of 150 mg has been ordered. The solution strength is 100 mg per mL.   _____

7. A strength of 3 mL containing 750 mcg is available to prepare 600 mcg.   _____

8. If the strength available is 1.5 g per mL, how many mL will a 4 g dosage require?   _____

9. Prepare a 0.25 mg dosage from a 0.5 mg per 1 mL strength solution. _____

10. Prepare a 3 g dosage from a 4 g in 2.7 mL strength solution. _____

Answers 1. 2.9 mL **2.** 1.9 mL **3.** 0.4 mL **4.** 1.3 mL **5.** 0.6 mL **6.** 1.5 mL **7.** 2.4 mL **8.** 2.7 mL
9. 0.5 mL **10.** 2 mL

Note: If you did not include the units of measure, your answers are incorrect.

Turn now to page 176, "Calculations When Dosages Are in Different Units of Measure," to complete the chapter.

RATIO AND PROPORTION EXPRESSED USING COLONS

Whereas a ratio is an expression of a significant relationship between two numbers, **a proportion** is used **to show the relationship between two ratios**. In a proportion, the ratios are separated by an **equal (=) sign**.

$$50 : 1 = 100 : 2$$

 KEYpoint: A true proportion contains two ratios that are equal.

The previous example is a true proportion.

$$50 : 1 = 100 : 2$$

By using our previous drug strength examples, we can mentally verify that these ratios are equal and that the proportion is true.

EXAMPLE 1   50 mg : 1 **tab** = 100 mg : 2 **tab**

If 1 tablet contains 50 mg, 2 tablets will contain 100 mg.

EXAMPLE 2   50 mg : 1 **mL** = 100 mg : 2 **mL**

If 1 mL contains 50 mg, 2 mL will contain 100 mg.

You can also prove mathematically that these ratios are equal and that the proportion is true. Look again at Example 1.

50 mg : 1 tab = 100 mg : 2 tab

The numbers on the **ends** of the proportion (50, 2) are called the **extremes**, whereas those in the **middle** (1, 100) are called the **means**.

 KEYpoint: It is critical in all math involving proportions that the means and extremes not be mixed up or an incorrect answer will be obtained.

Here is a memory cue that you can use to prevent confusion. Notice that the **means** are in the **middle** of a proportion. Both of these words begin with an "**m**" (**m**eans, **m**iddle). The **extremes** are on the **ends** of the proportion. Both of these words begin with an "**e**" (**e**xtremes, **e**nds). Use these cues to prevent mix-ups.

 KEY_point:_ In a true proportion, the product of the means equals the product of the extremes.

If you multiply the means, then the extremes—their products (answers)—will be equal.

EXAMPLE 1   50 mg : 1 tab = 100 mg : 2 tab

$$50 : 1 = 100 : 2$$

(extremes / means)

$$50 \times 2 = 100 \times 1$$

$$100 = 100$$

The product of the means, 100, equals the product of the extremes, 100. We have now proved mathematically what we previously proved mentally: The ratios are equal and the proportion is true.

EXAMPLE 2   500 mg : 2 mL = 250 mg : 1 mL

$$500 : 2 = 250 : 1$$

$$500 \times 1 = 2 \times 250$$

$$500 = 500$$

The product of the means, 500, equals the product of the extremes, 500. This is a true proportion; the ratios are equal.

EXAMPLE 3   10 units : 1 mL = 20 units : 2 mL

$$10 \times 2 = 20 \times 1$$

$$20 = 20$$

This is a true proportion.

▶ ▶ ▶ PROBLEMS 12.4

Determine mathematically if these proportions are true.

1. 34 mg : 2 mL = 51 mg : 3 mL   _____

2. 15 mg : 4 mL = 45 mg : 12 mL   _____

3. 46 mg : 1.3 mL = 23 mg : 0.65 mL   _____

4. 150 units : 2.3 mL = 130 units : 1.9 mL   _____

5. 40 mg : 1.1 mL = 80 mg : 2.2 mL   _____

Answers **1.** true (2 × 51 = 102 and 34 × 3 = 102) **2.** true (4 × 45 = 180 and 15 × 12 = 180)
3. true (46 × 0.65 = 29.9 and 1.3 × 23 = 29.9) **4.** not true (150 × 1.9 = 285 and 2.3 × 130 = 299)
5. true (40 × 2.2 = 88 and 1.1 × 80 = 88)

DOSAGE CALCULATION USING RATIO AND PROPORTION EXPRESSED WITH COLONS

Ratio and proportion are important in dosage calculations because they can be used when only **one ratio is known**, or **complete**, and **the second is incomplete**. Look carefully at the following examples for mL parenteral dosages, which is where calculations are most often required.

EXAMPLE 1 ▸   A solution strength of **8 mg per mL** will be used to prepare a dosage of **10 mg**.

The **known ratio** is provided by the **solution strength available**, 8 mg per mL. The **incomplete ratio** is the **dosage to be given**, 10 mg, and X is used to represent the mL which will contain 10 mg.

$$
\underset{\left(\substack{\text{complete ratio} \\ \text{drug strength}}\right)}{8\ \text{mg} : 1\ \text{mL}} \quad = \quad \underset{\left(\substack{\text{incomplete ratio} \\ \text{dosage to give}}\right)}{10\ \text{mg} : X\ \text{mL}}
$$

 KEY*point:* The ratios in a proportion are written in the same sequence of measurement units.

In the previous example, they are: mg : mL = mg : mL

Next, let's look at the math steps used to determine the value of the unknown, X mL. The math will be familiar because it was covered earlier in the refresher math section.

8 mg : 1 mL = 10 mg : X mL	Check the sequence of measurement units: mg : mL = mg : mL
8 : 1 = 10 : X	Drop the measurement units
8X = 10	Multiply the extremes, then the means, keeping X on the left of the equation
$X = \dfrac{10}{8}$	Divide 10 by the number in front of X
$= \dfrac{\overset{5}{\cancel{10}}}{\underset{4}{\cancel{8}}}$	Reduce the numbers by their highest common denominator, 2. Divide the final fraction. Divide 5 by 4.
$= \mathbf{1.25\ mL}$	The X in the original proportion was **mL**, so the answer is 1.25 **mL**

The ordered dosage of 10 mg is contained in 1.25 mL.

It is routine to check your math twice in dosage calculations. However, it is also necessary to **assess each answer to determine if it seems logical**, and here is where the previous review of the relative value of numbers is put to use. Consider the answer just obtained in Example 1.

$$8 \text{ mg} : 1 \text{ mL} = 10 \text{ mg} : X \text{ mL}$$

$$X = \textbf{1.25 mL}$$

If **1 mL** contains **8 mg**, you will need a **larger** volume than **1 mL** to obtain **10 mg**. The answer obtained, **1.25 mL**, **is** larger; therefore, it is logical. This routine check does not guarantee that your math is correct, but it does indicate that you have not mixed up the means and extremes in your calculations.

 KEY_point:_ Assess each answer obtained to determine if it is logical.

EXAMPLE 2 ▸   The dosage strength available is **25 mg in 1.5 mL**. A dosage of **20 mg** has been ordered.

$$25 \text{ mg} : 1.5 \text{ mL} = 20 \text{ mg} : X \text{ mL}$$ Make sure the units are written in the same sequence: mg : mL = mg: mL

$$25 : 1.5 = 20 : X$$ Drop the measurement units

$$25X = 1.5 \times 20$$ Multiply the extremes, then the means, keeping X on the left

$$= \frac{30}{25}$$ Divide by the number in front of X

$$= \frac{\overset{6}{\cancel{30}}}{\underset{5}{\cancel{25}}} = 1.2$$ Reduce the common denominator by 5, then divide the final fraction, 6 by 5

$$X = \textbf{1.2 mL}$$

The dosage ordered, 20 mg, is a smaller amount of drug than the strength available, 25 mg in 1.5 mL. So, the answer should be smaller than 1.5 mL, and 1.2 mL is smaller. This answer is logical.

EXAMPLE 3 ▸   A dosage of **200 mg** must be prepared from a solution strength of **80 mg per mL**.

$$80 \text{ mg} : 1 \text{ mL} = 200 \text{ mg} : X \text{ mL}$$

$$80X = 200$$

$$\frac{\overset{5}{\cancel{200}}}{\underset{2}{\cancel{80}}} = \frac{5}{2} = \textbf{2.5 mL}$$

The unknown, X, was mL, so the answer must be mL. The dosage ordered, 200 mg, is larger than the 80 mg per mL strength used, so it must be contained in more than 1 mL. The answer, 2.5 mL, is larger. Therefore, it is logical.

As soon as you are comfortable with the math for ratio and proportion, you can combine several steps and work even more efficiently. You may have already been doing this, but here are a few examples to demonstrate the shortcuts.

EXAMPLE 4   A **300 mg in 1.2 mL** solution will be used to prepare a dosage of **120 mg**.

$300 \text{ mg} : 1.2 \text{ mL} = 120 \text{ mg} : X \text{ mL}$ Set up the proportion, with the known ratios written first

$$X = \frac{1.2 \times 120}{300}$$ Multiply the means, and **immediately** divide by the number in front of X

$$= \frac{1.2 \times \cancel{120}^{2}}{\cancel{300}^{5}}$$ Reduce by the common denominator, 60.

$$= \frac{2.4}{5} = 0.48 \times \mathbf{0.5 \text{ mL}}$$ Do final division: 2.4 by 5. Round to the nearest tenth.

The required dosage, 120 mg, is smaller than the 300 mg per 1.2 mL available strength. Therefore, the smaller 0.5 mL answer is logical.

EXAMPLE 5   Prepare a **2 mg** dosage using a **1.5 mg in 0.5 mL** solution.

$1.5 \text{ mg} : 0.5 \text{ mL} = 2 \text{ mg} : X \text{ mL}$

$$X = \frac{\cancel{0.5}^{1} \times 2}{\cancel{1.5}_{3}} = 0.66 = \mathbf{0.7 \text{ mL}}$$

The dosage ordered, 2 mg, is larger than the 1.5 mg in 0.5 mL dosage available. The 0.7 mL answer is logical.

EXAMPLE 6   A **120 mg** dosage is ordered. The solution available is labeled **80 mg per mL**.

$80 \text{ mg} : 1 \text{ mL} = 120 \text{ mg} : X \text{ mL}$

$$X = \frac{\cancel{120}^{3}}{\cancel{80}^{2}} = \mathbf{1.5 \text{ mL}}$$

The 1.5 mL answer is logical because the 120 mg ordered is larger than the 80 mg per mL dosage strength available.

▶▶▶ PROBLEMS 12.5

Calculate these dosages. Express answers to the nearest tenth. Assess answers to determine if they are logical.

1. A dosage of 24 mg has been ordered. The solution strength available is 12.5 mg in 1.5 mL.   _____

2. A 40 mg in 2.5 mL solution will be used to prepare a 30 mg dosage.   _____

3. Prepare 0.3 mg from a solution strength of 0.6 mg in 0.8 mL.   _____

4. A 36 mg per 2 mL strength solution is used to prepare 24 mg.   _____

5. A dosage of 52 mg is to be prepared from a 78 mg in 0.9 mL solution.   _____

6. A dosage of 150 mg has been ordered. The solution strength is 100 mg per mL.   _____

7. A strength of 3 mL containing 750 mcg is available to prepare 600 mcg.   _____

8. If the strength available is 1.5 g per mL, how many mL will a 4 g dosage require?   _____

9. Prepare a 0.25 mg dosage from a 0.5 mg per 1 mL strength solution.   _____

10. Prepare a 3 g dosage from a 4 g in 2.7 mL strength solution.   _____

Answers 1. 2.9 mL **2.** 1.9 mL **3.** 0.4 mL **4.** 1.3 mL **5.** 0.6 mL **6.** 1.5 mL **7.** 2.4 mL **8.** 2.7 mL **9.** 0.5 mL
10. 2 mL

Note: If you did not include the units of measure, your answers are incorrect.

CALCULATIONS WHEN DOSAGES ARE IN DIFFERENT UNITS OF MEASURE

Consider the following dosage calculations. Refer to the ratio and proportion format you chose earlier.

EXAMPLE 1   The order is to give **0.15 g** of medication. The dosage strength available is **200 mg per mL**.

This problem cannot be solved as it is now written because **the dosages are in different units of measure: g and mg.** You learned that it may be safer to convert from larger to smaller units of measure to eliminate/avoid decimal points. **Convert the g to mg.**

As a common fraction		Separated by a colon
$\dfrac{200 \text{ mg}}{1 \text{ mL}} = \dfrac{0.15 \text{ g}}{X \text{ mL}}$	or	$200 \text{ mg} : 1 \text{ mL} = \textbf{0.15 g} : X \text{ mL}$
$\dfrac{200 \text{ mg}}{1 \text{ mL}} = \dfrac{\textbf{150 mg}}{X \text{ mL}}$	or	$200 \text{ mg} : 1 \text{ mL} = \textbf{150 mg} : X \text{ mL}$
$200X = 1 \times 150$		$200X = 1 \times 150$

$$X = \frac{150}{200} = 0.75$$ $$X = \frac{150}{200} = 0.75$$

$$= \textbf{0.8 mL}$$ $$= \textbf{0.8 mL}$$

150 mg is a smaller dosage than 200 mg, so it must be contained in a smaller volume than 1 mL. The answer, 0.8 mL, is logical.

EXAMPLE 2   You have a dosage strength of **200 mcg per mL**. The order is to give **0.5 mg**.

$$\frac{200 \text{ mcg}}{1 \text{ mL}} = \frac{\textbf{0.5 mg}}{X \text{ mL}}$$ **or** $200 \text{ mcg} : 1 \text{ mL} = \textbf{0.5 mg} : X \text{ mL}$

$$\frac{200 \text{ mcg}}{1 \text{ mL}} = \frac{\textbf{500 mcg}}{X \text{ mL}}$$ **or** $200 \text{ mcg} : 1 \text{ mL} = \textbf{500 mcg} : X \text{ mL}$

$$200X = 500$$ $$200X = 500$$

$$X = \textbf{2.5 mL}$$ $$X = \textbf{2.5 mL}$$

500 mcg is a larger quantity than 200 mcg, so it must be contained in a larger quantity than 1 mL. The answer, 2.5 mL, is logical.

Ratio and proportion is also used to solve calculations for **unit and mEq dosages**.

EXAMPLE 3   The order is to give **1200 units**. The available dosage strength is **1000 units per 1.5 mL**.

$$\frac{1000 \text{ units}}{1.5 \text{ mL}} = \frac{1200 \text{ units}}{X \text{ mL}}$$ **or** $1000 \text{ units} : 1.5 \text{ mL} = 1200 \text{ units} : X \text{ mL}$

$$1000X = 1.5 \times 1200$$ $$1000X = 1.5 \times 1200$$

$$X = \frac{1.5 \times 1200}{1000}$$ $$X = \frac{1.5 \times 1200}{1000}$$

$$= \textbf{1.8 mL}$$ $$= \textbf{1.8 mL}$$

1200 units is a larger dosage than 1000 units, so the answer in mL should be larger than 1.5 mL, which it is.

EXAMPLE 4   A drug has a dosage strength of **2 mEq per mL**. You are to give **10 mEq**.

$$\frac{2 \text{ mEq}}{1 \text{ mL}} = \frac{10 \text{ mEq}}{X \text{ mL}}$$ **or** $2 \text{ mEq} : 1 \text{ mL} = 10 \text{ mEq} : X \text{ mL}$

$$2X = 10$$ $$2X = 10$$

$$X = \textbf{5 mL}$$ $$X = \textbf{5 mL}$$

10 mEq is considerably larger than 2 mEq, so the answer should also be significantly larger, and it is.

▶▶▶ PROBLEMS 12.6

Solve these dosage problems. Express answers to the nearest tenth.

1. The drug label reads 1000 mcg in 2 mL. The order is 0.4 mg. _____

2. The ordered dosage is 275 mg. The available drug
   is labeled 0.5 g per 2 mL. _____

3. A dosage strength of 0.2 mg in 1.5 mL is available. Give 0.15 mg. _____

4. The strength available is 1 g in 3.6 mL. Prepare a 600 mg dosage. _____

5. A 10,000 units dosage has been ordered. The dosage strength
   available is 8000 units in 1 mL. _____

6. The dosage available is 20 mEq per 20 mL. You are
   to prepare 15 mEq. _____

7. The order is for 200,000 units. The strength available is
   150,000 units per 2 mL. _____

Answers   1. 0.8 mL   **2.** 1.1 mL   **3.** 1.1 mL   **4.** 2.2 mL   **5.** 1.3 mL   **6.** 15 mL   **7.** 2.7 mL

Summary

This concludes the introductory chapter on ratio and proportion and its uses in dosage calculations. The important points to remember from this chapter are:

▽ A ratio is composed of two numbers that have a significant relationship to each other.

▽ In medication dosages, ratios are used to express the amount of drug contained in a tablet or capsule, or in a certain volume of solution.

▽ A proportion consists of two ratios with a significant relationship to each other.

▽ If one number in a proportion is missing, it can be determined mathematically by solving an equation to determine the value of X.

▽ The available dosage strength provides the complete or known ratio for calculations.

▽ The dosage to be given provides the incomplete or unknown ratio.

▽ Ratios in a proportion are set up in the same sequence of measurement units; for example, mg, mL and mg, mL.

▽ If the measurement units in a calculation are different—for example, mg and g—one of these must be converted before the problem can be solved.

▽ It may be safer to convert from larger to smaller metric units of measure to eliminate decimal points.

▽ The math of calculations is double checked, and the answer is assessed to determine if X is appropriately larger or smaller than the dosage strength available.

Summary Self-Test

Calculate these dosages using ratio and proportion. Express mL answers to the nearest tenth (or hundredth where indicated) using the medication labels provided. Measure the dosages you calculate on the syringes provided. Have your answers checked by your instructor to be sure you have calculated and measured the dosages correctly.

Dosage Ordered   **mL Needed**

1. terbutaline sulfate 800 mcg   _____

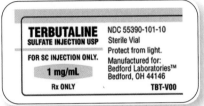

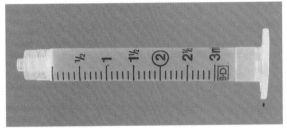

2. furosemide 15 mg   _____

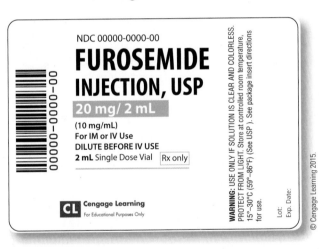

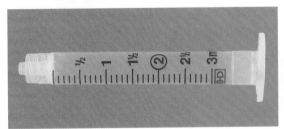

3. Vistaril® 70 mg   _____

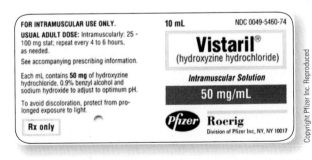

Dosage Ordered

mL Needed

4. fentanyl citrate 0.15 mg

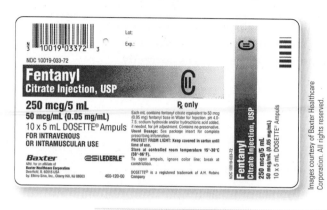

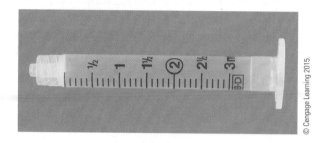

5. naloxone 350 mcg

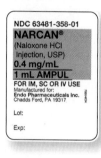

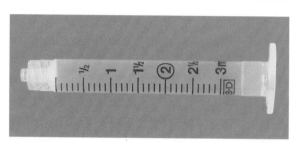

6. clindamycin 225 mg

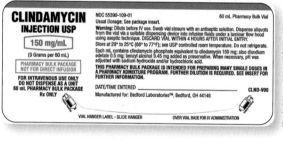

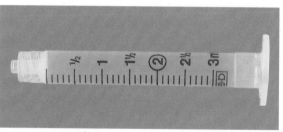

7. Robinul® 75 mcg (calculate to the nearest hundredth)

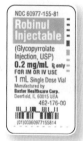

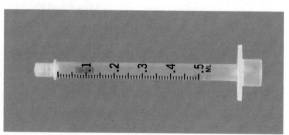

Dosage Ordered

mL Needed

8. midazolam HCI 4 mg _____

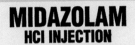
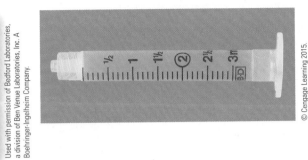

MIDAZOLAM
HCI INJECTION

NDC 55390-126-05   5 mL vial

USUAL DOSAGE: See package insert.

Store at controlled room temperature
15° to 30°C (59° to 86°F).

DISCARD UNUSED PORTION.

25 mg/5 mL*   C IV

*Midazolam 5 mg/mL (as the hydrochloride)

FOR IM OR IV USE ONLY

Contains Benzyl Alcohol   Rx ONLY

Mfg by: Ben Venue Labs, Inc.
Bedford, OH 44146

Mfg for: Bedford Laboratories™
Bedford, OH 44146

KC-MDZ-VB02

Used with permission of Bedford Laboratories, a division of Ben Venue Laboratories, Inc. A Boehringer-Ingelheim Company.

© Cengage Learning 2015.

9. Inapsine® 3 mg _____

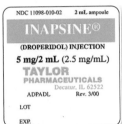
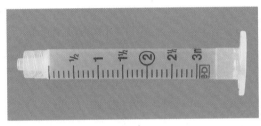

NDC 11098-010-02   2 mL ampoule

INAPSINE®

(DROPERIDOL) INJECTION

5 mg/2 mL (2.5 mg/mL)

TAYLOR
PHARMACEUTICALS
Decatur, IL 62522

ADPADL   Rev. 3/00

LOT

EXP.

Used with permission from Akorn Inc. and Taylor Pharmaceuticals.

© Cengage Learning 2015.

10. cyanocobalamin 800 mcg _____

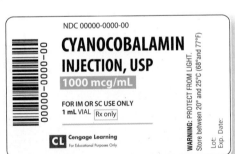

NDC 00000-0000-00

CYANOCOBALAMIN

INJECTION, USP

1000 mcg/mL

FOR IM OR SC USE ONLY

1 mL VIAL   Rx only

CL Cengage Learning
For Educational Purposes Only

WARNING: PROTECT FROM LIGHT.
Store between 20° and 25°C (68° and 77°F)

Lot:
Exp. Date:

© Cengage Learning 2015.

11. potassium acetate 16 mEq for IV additive _____

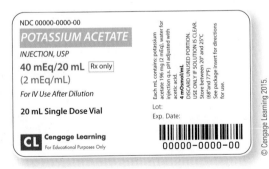
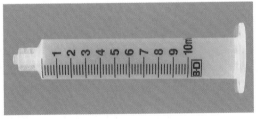

NDC 00000-0000-00

POTASSIUM ACETATE

INJECTION, USP

40 mEq/20 mL   Rx only

(2 mEq/mL)

For IV Use After Dilution

20 mL Single Dose Vial

CL Cengage Learning
For Educational Purposes Only

Each mL contains: potassium acetate 196 mg (2 mEq), water for injection q.s. pH adjusted with acetic acid.
4 mOsmol/mL.
DISCARD UNUSED PORTION.
USE ONLY IF SOLUTION IS CLEAR.
Store between 20° and 25°C (68° and 77°F)
See package insert for directions for use.

Lot:
Exp. Date:

00000-0000-00

© Cengage Learning 2015.

SECTION 4

Dosage Ordered

mL Needed

12. calcium gluconate 0.93 mEq for an IV additive

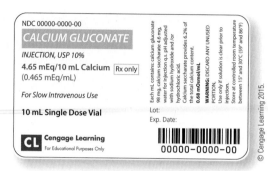

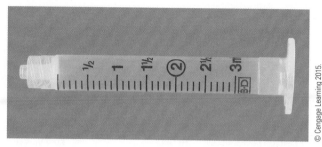

13. morphine sulfate 1.5 mg

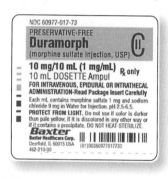

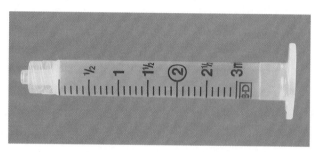

14. heparin sodium 450 units (calculate to the nearest hundredth)

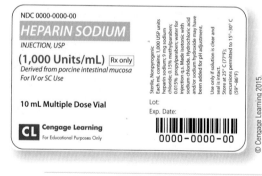

15. droperidol 4 mg

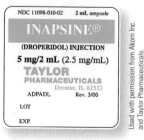

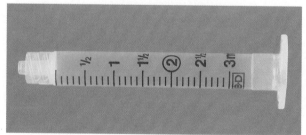

Dosage Ordered   **mL Needed**

16. Dilantin® 0.1 g

_____

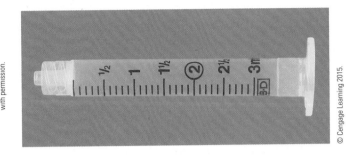

17. medroxyprogesterone 0.9 g

_____

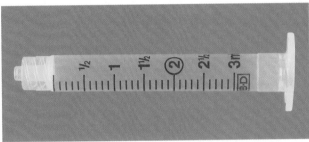

18. Ativan 7 mg

_____

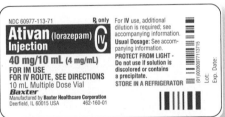

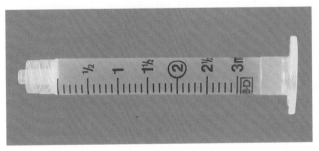

Dosage Ordered   **mL Needed**

19. Vistaril® 120 mg   _____

FOR INTRAMUSCULAR USE ONLY.

USUAL ADULT DOSE: Intramuscularly: 25 - 100 mg stat; repeat every 4 to 6 hours, as needed.

See accompanying prescribing information.

Each mL contains **50 mg** of hydroxyzine hydrochloride, 0.9% benzyl alcohol and sodium hydroxide to adjust to optimum pH.

To avoid discoloration, protect from prolonged exposure to light.

Rx only

10 mL   NDC 0049-5460-74

Vistaril®
(hydroxyzine hydrochloride)

Intramuscular Solution

50 mg/mL

Pfizer Roerig
Division of Pfizer Inc, NY, NY 10017

Store below 86°F (30°C).
PROTECT FROM FREEZING.

PATIENT: _____

ROOM NO.: _____

05-1111-32-4
MADE IN USA   **9249**

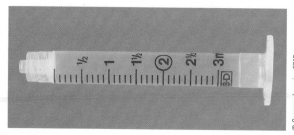

20. sodium chloride 60 mEq for an IV additive   _____

NDC 0000-0000-00

SODIUM CHLORIDE

INJECTION, USP

CONCENTRATED

PHARMACY BULK PACKAGE– Not for direct infusion

23.4% 4 mEq/mL
FOR IV USE ONLY
AFTER DILUTION

100 mL
Multiple Dose Vial   **Rx only**

CL Cengage Learning
For Educational Purposes Only

0000-0000-00

Preservative Free

Each mL contains: sodium chloride 234 mg; water for injection q.s. pH may have been adjusted with hydrochloric acid. 8008 mOsmol/L 4,000 mEq/L
Directions for pharmacy bulk package: Swab stopper with an antiseptic solution. Withdraw contents of the vial using a sterile dispensing set. If prompt fluid transfer is not possible, a maximum time of 4 hours from the time of initial entry is allowed to complete the transferring operations. Discard the container no later than 4 hours after initial closure.

Use only if solution is clear and seal is intact.
Store at controlled room temperature
15° to 30°C (59°–86°F). Do not freeze.

Lot:
Exp. Date:

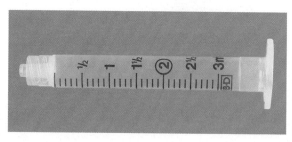

21. atropine sulfate 150 mcg   _____

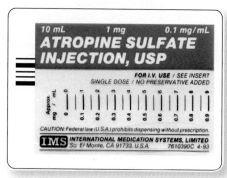

10 mL   1 mg   0.1 mg/mL

ATROPINE SULFATE INJECTION, USP

FOR I.V. USE / SEE INSERT
SINGLE DOSE / NO PRESERVATIVE ADDED

Approx. mg / mL
0 0.1 0.2 0.3 0.4 0.5 0.6 0.7 0.8 0.9

CAUTION: Federal law (U.S.A.) prohibits dispensing without prescription.

IMS INTERNATIONAL MEDICATION SYSTEMS, LIMITED
So. El Monte, CA 91733, U.S.A.   7610390C 4-93

22. meperidine 75 mg   _____

NDC 10019-162-44

Meperidine
HCl Injection, USP

100 mg/mL
1 mL
DOSETTE Vial   Rx only
FOR IM, SC OR SLOW IV USE
DO NOT USE
IF PRECIPITATED
Baxter Healthcare Corp.
Deerfield, IL 60015 USA

462 - 083 - 00

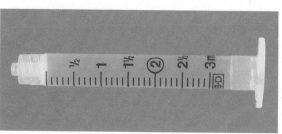

Dosage Ordered

mL Needed

23. fentanyl citrate 80 mcg

_____

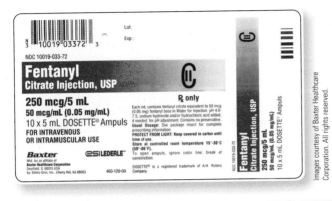

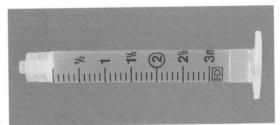

24. antibiotic solution 10 mg

_____

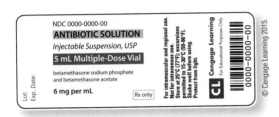

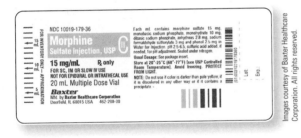

25. morphine sulfate 20 mg

_____

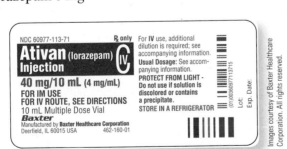

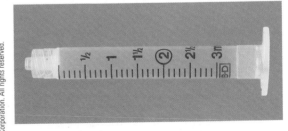

26. lorazepam 6 mg

_____

Dosage Ordered

mL Needed

27. Dilantin® 0.15 g

_____

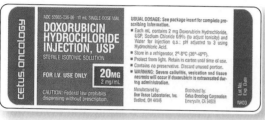

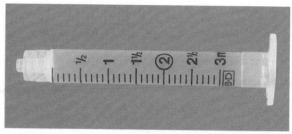

28. doxorubicin HCl 16 mg for an IV additive

_____

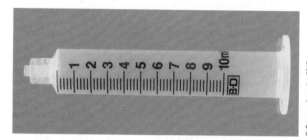

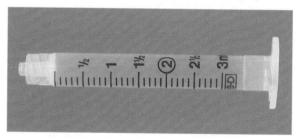

29. meperidine HCl 30 mg

_____

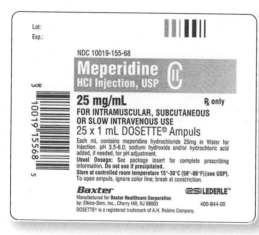

30. methotrexate 40 mg

_____

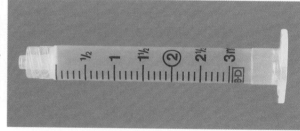

Dosage Ordered   **mL Needed**

31. midazolam HCl 3 mg   _____

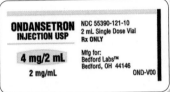

NDC 55390-126-05   5 mL vial
USUAL DOSAGE: See package insert.
Store at controlled room temperature
15° to 30°C (59° to 86°F).
DISCARD UNUSED PORTION.
Mfg by: Ben Venue Labs, Inc.
Bedford, OH 44146
Mfg for: Bedford Laboratories™
Bedford, OH 44146
KC-MDZ-VB02

MIDAZOLAM
HCl INJECTION

25 mg/5 mL* **C**ɪᵥ

*Midazolam 5 mg/mL (as the hydrochloride)
FOR IM OR IV USE ONLY
Contains Benzyl Alcohol   Rx ONLY

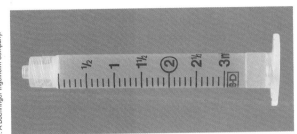

32. ondansetron 3 mg   _____

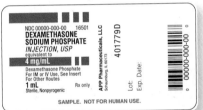

ONDANSETRON
INJECTION USP

NDC 55390-121-10
2 mL Single Dose Vial
Rx ONLY

4 mg/2 mL

2 mg/mL

Mfg for:
Bedford Labs™
Bedford, OH 44146
OND-V00

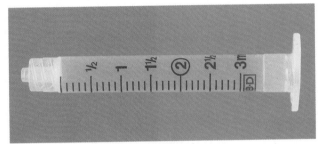

33. dexamethasone 5 mg   _____

NDC 00000-000-00   16501
DEXAMETHASONE
SODIUM PHOSPHATE
INJECTION, USP
equivalent to
4 mg/mL
Dexamethasone Phosphate
For IM or IV Use, See Insert
For Other Routes
1 mL   Rx only
Sterile, Nonpyrogenic

APP Pharmaceuticals, LLC
Schaumburg, IL 60173

401779D

Lot:
Exp. Date:

0 00000-000-00

SAMPLE. NOT FOR HUMAN USE.

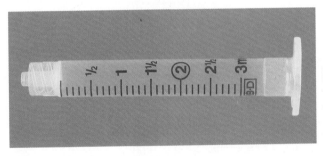

34. hydroxyzine HCl 40 mg   _____

FOR INTRAMUSCULAR USE ONLY
USUAL ADULT DOSE: Intramuscularly: 25 -
100 mg stat; repeat every 4 to 6 hours, as
needed. See accompanying prescribing
information.
Each mL contains **25 mg** of hydroxyzine
hydrochloride, 0.9% benzyl alcohol and
sodium hydroxide to adjust to optimum pH.
To avoid discoloration, protect from prolonged exposure to light.
CAUTION: Federal law prohibits
dispensing without prescription.

10 mL   NDC 0049-5450-74

Vistaril®
(hydroxyzine hydrochloride)

Intramuscular Solution
25 mg/mL

Pfizer **Roerig**
Division of Pfizer Inc, NY, NY 10017

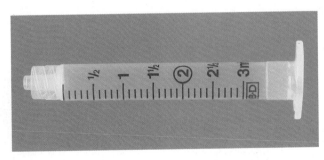

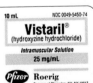
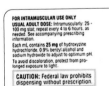

Dosage Ordered   **mL Needed**

35. ketorolac tromethamine 20 mg

_____

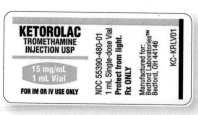

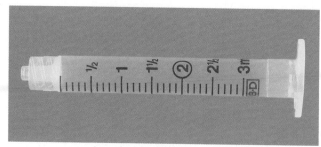

36. nalbuphine HCl 30 mg

_____

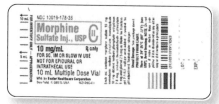

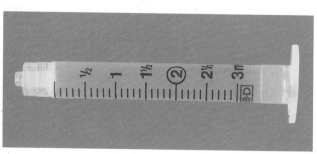

37. morphine 15 mg

_____

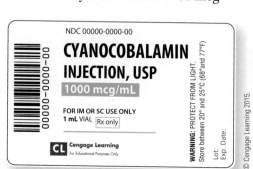

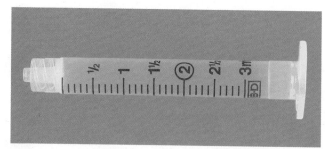

38. cyanocobalamin 750 mcg

_____

NDC 00000-0000-00

CYANOCOBALAMIN

INJECTION, USP

1000 mcg/mL

FOR IM OR SC USE ONLY
1 mL VIAL Rx only

CL Cengage Learning
For Educational Purposes Only

WARNING: PROTECT FROM LIGHT.
Store between 20° and 25°C (68° and 77°F).

Lot:
Exp. Date:

Dosage Ordered

mL Needed

39. aminophylline 0.4 g for an IV additive

_____

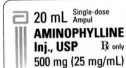

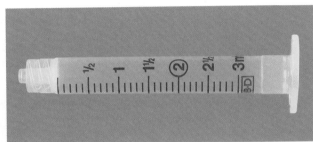

40. Dilantin® 125 mg

_____

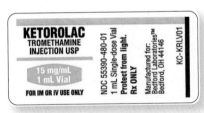

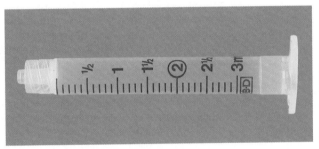

41. ketorolac 25 mg

_____

42. Vistaril® 50 mg

_____

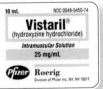

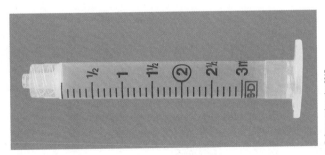

Dosage Ordered   **mL Needed**

43. Ativan 10 mg

_____

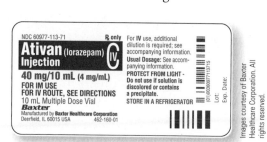

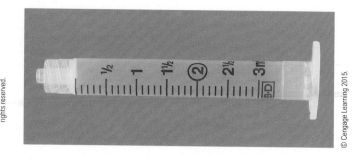

44. Robinul® 180 mcg

_____

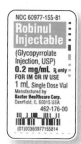

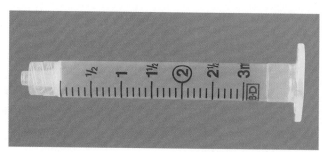

45. hydroxyzine HCl 70 mg

_____

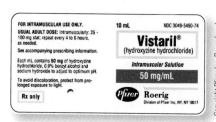

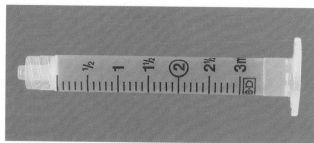

46. penicillin 400,000 units

_____

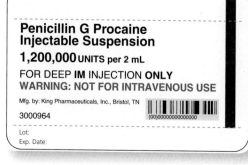

Penicillin G Procaine Injectable Suspension
1,200,000 UNITS per 2 mL
FOR DEEP IM INJECTION ONLY
WARNING: NOT FOR INTRAVENOUS USE
Mfg. by: King Pharmaceuticals, Inc., Bristol, TN
3000964
Lot:
Exp. Date:

Dosage Ordered

mL Needed

47. heparin sodium 1500 units (calculate to the nearest hundredth) _____

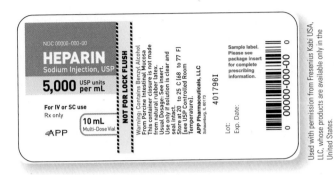

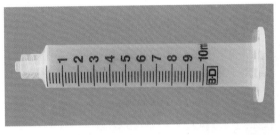

48. potassium chloride 20 mEq for an IV additive _____

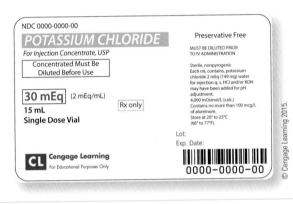

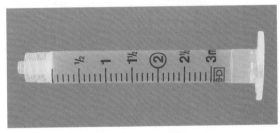

49. Inapsine® 4.5 mg _____

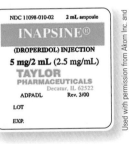

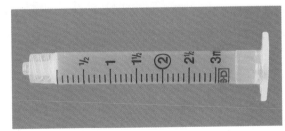

50. epinephrine 1.4 mg _____

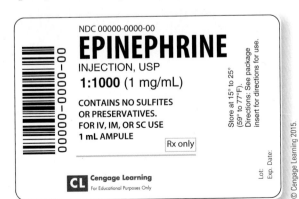

Dosage Ordered

mL Needed

51. Nubain® 15 mg

_____

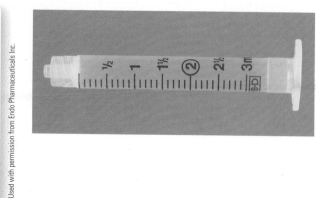

NDC 63481-509-05

NUBAIN®
(Nalbuphine HCl) **Rₓ only**
20 mg/mL injection

10 mL Multiple Dose Vial

Each mL contains: 20 mg nalbuphine HCl, 0.94% sodium citrate hydrous, 1.26% citric acid anhydrous, and 0.2% of a 9:1 mixture of methyl and propylparaben, as preservatives. pH is adjusted, if necessary, to 3.5 to 3.7 with hydrochloric acid.

FOR IM, SC OR IV USE
Usual Dosage: See package insert for complete prescribing information.
Store at 25°C (77°F); excursions permitted to 15°-30°C (59°-86°F).
PROTECT FROM EXCESSIVE LIGHT.

Manufactured for:
Endo Pharmaceuticals Inc.
Chadds Ford, PA 19317

Used with permission from Endo Pharmaceuticals Inc.

© Cengage Learning 2015.

52. furosemide 15 mg

_____

NDC 00000-0000-00

FUROSEMIDE
INJECTION, USP

20 mg/ 2 mL

(10 mg/mL)
For IM or IV Use
DILUTE BEFORE IV USE
2 mL Single Dose Vial Rx only

CL Cengage Learning
For Educational Purposes Only

WARNING: USE ONLY IF SOLUTION IS CLEAR AND COLORLESS. PROTECT FROM LIGHT. Store at controlled room temperature, 15°-30°C (59°-86°F) (See USP). See package insert directions for use.

Lot:
Exp. Date:

© Cengage Learning 2015.

© Cengage Learning 2015.

53. dexamethasone 6000 mcg

_____

NDC 00000-000-00 16501

DEXAMETHASONE
SODIUM PHOSPHATE
INJECTION, USP
equivalent to
4 mg/mL
Dexamethasone Phosphate
For IM or IV Use, See Insert
For Other Routes
1 mL
Sterile, Nonpyrogenic

APP Pharmaceuticals, LLC
Schaumburg, IL 60173

401779D

Rx only

Lot:
Exp. Date:

SAMPLE. NOT FOR HUMAN USE.

Used with permission from Fresenius Kabi USA, LLC, whose products are available only in the United States.

© Cengage Learning 2015.

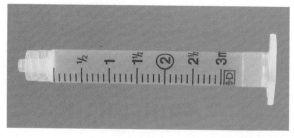

Dosage Ordered

mL Needed

54. phenytoin Na 75 mg

_____

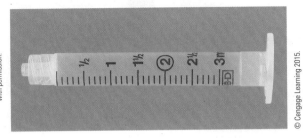

55. lidocaine HCl 15 mg

_____

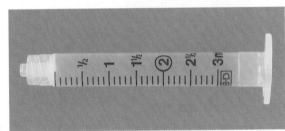

Answers				
1. 0.8 mL	**12.** 2 mL	**24.** 1.7 mL	**36.** 1.5 mL	**48.** 10 mL
2. 1.5 mL	**13.** 1.5 mL	**25.** 1.3 mL	**37.** 1.5 mL	**49.** 1.8 mL
3. 1.4 mL	**14.** 0.45 mL	**26.** 1.5 mL	**38.** 0.8 mL	**50.** 1.4 mL
4. 3 mL	**15.** 1.6 mL	**27.** 3 mL	**39.** 16 mL	**51.** 0.8 mL
5. 0.9 mL	**16.** 2 mL	**28.** 8 mL	**40.** 2.5 mL	**52.** 1.5 mL
6. 1.5 mL	**17.** 2.3 mL	**29.** 1.2 mL	**41.** 1.7 mL	**53.** 1.5 mL
7. 0.38 mL	**18.** 1.8 mL	**30.** 1.6 mL	**42.** 2 mL	**54.** 1.5 mL
8. 0.8 mL	**19.** 2.4 mL	**31.** 0.6 mL	**43.** 2.5 mL	**55.** 0.8 mL
9. 1.2 mL	**20.** 15 mL	**32.** 1.5 mL	**44.** 0.9 mL	
10. 0.8 mL	**21.** 1.5 mL	**33.** 1.3 mL	**45.** 1.4 mL	
11. 8 mL	**22.** 0.8 mL	**34.** 1.6 mL	**46.** 0.7 mL	
	23. 1.6 mL	**35.** 1.3 mL	**47.** 0.3 mL	

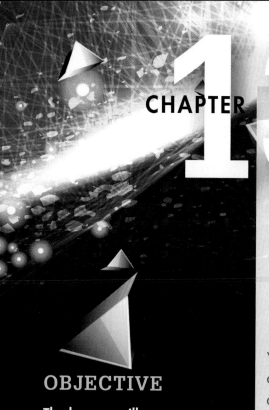

13

DIMENSIONAL ANALYSIS/UNITS CONVERSION

OBJECTIVE

The learner will:

1. use dimensional analysis to calculate dosages.

PREREQUISITES

Chapters 1–10

You may already be familiar with dimensional analysis (DA) under its official name: **units conversion**, which is used in chemistry, physics, and other scientific calculations. DA was first introduced for dosage calculations in the 1950s using the name dimensional analysis, but it has had several other names along the way: the label factor and factor label methods being two.

DA is actually ratio and proportion made simple. Its great virtue is that **it reduces multiple-step calculations to a single equation.** However, to understand the simplicity of DA, it is necessary to look at clinical ratios from a different perspective.

CLINICAL RATIOS

Clinical ratios provide the components for **all** the calculations you have already learned and will be learning in the remainder of this text. Some examples of ratios you are already familiar with from previous chapters include the following:

> **oral dosages:** 1 tab = 250 mg; 5 mL = 125 mg
> **IM and subcutaneous dosages:** 2 g = 1.5 mL;
> 1 mL = 10 units; 10 mL = 20 mEq
> **metric conversions:** 1000 mcg = 1 mg; 1 g = 1000 mg

In addition, you will be using the following ratios, although it isn't necessary for you to memorize them at this time.

> **IV flow rates:** 80 gtt per min; 100 mL per hr
> **IV set calibrations:** 10 gtt per mL; 15 gtt per mL; 60 gtt per mL
> **time conversions:** 60 min = 1 hr; 1 hr = 60 min

In DA, ratios are written as common fractions.

$$\frac{1 \text{ tab}}{250 \text{ mg}} \qquad \frac{125 \text{ mg}}{5 \text{ mL}} \qquad \frac{2 \text{ g}}{1.5 \text{ mL}}$$

$$\frac{10 \text{ units}}{1 \text{ mL}} \qquad \frac{20 \text{ mEq}}{10 \text{ mL}} \qquad \frac{1000 \text{ mcg}}{1 \text{ mg}}$$

THE BASIC DA EQUATION

The first step in setting up a DA equation is to **write the unit of measure being calculated**. One commonly calculated measure is mL, so let's begin by using a mL calculation to illustrate the steps involved. Notice that color is used in the first DA examples to help you learn the sequence of ratio entry.

EXAMPLE 1 ▪   The available dosage strength is **750 mg in 2.5 mL**. How many mL will be needed to prepare a **600 mg** dosage?

Write the mL unit of measure being calculated, followed by an equal sign.

$$mL =$$

There are two important reasons for identifying the unit of measure being calculated first: It eliminates any confusion over exactly **which** measure is being calculated, and it dictates how the first or "starting" clinical ratio is entered in the equation.

 KEYpoint: In a DA equation, the unit of measure being calculated is written first, followed by an equal sign.

Next, go back to the problem to **identify the complete clinical ratio that contains mL**. This is provided by the **dosage strength available**, which is **750 mg in 2.5 mL**. Enter this as a common fraction so that **the 2.5 mL *numerator* matches the mL unit of measure being calculated; 750 mg** becomes **the *denominator***.

$$mL = \frac{2.5 \ mL}{750 \ mg}$$

 KEYpoint: In a DA equation, the unit of measure being calculated is matched in the numerator of the first clinical ratio entered.

All additional ratios are entered so that **each *denominator* is matched in its successive *numerator*.** The **denominator in the first ratio is mg**, so the **next numerator must be mg**. Go back to the problem to discover that this is provided by the **600 mg** dosage to be given. Enter this now as the next numerator to complete this single-step equation.

$$mL = \frac{2.5 \ mL}{750 \ mg} \times \frac{600 \ mg}{}$$

 KEYpoint: The unit of measure in each denominator of a DA equation is matched in the successive numerator entered.

All the pertinent clinical ratios have now been entered in this one-step DA equation. The next step is to **cancel the alternate denominator/numerator measurement units (but not their quantities) to be sure they match**. This ensures that the clinical ratios were entered correctly. **After cancellation, only the unit of measure being calculated may remain in the equation**. The denominator/numerator mg/mg units cancel, leaving only the mL unit being calculated remaining in the equation.

$$mL = \frac{2.5 \text{ mL}}{750 \text{ m\cancel{g}}} \times \frac{600 \text{ m\cancel{g}}}{}$$

 KEY_point:_ Only the unit of measure being calculated may remain in the equation after the denominator/numerator units of measure are cancelled.

Only the mL being calculated remains in the equation. The math can now be done.

$$mL = \frac{2.5 \text{ mL}}{750 \text{ m\cancel{g}}} \times \frac{600 \text{ m\cancel{g}}}{}$$

$$mL = \frac{2.5 \text{ mL}}{\cancel{750}_{\,5} \text{ m\cancel{g}}} \times \frac{\cancel{600}^{\,4} \text{ m\cancel{g}}}{} \qquad \text{Divide by 150}$$

$$mL = \frac{\cancel{10}^{\,2}}{\cancel{5}_{\,1}} = \textbf{2 mL}$$

To obtain a dosage of 600 mg from an available dosage strength of 750 mg in 2.5 mL, you would give 2 mL.

DA works exactly the same way for every calculation **regardless of the number of ratios entered**. As you can see, there are no complicated rules to memorize. In these simple steps, you have already learned how to use DA for all clinical calculations.

EXAMPLE 2 ▸   A dosage of **50,000 units** is ordered to be added to an IV solution. The strength available is **10,000 units in 1.5 mL**. Calculate how many **mL** will contain this dosage.

Write the mL being calculated to the left of the equation followed by an equal sign.

$$mL =$$

Locate the complete ratio containing mL, the 10,000 units in 1.5 mL dosage strength available. Enter this now, with **1.5 mL as the numerator to match the mL being calculated**; 10,000 units becomes the denominator.

$$mL = \frac{1.5 \text{ mL}}{10,000 \text{ units}}$$

The units denominator must be matched in the next numerator. This is provided by the 50,000 units ordered. Enter this now to complete this one-step equation.

$$mL = \frac{1.5 \text{ mL}}{10,000 \text{ units}} \times \frac{50,000 \text{ units}}{}$$

Cancel the alternate denominator/numerator units/units entries to double-check for correct ratio entry. Only the mL being calculated remains in the equation. Do the math.

$$\text{mL} = \frac{1.5 \ \text{mL}}{10,000 \ \cancel{\text{units}}} \times \frac{50,000 \ \cancel{\text{units}}}{}$$

$$\text{mL} = \frac{15 \ \text{mL}}{\cancel{100,000}_{\,2} \ \text{units}} \times \frac{\cancel{50,000}^{\,1} \ \text{units}}{}$$

Eliminate the decimal point in 1.5, then reduce the numbers as much as possible; divide the final fraction.

$$\text{mL} = \frac{15}{2} = \textbf{7.5 mL}$$

It will require a 7.5 mL volume of the 10,000 units in 1.5 mL solution to prepare the 50,000 units ordered for this IV additive.

EXAMPLE 3   Tablet calculations are not common but would be done the same way using DA.

Scored (breakable) **tablets** with a strength of **0.5 mg** are available to prepare a dosage of **1.25 mg**. How many **tablets** must you give?

Enter the tab being calculated to the left of the equation followed by an equal sign.

$$\text{tab} =$$

The tab unit being calculated is matched by the tab strength available, 0.5 mg in 1 tab. Enter this as the first ratio, with 1 tab as the numerator; 0.5 mg becomes the denominator.

$$\text{tab} = \frac{1 \ \text{tab}}{0.5 \ \text{mg}}$$

The mg denominator must be matched in the next numerator. This is provided by the 1.25 mg ordered. Enter this to complete the equation.

$$\text{tab} = \frac{1 \ \text{tab}}{0.5 \ \text{mg}} \times \frac{1.25 \ \text{mg}}{}$$

Cancel the alternate denominator/numerator mg units of measure to check that you have entered the ratios correctly. Only the tab being calculated remains in the equation. Do the math.

$$\text{tab} = \frac{1 \ \text{tab}}{0.5 \ \cancel{\text{mg}}} \times \frac{1.25 \ \cancel{\text{mg}}}{}$$

$$\text{tab} = \frac{1 \ \text{tab}}{\cancel{50}_{\,2} \ \cancel{\text{mg}}} \times \frac{\cancel{125}^{\,5} \ \cancel{\text{mg}}}{}$$

Eliminate the decimal points. Reduce the numbers.

$$\text{tab} = \frac{5}{2} = \textbf{2.5 tab}$$

To obtain the 1.25 mg dosage ordered, 2½ tab must be given.

Let's stop for a moment now and take a look at what happens if the ratios are incorrectly entered in a DA equation. We'll **assume that the units of measure have not been entered with their quantities** and that the **entries have been mixed up**. The correct equation will be shown alongside for comparison.

EXAMPLE 4   A drug label reads **100 mg per 2 mL**. The medication order is for **130 mg**. How many **mL** must you prepare?

Correct   **Incorrect**

$$\text{mL} = \frac{2 \text{ mL}}{100 \text{ mg}} \times \frac{130 \text{ mg}}{} = \textbf{2.6 mL} \quad \text{mL} = \frac{100}{2} \times \frac{130}{} = \textbf{6500 mL}$$

In the incorrect equation, the starting ratio is upside down, and because the units of measure were not entered with their quantities, there is no way to catch this. The safety step of cancellation to check ratio entry cannot be done. But notice something else: The answer, 6500 mL, is impossible. If the entries in a DA equation are mixed up, the numbers are often so outrageous that you will know instantly that you have made a mistake. **But mistakes are not always this obvious, so stick to the step-by-step calculation rules**. There is a reason for every one of them. Let's look at a few more examples.

EXAMPLE 5   How many **mL** will you draw up to prepare a **1.2 g** dosage if the solution available is labeled **2 g in 3 mL**?

Write the mL unit being calculated to the left of the equation followed by an equal sign. Enter the starting ratio, 2 g in 3 mL, with 3 mL as the numerator to match the mL being calculated; 2 g becomes the denominator.

$$\text{mL} = \frac{3 \text{ mL}}{2 \text{ g}}$$

Match the g denominator in the next numerator with the 1.2 g ordered to complete the equation.

$$\text{mL} = \frac{3 \text{ mL}}{2 \text{ g}} \times \frac{1.2 \text{ g}}{}$$

Cancel the alternate denominator/numerator g units of measure to double-check that the entries are correct. Only the mL being calculated remains.

$$\text{mL} = \frac{3 \text{ mL}}{2 \cancel{\text{ g}}} \times \frac{1.2 \cancel{\text{ g}}}{}$$

Do the math, expressing fractional answers to the nearest tenth.

$$\text{mL} = \frac{3 \text{ mL}}{2 \cancel{\text{ g}}} \times \frac{1.2 \cancel{\text{ g}}}{} = \textbf{1.8 mL}$$

The 1.2 g dosage ordered is contained in 1.8 mL of the 2 g in 3 mL solution available.

EXAMPLE 6   Medication with a strength of **0.75 mg per mL** is available to prepare a dosage of **2 mg**. Calculate the mL this will require.

Write the mL being calculated to the left of the equation followed by an equal sign.

$$\text{mL} =$$

The mL being calculated is provided for the first ratio by the 0.75 mg per mL dosage strength available. Enter 1 mL as the numerator and 0.75 mg as the denominator.

$$mL = \frac{1 \text{ mL}}{0.75 \text{ mg}}$$

The mg denominator must now be matched. This is provided by the 2 mg dosage ordered. Enter this now to complete this one-step equation.

$$mL = \frac{1 \text{ mL}}{0.75 \text{ mg}} \times \frac{2 \text{ mg}}{}$$

Cancel the alternate denominator/numerator mg units of measure to check for correct ratio entry, then do the math.

$$mL = \frac{1 \text{ mL}}{0.75 \text{ mg}} \times \frac{2 \text{ mg}}{} = 2.67 = \textbf{2.7 mL}$$

It will require 2.7 mL of the 0.75 mg in 1 mL dosage available to administer the 2 mg ordered.

▶▶▶ PROBLEMS 13.1

Calculate these dosages using DA. Express mL answers to the nearest tenth.

1. A dosage of 0.3 g has been ordered. The strength available is 0.4 g in 1.5 mL.   _____

2. A dosage strength of 0.8 mg in 2 mL is to be used to prepare a 0.5 mg dosage.   _____

3. Prepare a 1.8 mg dosage from a solution labeled 2 mg in 3 mL.   _____

4. The order is for 1500 mg. You have available a 1200 mg per mL solution.   _____

5. A dosage strength of 0.2 mg in 1.5 mL is available. Give 0.15 mg.   _____

6. The strength available is 1000 mg in 3.6 mL. Prepare a 600 mg dosage.   _____

7. A 10,000 units dosage has been ordered. The strength available is 8000 units in 1 mL.   _____

8. An IV additive has a dosage strength of 20 mEq per 20 mL. A dosage of 15 mEq has been ordered.   _____

9. A 200,000 units dosage must be prepared from a 150,000 units in 2 mL strength.   _____

10. An IV additive order is for 400 mg. The solution available has a strength of 500 mg in 20 mL.   _____

Answers **1.** 1.1 mL **2.** 1.3 mL **3.** 2.7 mL **4.** 1.3 mL **5.** 1.1 mL **6.** 2.2 mL **7.** 1.3 mL **8.** 15 mL
9. 2.7 mL **10.** 16 mL

You now know the basics of using DA in calculations. **But how do you know if the answer you obtain is correct?** The answer to this question is provided by the key points already covered.

- ▶ **If** the unit being calculated is correctly identified to the left of the equation
- ▶ **If** the starting ratio is entered so that its numerator matches the unit of measure being calculated
- ▶ **If** the unit of measure in each denominator is matched in each successively entered numerator
- ▶ **If** the only unit of measure remaining after cancellation is the same as the unit of measure being calculated
- ▶ **If** the quantities have been correctly entered
- ▶ **If** the math has been double-checked and is correct

Then the Answer Will Be Correct.

A tall order? Not really. You are doing a clinical dosage calculation. All you must do is carefully follow each step, and the answer will be correct.

In addition, **don't divorce your previous learning and reasoning from the calculation process.** You already know that **most IM dosages are contained in a 0.5–3 mL volume,** that **IV additives may be contained in larger volumes,** and that **large numbers of tab/cap are unusual** in dosages. **If you get an unreasonable answer to a calculation, you must question it.** In time, you will know the average dosages of all the drugs you give and another safety component will be added to your repertoire, but for now, concentrate on the simple mechanics of calculation you have just been taught. Don't shortcut these steps, and you'll do just fine.

EQUATIONS REQUIRING METRIC CONVERSIONS

The major advantage of DA is that it allows multiple ratios to be entered in a single equation. This is especially useful when a drug is ordered in one unit of measure—for example, mg—but is labeled in another—for example, g or mcg.

There are two ways to handle a conversion. Sometimes, it will be easier to do the conversion before setting up the equation. In other instances, you may elect to incorporate the conversion into an equation. For practice purposes, let's look at how **conversion ratios**—for example, **1 g = 1000 mg** or **1 mg = 1000 mcg**—are entered in a DA equation.

EXAMPLE 1   The IM dosage ordered is **275 mg**. The drug available is labeled **0.5 g per 2 mL**. How many **mL** must you give?

Enter the mL to be calculated to the left of the equation. Locate the ratio containing mL, the 0.5 g per 2 mL dosage strength, and enter it, with 2 mL as the numerator; 0.5 g becomes the denominator.

$$\text{mL} = \frac{2 \text{ mL}}{0.5 \text{ g}}$$

When you refer back to the problem, you will not find a g measure to match the starting ratio g denominator. The dosage to be given is in mg. So, a **conversion ratio between g and mg** is needed: 1 g = 1000 mg. Enter this now, with **1 g as the numerator to match the g of the previous denominator**; 1000 mg becomes the new denominator.

$$\text{mL} = \frac{2 \text{ mL}}{0.5 \text{ g}} \times \frac{1 \text{ g}}{1000 \text{ mg}}$$

The final entry, the 275 mg dosage to be given, will automatically fall into its correct position as it is entered as the final numerator to match the mg of the previous denominator. The equation is now complete.

$$mL = \frac{2\ mL}{0.5\ g} \times \frac{1\ g}{1000\ mg} \times \frac{275\ mg}{}$$

Cancel the alternate denominator/numerator g/g and mg/mg units of measure to double-check the ratio entry. Only the mL being calculated remains. Do the math.

$$mL = \frac{2\ mL}{0.5\ \cancel{g}} \times \frac{1\ \cancel{g}}{1000\ \cancel{mg}} \times \frac{275\ \cancel{mg}}{} = \textbf{1.1 mL}$$

To give a dosage of 275 mg, you must prepare 1.1 mL of the 0.5 g in 2 mL strength solution.

EXAMPLE 2   The drug label reads **800 mcg in 1.5 mL**. The IM order is for **0.6 mg**. Enter the mL to be calculated followed by an equal sign to the left of the equation. Locate the ratio containing mL, 800 mcg in 1.5 mL. Enter 1.5 mL as the numerator to match the mL being calculated; 800 mcg becomes the denominator.

$$mL = \frac{1.5\ mL}{800\ mcg}$$

There is no mcg measure in the problem, which is your clue to the necessity for a conversion ratio. Enter the 1000 mcg = 1 mg conversion ratio, with 1000 mcg as the numerator to match the mcg of the previous denominator; 1 mg becomes the denominator.

$$mL = \frac{1.5\ mL}{800\ mcg} \times \frac{1000\ mcg}{1\ mg}$$

The mg denominator is now matched by the 0.6 mg dosage to be given, and completes the equation.

$$mL = \frac{1.5\ mL}{800\ mcg} \times \frac{1000\ mcg}{1\ mg} \times \frac{0.6\ mg}{}$$

Cancel the alternate denominator/numerator mcg/mcg and mg/mg units of measure to check for correct ratio entry. Only the mL being calculated should remain in the equation. Do the math.

$$mL = \frac{1.5\ mL}{800\ \cancel{mcg}} \times \frac{1000\ \cancel{mcg}}{1\ \cancel{mg}} \times \frac{0.6\ \cancel{mg}}{} = 1.12 = \textbf{1.1 mL}$$

To give a dosage of 0.6 mg from the available 1.5 mL per 800 mcg strength, you must prepare 1.1 mL.

EXAMPLE 3   Prepare a **0.5 mg** dosage from an available strength of **200 mcg per mL**. Enter the mL being calculated to the left of the equation followed by an equal sign. Enter the 1 mL in 200 mcg dosage as the starting ratio, with 1 mL as the numerator to match the mL being calculated; 200 mcg becomes the denominator.

$$mL = \frac{1 \text{ mL}}{200 \text{ mcg}}$$

A mcg to mg conversion ratio is needed. Enter 1000 mcg as the numerator to match the mcg in the previous denominator; 1 mg becomes the new denominator.

$$mL = \frac{1 \text{ mL}}{200 \text{ mcg}} \times \frac{1000 \text{ mcg}}{1 \text{ mg}}$$

The mg denominator is now matched by the 0.5 mg dosage ordered to complete the equation.

$$mL = \frac{1 \text{ mL}}{200 \text{ mcg}} \times \frac{1000 \text{ mcg}}{1 \text{ mg}} \times \frac{0.5 \text{ mg}}{}$$

Cancel the alternate mcg/mcg and mg/mg units of measure to double-check for correct ratio entry. Only the mL unit being calculated remains in the equation. Do the math.

$$mL = \frac{1 \text{ mL}}{200 \text{ mcg}} \times \frac{1000 \text{ mcg}}{1 \text{ mg}} \times \frac{0.5 \text{ mg}}{} = \textbf{2.5 mL}$$

A 0.5 mg dosage requires a 2.5 mL volume of the 200 mcg per mL strength solution available.

EXAMPLE 4 The medication has a strength of **0.5 g in 1.5 mL**. Prepare **750 mg**. Enter the mL to be calculated to the left of the equation followed by an equal sign. Enter the starting ratio, the 1.5 mL in 0.5 g dosage available, with 1.5 mL as the numerator, to match the mL being calculated; 0.5 g becomes the denominator.

$$mL = \frac{1.5 \text{ mL}}{0.5 \text{ g}}$$

There is no g dosage in the problem, which signals the need for a conversion ratio. Enter the 1 g = 1000 mg conversion ratio, with 1 g as the numerator, to match the g denominator of the starting ratio; 1000 mg becomes the new denominator.

$$mL = \frac{1.5 \text{ mL}}{0.5 \text{ g}} \times \frac{1 \text{ g}}{1000 \text{ mg}}$$

Enter the dosage ordered, 750 mg, as the final numerator to match the mg in the previous denominator. The equation is complete.

$$mL = \frac{1.5 \text{ mL}}{0.5 \text{ g}} \times \frac{1 \text{ g}}{1000 \text{ mg}} \times \frac{750 \text{ mg}}{}$$

Cancel the alternate g/g and mg/mg units of measure to check the accuracy of ratio entry, then complete the math.

$$mL = \frac{1.5 \text{ mL}}{0.5 \text{ g}} \times \frac{1 \text{ g}}{1000 \text{ mg}} \times \frac{750 \text{ mg}}{} = 2.25 = \textbf{2.3 mL}$$

A 750 mg dosage requires 2.3 mL of the 0.5 g in 1.5 mL medication.

▶▶▶ PROBLEMS 13.2

Calculate these dosages using DA. Express mL answers to the nearest tenth.

1. Prepare 0.1 g of an IM medication from a strength of
   200 mg per mL.   _____

2. A drug label reads 0.1 g in 2 mL. Prepare a 130 mg dosage.   _____

3. An oral solution has a strength of 500 mg in 5 mL. Prepare
   a 0.6 g dosage.   _____

4. Prepare a 0.75 g dosage from a 250 mg per mL strength solution.   _____

5. Prepare 500 mg for IM injection from an available strength of
   1 g per 3 mL.   _____

6. A dosage of 85 mg is ordered, and the drug available is labeled
   0.1 g in 1.5 mL.   _____

7. The strength available is 500 mcg in 1.5 mL. Prepare
   a 0.75 mg dosage.   _____

8. A dosage of 1500 mg has been ordered. The solution available
   is 0.5 g per mL.   _____

9. The dosage strength available is 200 mcg per mL. A 0.5 mg dosage
   has been ordered.   _____

10. The dosage ordered is 0.2 g. Tablets available are labeled 80 mg. _____

> **Answers 1.** 0.5 mL **2.** 2.6 mL **3.** 6 mL **4.** 3 mL **5.** 1.5 mL **6.** 1.3 mL **7.** 2.3 mL **8.** 3 mL
> **9.** 2.5 mL **10.** 2½ tab

Summary

**This ends your introduction to clinical calculations using dimensional analysis. The
important points to remember from this chapter are:**

▽ The unit of measure being calculated is written first to the left of the equation,
   followed by an equal sign.

▽ All ratios entered must include the quantity and the unit of measure.

▽ The numerator in the starting ratio must be in the same measurement unit as the
   unit of measure being calculated.

▽ The unit of measure in each denominator must be matched in the numerator of
   each successive ratio entered.

▽ Metric system conversions can be made by incorporating a conversion ratio
   directly into the DA equation.

▽ The unit of measure in each alternate denominator and numerator must cancel,
   leaving only the unit of measure being calculated remaining in the equation.

▽ The numerator of the starting ratio is never cancelled.

Summary Self-Test

Calculate these dosages using DA. Express mL answers to the nearest tenth (or hundredth where indicated) using the medication labels provided. Measure the dosages you calculate on the syringes provided. Have your answers checked by your instructor to be sure you have calculated and measured the dosages correctly.

Dosage Ordered   **mL Needed**

1. terbutaline sulfate 800 mcg   _____

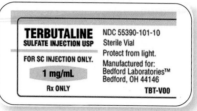

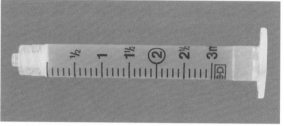

2. furosemide 15 mg   _____

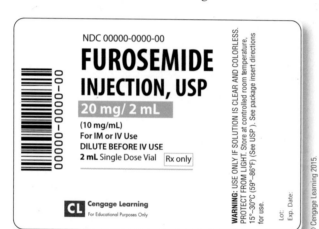

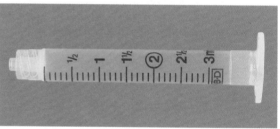

3. Vistaril® 70 mg   _____

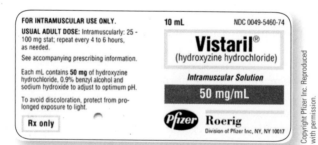

Dosage Ordered   **mL Needed**

4. fentanyl citrate 0.15 mg   _____

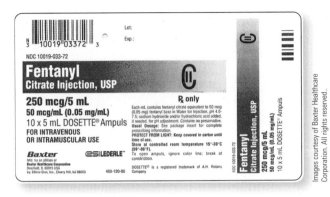

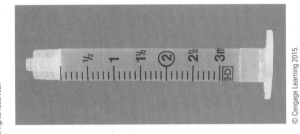

5. naloxone 350 mcg   _____

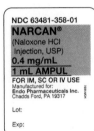

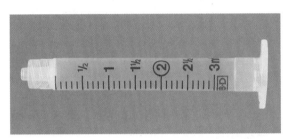

6. clindamycin 225 mg   _____

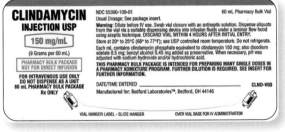

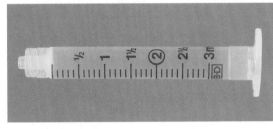

7. Robinul® 75 mcg (calculate to the nearest hundredth)   _____

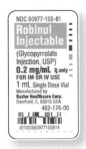

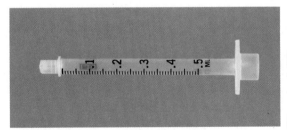

Dosage Ordered

mL Needed

8. midazolam HCl 4 mg

_____

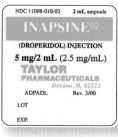
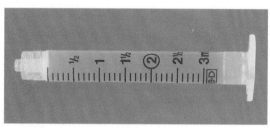

9. Inapsine® 3 mg

_____

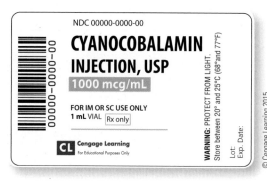
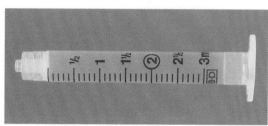

10. cyanocobalamin 800 mcg

_____

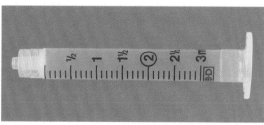

11. potassium acetate 16 mEq for IV additive

_____

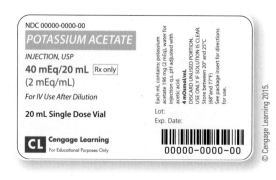

Dosage Ordered

mL Needed

12. calcium gluconate 0.93 mEq for an IV additive   _____

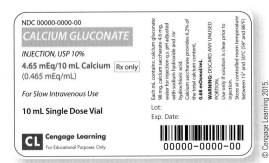

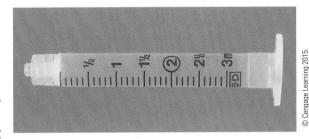

13. morphine sulfate 1.5 mg   _____

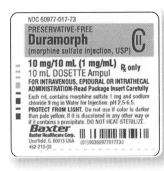

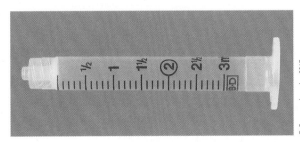

14. heparin sodium 450 units (calculate to the nearest hundredth)   _____

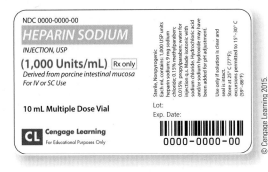

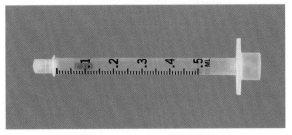

15. droperidol 4 mg   _____

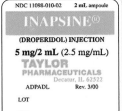

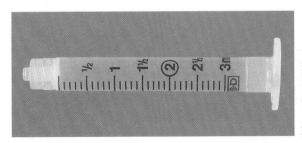

Dosage Ordered   **mL Needed**

16. Dilantin® 0.1 g   _____

Dosage–See package insert.
Rx only
Manufactured by:
Parkedale Pharmaceuticals, Inc.
Rochester, MI 48307
For:
PARKE-DAVIS
Div of Warner-Lambert Co
Morris Plains, NJ 07950 USA

N 0071-4475-45
STERI-VIAL®
Dilantin®
(Phenytoin Sodium
Injection, USP)
ready/mixed
250 mg in 5 mL
5 mL

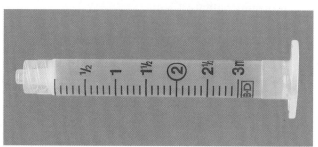

17. medroxyprogesterone 0.9 g   _____

See package insert for complete product information.
Shake vigorously immediately before each use. Store at controlled room temperature 20° to 25°C (68° to 77°F) (see USP).
Each mL contains: Medroxy-progesterone acetate, 400 mg. Also, polyethylene glycol 3350, 20.3 mg; sodium sulfate anhydrous, 11 mg; myristyl-gamma-picolinium chloride, 1.69 mg added as preservative. When necessary, pH was adjusted with sodium hydroxide and/or hydrochloric acid.

Pharmacia & Upjohn Company
Kalamazoo, Michigan 49001, USA

NDC 0009-0626-02   10 mL Vial

Depo-Provera®

medroxyprogesterone
acetate injectable
suspension, USP

400 mg/mL

For intramuscular use only
Rx only

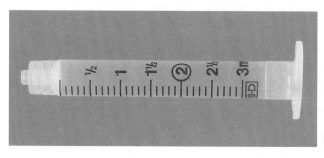

18. Ativan 7 mg   _____

NDC 60977-113-71   Rx only
Ativan (lorazepam) **C IV**
Injection
40 mg/10 mL (4 mg/mL)
FOR IM USE
FOR IV ROUTE, SEE DIRECTIONS
10 mL Multiple Dose Vial
Baxter
Manufactured by **Baxter Healthcare Corporation**
Deerfield, IL 60015 USA   462-160-01

For **IV** use, additional dilution is required; see accompanying information.
Usual Dosage: See accompanying information.
PROTECT FROM LIGHT - Do not use if solution is discolored or contains a precipitate.
STORE IN A REFRIGERATOR
Lot:
Exp. Date:

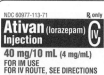

Dosage Ordered

mL Needed

19. Vistaril® 120 mg _____

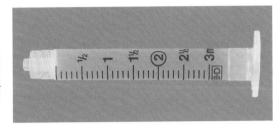

FOR INTRAMUSCULAR USE ONLY.
USUAL ADULT DOSE: Intramuscularly: 25 - 100 mg stat; repeat every 4 to 6 hours, as needed.

See accompanying prescribing information.

Each mL contains **50 mg** of hydroxyzine hydrochloride, 0.9% benzyl alcohol and sodium hydroxide to adjust to optimum pH.

To avoid discoloration, protect from prolonged exposure to light.

Rx only

10 mL   NDC 0049-5460-74

Vistaril®
(hydroxyzine hydrochloride)

Intramuscular Solution

50 mg/mL

Pfizer **Roerig**
Division of Pfizer Inc, NY, NY 10017

Store below 86°F (30°C).
PROTECT FROM FREEZING.

PATIENT: _____

ROOM NO.: _____

05-1111-32-4
MADE IN USA   9249

Copyright Pfizer Inc. Reproduced with permission.

© Cengage Learning 2015.

20. sodium chloride 60 mEq for an IV additive _____

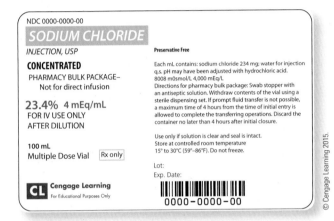

NDC 0000-0000-00

SODIUM CHLORIDE

INJECTION, USP

CONCENTRATED
PHARMACY BULK PACKAGE–
Not for direct infusion

23.4% 4 mEq/mL
FOR IV USE ONLY
AFTER DILUTION

100 mL
Multiple Dose Vial   Rx only

CL Cengage Learning
For Educational Purposes Only

0000-0000-00

Preservative Free

Each mL contains: sodium chloride 234 mg; water for injection q.s. pH may have been adjusted with hydrochloric acid. 8008 mOsmol/L 4,000 mEq/L
Directions for pharmacy bulk package: Swab stopper with an antiseptic solution. Withdraw contents of the vial using a sterile dispensing set. If prompt fluid transfer is not possible, a maximum time of 4 hours from the time of initial entry is allowed to complete the transferring operations. Discard the container no later than 4 hours after initial closure.

Use only if solution is clear and seal is intact.
Store at controlled room temperature
15° to 30°C (59°–86°F). Do not freeze.

Lot:
Exp. Date:

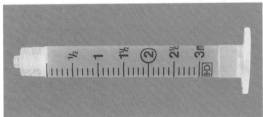

© Cengage Learning 2015.

© Cengage Learning 2015.

21. atropine sulfate 150 mcg _____

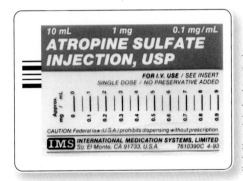

10 mL   1 mg   0.1 mg/mL

**ATROPINE SULFATE
INJECTION, USP**

FOR I.V. USE / SEE INSERT
SINGLE DOSE / NO PRESERVATIVE ADDED

Approx.
mg / mL

CAUTION: Federal law (U.S.A.) prohibits dispensing without prescription.

IMS INTERNATIONAL MEDICATION SYSTEMS, LIMITED
So. El Monte, CA 91733, U.S.A.   7610390C 4-93

Used with permission from International Medication Systems, Limited.

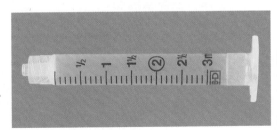

© Cengage Learning 2015.

22. meperidine 75 mg _____

NDC 10019-162-44

Meperidine
HCl Injection, USP

100 mg/mL
1 mL
DOSETTE Vial   Rx only
FOR IM, SC OR SLOW IV USE
DO NOT USE
IF PRECIPITATED
Baxter Healthcare Corp.
Deerfield, IL 60015 USA

462 · 083 · 00

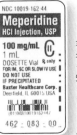

Images courtesy of Baxter Healthcare Corporation. All rights reserved.

© Cengage Learning 2015.

Dosage Ordered   **mL Needed**

23. fentanyl citrate 80 mcg _____

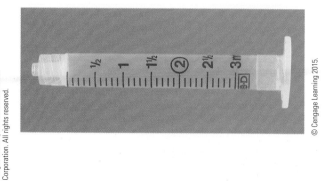

24. antibiotic solution 70 mg _____

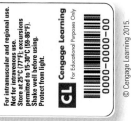

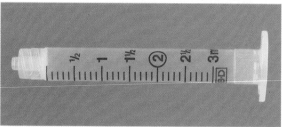

25. morphine sulfate 20 mg _____

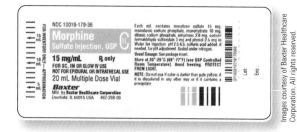

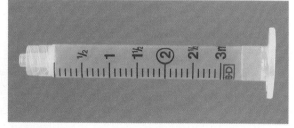

26. lorazepam 6 mg _____

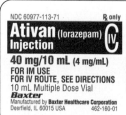

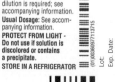

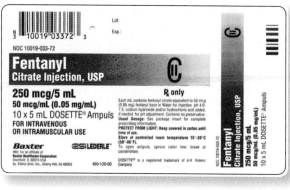

Dosage Ordered

mL Needed

27. Dilantin® 0.15 g

_____

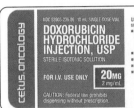

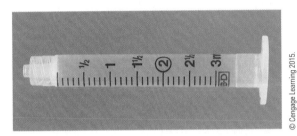

28. doxorubicin HCl 16 mg for an IV additive

_____

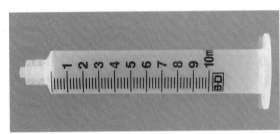

29. meperidine HCl 30 mg

_____

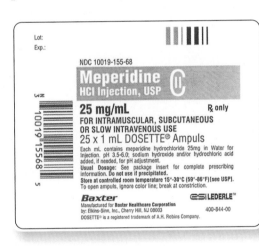

30. methotrexate 40 mg

_____

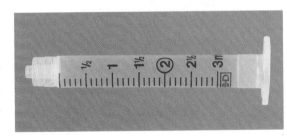

Dosage Ordered   **mL Needed**

31. midazolam HCl 3 mg

_____

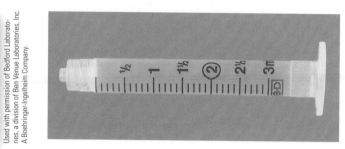

32. ondansetron 3 mg

_____

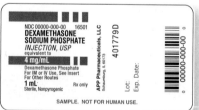

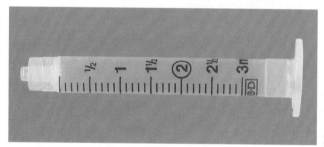

33. dexamethasone 5 mg

_____

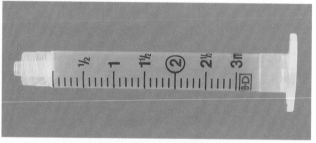

34. hydroxyzine HCl 40 mg

_____

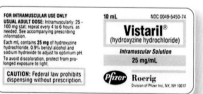

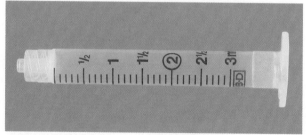

Dosage Ordered   **mL Needed**

35. ketorolac tromethamine 20 mg   _____

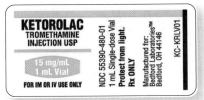

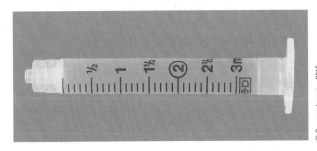

36. nalbuphine HCl 30 mg   _____

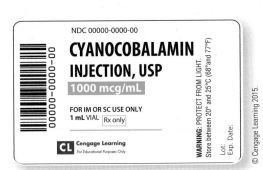

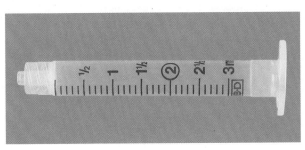

37. morphine 15 mg   _____

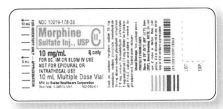

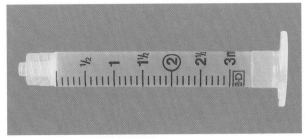

38. cyanocobalamin 750 mcg   _____

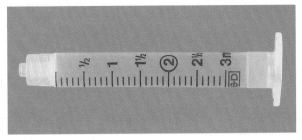

Dosage Ordered   **mL Needed**

39. aminophylline 0.4 g for an IV additive   _____

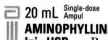

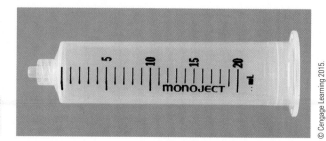

40. Dilantin® 125 mg   _____

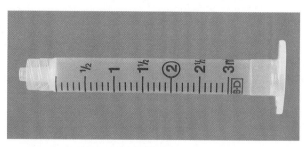

41. ketorolac 25 mg   _____

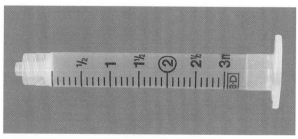

42. Vistaril® 50 mg   _____

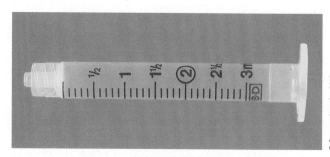

Dosage Ordered

mL Needed

43. Ativan 10 mg

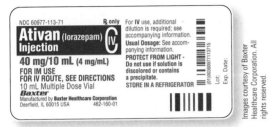

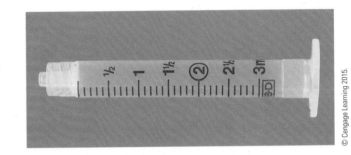

_____

44. Robinul® 180 mcg

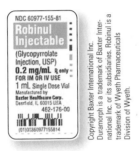

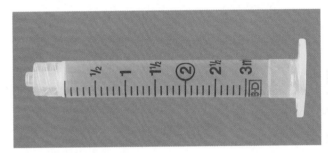

_____

45. hydroxyzine HCl 70 mg

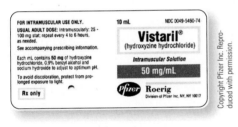

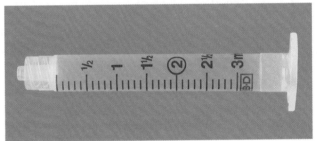

_____

46. penicillin 400,000 units

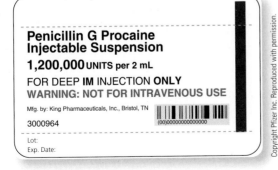

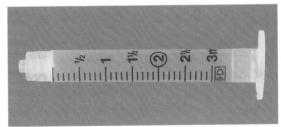

_____

Dosage Ordered   **mL Needed**

47. heparin sodium 1500 units (calculate to the nearest hundredth) _____

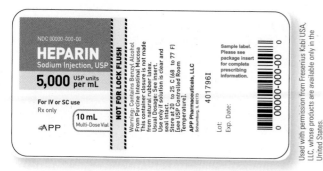

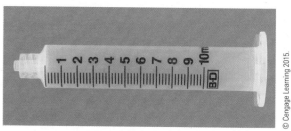

48. potassium chloride 20 mEq for an IV additive _____

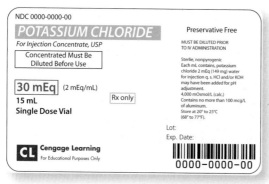

49. Inapsine® 4.5 mg _____

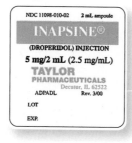

50. epinephrine 1.4 mg _____

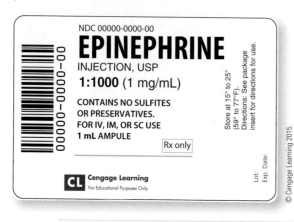

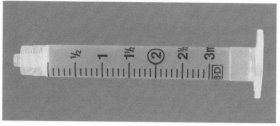

Dosage Ordered   **mL Needed**

51. Nubain® 15 mg   _____

NDC 63481-509-05

NUBAIN® R_x only
(Nalbuphine HCl)
20 mg/mL injection
10 mL Multiple Dose Vial

Each mL contains: 20 mg nalbuphine
HCl, 0.94% sodium citrate hydrous,
1.26% citric acid anhydrous, and
0.2% of a 9:1 mixture of methyl and
propylparaben, as preservatives. pH is
adjusted, if necessary, to 3.5 to 3.7
with hydrochloric acid.

FOR IM, SC OR IV USE
Usual Dosage: See package insert
for complete prescribing information.
Store at 25°C (77°F); excursions
permitted to 15°-30°C (59°-86°F).
PROTECT FROM EXCESSIVE LIGHT.

Manufactured for:
Endo Pharmaceuticals Inc.
Chadds Ford, PA 19317

Used with permission from Endo Pharmaceuticals Inc.

© Cengage Learning 2015.

52. furosemide 15 mg   _____

NDC 00000-0000-00

FUROSEMIDE
INJECTION, USP

20 mg/ 2 mL

(10 mg/mL)
For IM or IV Use
DILUTE BEFORE IV USE
2 mL Single Dose Vial   Rx only

CL **Cengage Learning**
For Educational Purposes Only

WARNING: USE ONLY IF SOLUTION IS CLEAR AND COLORLESS.
PROTECT FROM LIGHT. Store at controlled room temperature,
15°-30°C (59°-86°F) (See USP). See package insert directions
for use.
Lot:
Exp. Date:

© Cengage Learning 2015.

© Cengage Learning 2015.

53. dexamethasone 6000 mcg   _____

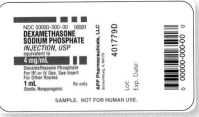

NDC 00000-000-00 16501
DEXAMETHASONE
SODIUM PHOSPHATE
INJECTION, USP
equivalent to
4 mg/mL
Dexamethasone Phosphate
For IM or IV Use, See insert
For Other Routes
1 mL   Rx only
Sterile, Nonpyrogenic

401779D

Lot:
Exp. Date:

SAMPLE. NOT FOR HUMAN USE.

APP Pharmaceuticals, LLC
Schaumburg, IL 60173

Used with permission from Fresenius
Kabi USA, LLC, whose products are
available only in the United States.

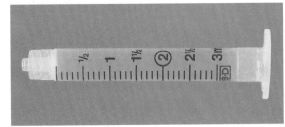

© Cengage Learning 2015.

SECTION 4

Dosage Ordered   **mL Needed**

54. phenytoin Na 75 mg   _____

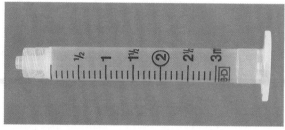

55. lidocaine HCl 15 mg   _____

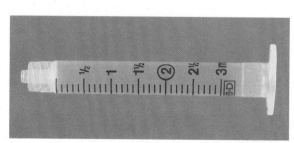

Answers

1. 0.8 mL	**12.** 2 mL	**24.** 1.8 mL	**36.** 1.5 mL	**48.** 10 mL
2. 1.5 mL	**13.** 1.5 mL	**25.** 1.3 mL	**37.** 1.5 mL	**49.** 1.8 mL
3. 1.4 mL	**14.** 0.45 mL	**26.** 1.5 mL	**38.** 0.8 mL	**50.** 1.4 mL
4. 3 mL	**15.** 1.6 mL	**27.** 3 mL	**39.** 16 mL	**51.** 0.8 mL
5. 0.9 mL	**16.** 2 mL	**28.** 8 mL	**40.** 2.5 mL	**52.** 1.5 mL
6. 1.5 mL	**17.** 2.3 mL	**29.** 1.2 mL	**41.** 1.7 mL	**53.** 1.5 mL
7. 0.38 mL	**18.** 1.8 mL	**30.** 1.6 mL	**42.** 2 mL	**54.** 1.5 mL
8. 0.8 mL	**19.** 2.4 mL	**31.** 0.6 mL	**43.** 2.5 mL	**55.** 0.8 mL
9. 1.2 mL	**20.** 15 mL	**32.** 1.5 mL	**44.** 0.9 mL	
10. 0.8 mL	**21.** 1.5 mL	**33.** 1.3 mL	**45.** 1.4 mL	
11. 8 mL	**22.** 0.8 mL	**34.** 1.6 mL	**46.** 0.7 mL	
	23. 1.6 mL	**35.** 1.3 mL	**47.** 0.3 mL	

14

FORMULA METHOD

The formula method may be used for one-step dosage calculations. It is really just a variation of ratio and proportion and in other texts has occasionally been presented using different initials. If you are familiar with different initials from those used in this chapter, by all means continue to use them. The important thing is the **answer**, not the initials used to obtain it.

BASIC FORMULA

The initials most commonly used in the formula method are as follows:

$$\frac{D}{H} \times Q = X$$

Here's what these initials mean.

D = **desired**	The dosage **ordered**, in mg, g, etc.
H = **have**	The dosage strength **available**, in mg, g, etc.
Q = **quantity**	The mL **volume** the dosage strength **available** is contained in
X = **the unknown**	The mL **volume** the **desired** dosage will be contained in

It is necessary to memorize this formula. Printing it several times will help you to remember it.

The same three precautions that governed previous calculations also apply to the use of the formula: (1) routinely double-check all math; (2) assess each answer to determine if it is logical; and (3) seek help if you have any doubt of your accuracy. Now let's look at some examples of how the formula is used so you can begin to be comfortable with it.

 KEYpoint: The unknown, *X*, will always be expressed in the same units of measure as *Q*, the mL volume the dosage available is contained in.

OBJECTIVE

The learner will:

1. use the formula method to solve dosage problems containing metric, unit, and mEq dosages.

EXAMPLE 1 A dosage of **80 mg** is ordered. The dosage strength available is **100 mg in 2 mL**. Calculate the mL necessary to administer this dosage.

The desired dosage (D) is 80 mg. You have (H) 100 mg in (Q) 2 mL available. Remember that X will always be expressed in the same units of measure as Q, which is mL in this problem. **Always set up the formula with the units of measure included.**

$$\frac{(D)\ 80\ \text{mg}}{(H)\ 100\ \text{mg}} \times (Q)\ 2\ \text{mL} = X\ \text{mL}$$

$$\frac{80}{100} \times 2 = X = \textbf{1.6 mL}$$

To give a dosage of 80 mg, you must administer 1.6 mL.

After you have double-checked your math, **look at your answer to see if it is logical.** The dosage strength available is 100 mg in 2 mL. **To prepare** 80 mg, which is **a smaller dosage, you will need a smaller volume.** Your answer, 1.6 mL, is smaller; therefore, it is logical.

EXAMPLE 2 The dosage ordered is **0.4 mg**. The strength available is **0.25 mg in 1.2 mL**.

The desired dosage (D) is 0.4 mg. You have (H) 0.25 mg in (Q) 1.2 mL.

$$\frac{0.4\ \text{mg}}{0.25\ \text{mg}} \times 1.2\ \text{mL} = X\ \text{mL}$$

$$\frac{0.4}{0.25} \times 1.2 = X = 1.92 = \textbf{1.9 mL}$$

To give a dosage of 0.4 mg, you must administer 1.9 mL.

The 0.4 mg ordered is a larger dosage than the 0.25 mg strength available, and the volume that contains it must be larger, which 1.9 mL is.

EXAMPLE 3 A dosage of **750 mcg** has been ordered. The strength available is **1000 mcg per mL**.

$$\frac{750\ \text{mcg}}{1000\ \text{mcg}} \times 1\ \text{mL} = X\ \text{mL}$$

$$\frac{750}{1000} \times 1 = X = 0.75 = \textbf{0.8 mL}$$

To give a dosage of 750 mcg, you must administer 0.8 mL.

The answer should be a smaller quantity than 1 mL, and 0.8 mL is.

▶▶▶ PROBLEMS 14.1

Calculate the dosages. Express answers to the nearest tenth.

1. A dosage of 0.8 g has been ordered. The strength available
   is 1 g in 2.5 mL.   _____

2. You have available a dosage strength of 250 mg in 1.5 mL.
   The order is for 200 mg.   _____

3. The strength available is 1 g in 5 mL. The order is for 0.2 g.   _____

4. A dosage of 300 mcg has been ordered. The strength available
   is 500 mcg in 1.2 mL.   _____

Answers 1. 2 mL **2.** 1.2 mL **3.** 1 mL **4.** 0.7 mL

USE WITH METRIC CONVERSIONS

Consider the following problem:

A dosage of 200 mcg is ordered. The strength available is 0.3 mg in 1.5 mL.

   This problem cannot be solved as it is now written because the drug strengths, *D* and *H*, are in different units of measure. One of them must be changed before the problem can be solved.

 KEY*point:* The drug strengths, **D** and **H**, must be expressed in the same units of measure.

EXAMPLE 1   A dosage of **200 mcg** is ordered. The strength available is **0.3 mg in 1.5 mL**.

- **Convert mg to mcg to eliminate the decimal point.**

   0.3 mg = 300 mcg

- **Use the formula for the calculation.**

$$\frac{200 \text{ mcg}}{300 \text{ mcg}} \times 1.5 \text{ mL} = X \text{ mL}$$

$$\frac{200}{300} \times 1.5 \text{ mL} = \textbf{1 mL}$$

To give 200 mcg, you must administer 1 mL.

Your answer must be a smaller quantity than 1.5 mL, which 1 mL is, because the dosage ordered is smaller than the strength available. Therefore, it is logical.

EXAMPLE 2   A dosage of **0.7 g** has been ordered. Available is a strength of **1000 mg in 1.5 mL**.

- **Convert g to mg to eliminate the decimal point.**

   0.7 g = 700 mg

SECTION 4

- **Use the formula for the calculation.**

$$\frac{700 \text{ mg}}{1000 \text{ mg}} \times 1.5 \text{ mL} = X \text{ mL}$$

$$\frac{700}{1000} \times 1.5 \text{ mL} = 1.05 \text{ mL} = \textbf{1.1 mL}$$

To give 0.7 g, you must administer 1.1 mL.

The answer should be less than 1.5 mL, which 1.1 mL is, because the 700 mg ordered is less than the 1000 mg strength available.

▶▶▶ PROBLEMS 14.2

Calculate the dosages. Express answers to the nearest tenth.

1. The dosage ordered is 780 mcg. The strength available is 1 mg per mL.   _____

2. The available dosage strength is 0.1 g per mL. The dosage ordered is 250 mg.   _____

3. Prepare a dosage of 0.6 mg from an available strength of 1000 mcg per 2 mL.   _____

4. A dosage of 0.4 g has been ordered. The strength available is 500 mg per 1.3 mL.   _____

Answers **1.** 0.8 mL **2.** 2.5 mL **3.** 1.2 mL **4.** 1 mL

USE WITH UNITS AND mEq CALCULATIONS

Dosages expressed in units or mEq are handled in exactly the same way as metric measures.

EXAMPLE 1   A dosage of **7500 units** is ordered. The available strength is **10,000 units per mL**.

$$\frac{7500 \text{ units}}{10,000 \text{ units}} \times 1 \text{ mL} = X \text{ mL}$$

$$\frac{7500}{10,000} \times 1 = 0.75 = \textbf{0.8 mL}$$

To give 7500 units, administer 0.8 mL.

The dosage ordered, 7500 units, is less than the strength available, 10,000 units, and must be contained in a smaller volume of solution than 1 mL, which 0.8 mL is.

EXAMPLE 2 A dosage strength of **40 mEq in 5 mL** is available. You are to pre-pare **30 mEq**.

$$\frac{30 \text{ mEq}}{40 \text{ mEq}} \times 5 \text{ mL} = X \text{ mL}$$

$$\frac{30}{40} \times 5 = 3.75 = \textbf{3.8 mL}$$

A volume of 3.8 mL is necessary to prepare a 30 mEq dosage.

The dosage ordered, 30 mEq, is less than the 40 mEq dosage strength available. It must be contained in a smaller volume than 5 mL, and the answer, 3.8 mL, indicates that it is.

▶▶▶ PROBLEMS 14.3

Calculate the dosages. Express answers to the nearest tenth.

1. A dosage strength of 1000 units per 1.5 mL is available.
   Prepare a 1250 units dosage.   _____

2. A dosage of 45 units has been ordered. The strength available
   is 80 units per mL.   _____

3. The IV solution available has a strength of 200 mEq per 20 mL.
   You are to prepare a 50 mEq dosage.   _____

4. The strength available is 80 mEq per 5 mL. Prepare 30 mEq. _____

Answers **1.** 1.9 mL **2.** 0.6 mL **3.** 5 mL **4.** 1.9 mL

Summary

This concludes the chapter on using the formula method to solve dosage calculations. The important points to remember from this chapter are:

▼ The formula method can be used to solve problems expressed in metric, unit, and mEq dosages.

▼ When the formula method is used, D and H, the dosage strengths, must be expressed in the same units of measure.

▼ The answer obtained, X, will always be in the same unit of measure as Q, the quantity.

▼ The math for all calculations is routinely double-checked.

▼ A logical assessment of the answer you obtain is a routine step in calculations.

Summary Self-Test

Calculate the dosages. Express answers as decimal fractions to the nearest tenth.

1. A 50 mg dosage has been ordered. The strength available is 60 mg in 1.5 mL.   _____

2. Prepare a 300 mcg dosage. The dosage available is 0.4 mg per mL.   _____

3. Prepare 0.45 g. The strength available is 300 mg per mL.   _____

4. The medication is labeled 5 mg per mL. An 8 mg dosage has been ordered.   _____

5. Prepare a 70 mg dosage from a solution labeled 250 mg in 5 mL.   _____

6. The drug is labeled 25 mg per mL; 30 mg has been ordered.   _____

7. The label reads 50 mg per mL. Prepare a 60 mg dosage.   _____

8. The order is for 12 mg. The vial is labeled 5 mg per mL.   _____

9. A dosage of 7 mg has been ordered. The vial label reads 10 mg per mL.   _____

10. The dosage strength is 10 mg in 1 mL; 8 mg has been ordered.   _____

11. Prepare a 0.3 g dosage from a medication labeled 900 mg per 6 mL.   _____

12. Prepare a 300 mg IV dosage from a vial labeled 0.5 g in 20 mL.   _____

13. The vial is labeled 0.5 g per 2 mL. A dosage of 750 mg has been ordered.   _____

14. Prepare a dosage of 0.2 mg from an available dosage of 250 mcg in 5 mL.   _____

15. The order is for 130 mg and the single-use ampule is labeled 0.1 g per 2 mL.   _____

16. Draw up a 12 mg dosage from a vial labeled 15 mg in 5 mL.   _____

17. The ampule is labeled 20 mg in 2 mL. Prepare 14 mg.   _____

18. The medication is labeled 1.2 g per 30 mL. Draw up an 800 mg dosage for IV administration.   _____

19. Prepare an 80 mg dosage of a medication labeled 100 mg in 2 mL.   _____

20. The solution strength is 0.4 mg per mL. A dosage of 300 mcg has been ordered.   _____

21. Prepare a 600 mg dosage from an available dosage strength of 0.4 g per mL.   _____

22. Draw up a 60 mEq dosage for addition to an IV from a solution labeled 40 mEq per 20 mL.   _____

23. The label reads 400 mcg per mL; 0.6 mg has been ordered.   _____

24. Prepare a 60 mg dosage from a 75 mg per mL strength.   _____

25. Prepare a 0.1 g dosage from a vial labeled 40 mg per mL.   _____

26. The drug is labeled 50 mg in 10 mL. The order is for 8 mg.   _____

27. Measure a 0.8 mg dosage from an available strength of 1000 mcg per mL.   _____

28. Prepare 40 mg from a vial labeled 25 mg per mL.   _____

29. A dosage of 10 mg has been ordered. You have available a strength of 4000 mcg per mL. _____

30. Prepare 200 mg for IV use of a medication labeled 0.25 g per 25 mL. _____

31. The dosage strength available is 15 mg in 1 mL; 10 mg has been ordered. _____

32. Prepare a 4 mg dosage from a strength available of 5 mg per mL. _____

33. A dosage of 75 units has been ordered from an available strength of 90 units in 1.5 mL. _____

34. You are to prepare 100 mEq for addition to an IV solution. The solution available is labeled 80 mEq per 20 mL. _____

35. Prepare a dosage of 180 mg from a 0.15 g in 1 mL solution. _____

36. Prepare a 750-unit dosage from an available strength of 1000 units per mL. _____

37. Prepare a 20 mEq dosage of an IV additive from a vial labeled 40 mEq per 20 mL. _____

38. 400,000 units have been ordered and you have available 300,000 units in 1 mL. _____

39. A dosage of 0.2 mg per 2 mL is available. Prepare a 250 mcg dosage. _____

40. A dosage of 35 mEq has been ordered for addition to an IV solution. The solution is labeled 50 mEq per 50 mL. _____

Answers				
1. 1.3 mL	**9.** 0.7 mL	**18.** 20 mL	**27.** 0.8 mL	**36.** 0.8 mL
2. 0.8 mL	**10.** 0.8 mL	**19.** 1.6 mL	**28.** 1.6 mL	**37.** 10 mL
3. 1.5 mL	**11.** 2 mL	**20.** 0.8 mL	**29.** 2.5 mL	**38.** 1.3 mL
4. 1.6 mL	**12.** 12 mL	**21.** 1.5 mL	**30.** 20 mL	**39.** 2.5 mL
5. 1.4 mL	**13.** 3 mL	**22.** 30 mL	**31.** 0.7 mL	**40.** 35 mL
6. 1.2 mL	**14.** 4 mL	**23.** 1.5 mL	**32.** 0.8 mL	
7. 1.2 mL	**15.** 2.6 mL	**24.** 0.8 mL	**33.** 1.2 mL	
8. 2.4 mL	**16.** 4 mL	**25.** 2.5 mL	**34.** 25 mL	
	17. 1.4 mL	**26.** 1.6 mL	**35.** 1.2 mL	

SECTION

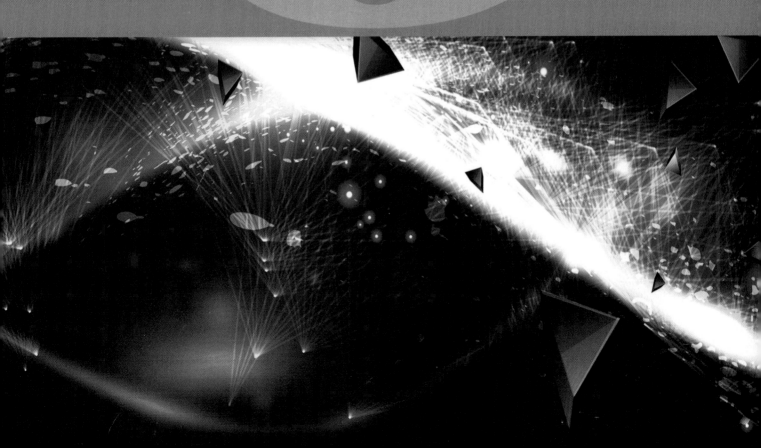

Dosage Calculation from Body Weight and Body Surface Area

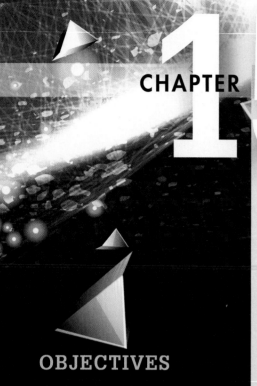

15

ADULT AND PEDIATRIC DOSAGES BASED ON BODY WEIGHT

OBJECTIVES

The learner will:

1. convert body weight from lb to kg.

2. convert body weight from kg to lb.

3. calculate dosages using mcg/mg per kg, or per lb.

4. determine if dosages ordered are within the normal range.

Body weight is a major factor in calculating drug dosages for both adults and children. It is the **most** important determiner of dosages for infants and neonates, whose ability to metabolize drugs is not fully developed. The dosage that will produce optimum therapeutic results for any particular individual, either child or adult, depends not only on dosage but on individual variables, including drug sensitivities and tolerance, age, weight, sex, and metabolic, pathologic, or psychologic conditions.

The prescriber will order the drug and dosage. However, it is a nursing responsibility to check each dosage to be sure the order is correct. Each drug label or drug package insert provides specific dosage details, but more complete information is readily available in drug formularies, the *Physicians' Desk Reference (PDR)*, and other medical references. The hospital pharmacist is the ultimate resource for information.

Individualized dosages may be calculated in terms of mcg or mg per kg or lb per day. The total daily dosage may be administered in divided (more than one) dosages; for example, every 6 hours or every 8 hours.

Because body weight is critical in calculating infant and neonatal dosages, measurement is usually done using a weight scale calibrated in kg. Adult weights may be recorded in either kg or lb; occasionally, conversions between these two measures are necessary.

CONVERTING lb TO kg

If body weight is recorded in lb, but the drug literature lists dosage per kg, a conversion from lb to kg will be necessary. There are 2.2 lb in 1 kg. This means that **kg body weights are smaller than lb weights**, so **the conversion from lb to kg is made by dividing body weight by 2.2.** For ease of calculation, fractional lb may be converted to the nearest quarter and written as decimal fractions instead of oz: ¼ lb (4 oz) as 0.25, ½ lb (8 oz) as 0.5, and ¾ lb (12 oz) as 0.75. If this kind of accuracy is critical, the prescribing orders should so indicate.

EXAMPLE 1   A child weighs 41 lb 12 oz. Convert to kg.

41 lb 12 oz = 41.75 ÷ 2.2 = 18.97 = **19 kg**

The kg weight should be a smaller number than 41.75 because you are dividing, and 19 kg is smaller.

EXAMPLE 2   Convert the weight of a 144½ lb adult to kg.

144½ lb = 144.5 ÷ 2.2 = 65.68 = **65.7 kg**

EXAMPLE 3   Convert the weight of a 27¼ lb child to kg.

27¼ lb = 27.25 ÷ 2.2 = 12.38 = **12.4 kg**

▶▶▶ PROBLEMS 15.1

Convert these body weights. Round to the nearest tenth kg.

1. 58¾ lb = _____ kg   6. 134½ lb = _____ kg

2. 63½ lb = _____ kg   7. 112¾ lb = _____ kg

3. 163¼ lb = _____ kg   8. 73¼ lb = _____ kg

4. 39¾ lb = _____ kg   9. 121½ lb = _____ kg

5. 100¼ lb = _____ kg   10. 92¾ lb = _____ kg

Answers **1.** 26.7 kg **2.** 28.9 kg **3.** 74.2 kg **4.** 18.1 kg **5.** 45.6 kg **6.** 61.1 kg **7.** 51.3 kg **8.** 33.3 kg **9.** 55.2 kg **10.** 42.2 kg

CONVERTING kg TO lb

There are 2.2 lb in 1 kg. To convert from kg to lb, **multiply by 2.2**. Because you are multiplying, **the answer in lb will be larger than the kg** being converted. Express weight to the nearest tenth lb.

EXAMPLE 1   A child weighs 23.3 kg. Convert to lb.

23.3 kg = 23.3 × 2.2 = 51.26 = **51.3 lb**

The answer must be larger because you are multiplying, and it is larger.

EXAMPLE 2   Convert an adult weight of 73.4 kg to lb.

73.4 kg = 73.4 × 2.2 = 161.48 = **161.5 lb**

EXAMPLE 3   Convert the weight of a 14.2 kg child to lb.

14.2 kg = 14.2 × 2.2 = 31.24 = **31.2 lb**

▶▶▶ PROBLEMS 15.2

Convert kg to lb. Round to the nearest tenth lb.

1. 21.3 kg = _____ lb

2. 99.2 kg = _____ lb

3. 28.7 kg = _____ lb

4. 71.4 kg = _____ lb

5. 30.8 kg = _____ lb

6. 43.7 kg = _____ lb

7. 63.8 kg = _____ lb

8. 57.1 kg = _____ lb

9. 84.2 kg = _____ lb

10. 34.9 kg = _____ lb

Answers   **1.** 46.9 lb   **2.** 218.2 lb   **3.** 63.1 lb   **4.** 157.1 lb   **5.** 67.8 lb   **6.** 96.1 lb   **7.** 140.4 lb
8. 125.6 lb   **9.** 185.2 lb   **10.** 76.8 lb

CALCULATING DOSAGES FROM DRUG LABEL INFORMATION

Information you will need to calculate dosages from body weight will be on the actual drug label or on the drug package insert.

Calculating the dosage is a two-step procedure. First, the **total daily dosage** is calculated. Then it is **divided by the number of doses per day** to obtain the actual dose administered at one time.

Let's start by looking at some oral antibiotic labels that contain the mg/kg/day dosage guidelines.

EXAMPLE 1 ▌

Refer to the information written sideways on the right of the sample antibiotic label in Figure 15-1 for children's dosages. Notice that the dosage is **20 mg/kg/day (or 40 mg/kg/day in otitis media)**. This dosage is to be given in **divided doses every 8 hours**—or a total of 3 doses (24 hr ÷ 8 hr = 3 doses).

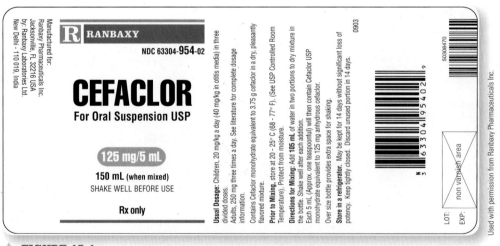

▲ FIGURE 15-1

Once you have located the dosage information, you can move ahead and calculate the dosage. Let's assume you are checking the dosage ordered for an **18.2 kg** child. Start by calculating the **recommended daily dosage range**.

Lower daily dosage = 20 mg/kg

20 mg × 18.2 kg (weight of child) = **364 mg/day**

Upper daily dosage = 40 mg/kg

40 mg × 18.2 kg = **728 mg/day**

The recommended range for this 18.2 kg child is 364–728 mg/day.

The drug is to be given in three divided doses.

Lower dosage 364 mg ÷ 3 = **121 mg per dose**

Upper dosage 728 mg ÷ 3 = **243 mg per dose**

The per dose dosage range is 121–243 mg per dose every 8 hours.

Now that you have the dosage range for this child, you are able to assess the accuracy of physician orders. Let's look at some orders and see how you can use the dosage range you just calculated.

1. **If the order is to give 125 mg every 8 hours, is this within the recommended dosage range?**
   Yes, 125 mg is within the average range of 121–243 mg per dose.

2. **If the order is to give 375 mg every 8 hours, is this within the recommended dosage range?**
   No, this is an overdosage. The maximum recommended dosage is 243 mg per dose. The 375 mg dose should not be given; the prescriber must be called and the order questioned.

3. **If the order is for 75 mg every 8 hours, is this an accurate dosage?**
   The recommended lower limit for an 18.2 kg child is 121 mg. Although 75 mg might be **safe**, it will probably be **ineffective**. Notify the prescriber that the dosage appears to be too low.

4. **If the order is for 250 mg every 8 hours, is this accurate?**
   Because 243 mg per dose is the recommended upper limit, 250 mg is essentially within normal range. The drug strength is 125 mg per 5 mL, and a 250 mg dosage is 10 mL. The prescriber has probably ordered this dosage based on the available dosage strength and for ease of preparation.

5. **If the dosage ordered is 125 mg every 4 hours, is this an accurate dosage?**
   In this order, the **frequency of administration** does not match the recommended dosage of every 8 hours. The total daily dosage of 750 mg (125 mg × 6 doses = 750 mg) is slightly, but not significantly, higher than the 728 mg maximum. There may be a reason the prescriber ordered the dosage every 4 hours, but call to verify it.

 KEYpoint: To determine the safety of an ordered dosage, use body weight to calculate the dosage range ordered, and compare this with the recommended dosage range in mg/kg/day (or mg/lb/day). Assessment must also include the frequency of dosage ordered.

The difference between 4 and 6 mg is much more critical than the difference between 243 and 250 mg because the drug potency is obviously greater.

Additional factors that must be considered are age, weight, and medical condition. Although these factors cannot be dealt with at length, keep in mind that **the younger, the older, or the more compromised by illness an individual is, the more critical a discrepancy is likely to be.**

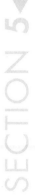

KEY_point:_ Discrepancies in dosages are much more significant if the number of mg or mcg ordered is small.

▶▶▶ PROBLEMS 15.3

Refer to the Biaxin® Granules label in Figure 15-2 to answer the questions for a 20 lb child.

1. What is the child's body weight in kg to the nearest tenth? _____
2. What is the recommended dosage in mg per day for this child? _____
3. How many mg will this be per dose? _____
4. The order is to give 62.5 mg twice a day. Is this dosage reasonable? _____
5. How many mL would you need to administer this dosage? _____
6. How much water must you add as diluent to prepare this oral suspension? _____

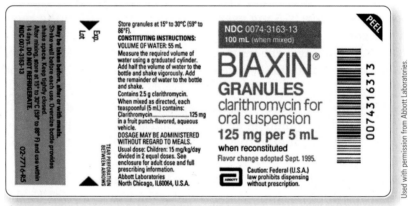

▲ FIGURE 15-2

Answers **1.** 9.1 kg **2.** 136.5 mg/day **3.** 68.3 mg/dose **4.** yes **5.** 2.5 mL **6.** 55 mL

CALCULATING DOSAGES FROM DRUG LITERATURE

The labels you have just been reading were from oral syrups and suspensions, but the same calculation steps are necessary for dosages to be administered by the IV or IM route. Parenteral labels are much smaller in size and usually do not include dosage recommendations. To obtain these, you will have to refer to the **drug package inserts**, the **_PDR_**, or **similar references**. These references will contain extensive details about each drug's chemistry, actions, adverse reactions, recommended administration, and so on, so it will be necessary for you to search for and select the information you need under the heading **Dosage and Administration**. In the following exercises, the searching has been done for you, and only those excerpts necessary for your calculations are shown.

▶▶▶ PROBLEMS 15.4

Refer to the cefazolin package insert in Figure 15-3 to locate the information for pediatric dosages.

1. What is the dosage range in mg/kg/day for mild-to-moderate infections?   _____

2. What is the dosage range for mild-to-moderate infections in mg/lb/day?   _____

3. The total dosage will be divided into how many doses per day?   _____

4. In severe infections, what is the maximum daily dosage recommended in mg/kg? In mg/lb?   _____

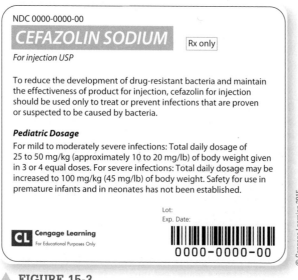

NDC 0000-0000-00

CEFAZOLIN SODIUM   [Rx only]

For injection USP

To reduce the development of drug-resistant bacteria and maintain the effectiveness of product for injection, cefazolin for injection should be used only to treat or prevent infections that are proven or suspected to be caused by bacteria.

Pediatric Dosage
For mild to moderately severe infections: Total daily dosage of 25 to 50 mg/kg (approximately 10 to 20 mg/lb) of body weight given in 3 or 4 equal doses. For severe infections: Total daily dosage may be increased to 100 mg/kg (45 mg/lb) of body weight. Safety for use in premature infants and in neonates has not been established.

Lot:
Exp. Date:

CL Cengage Learning
For Educational Purposes Only

0000-0000-00

© Cengage Learning 2015.

▲ FIGURE 15-3

Answers 1. 25–50 mg **2.** 10–20 mg **3.** 3–4 doses per day **4.** 100 mg/kg; 45 mg/lb

▶▶▶ PROBLEMS 15.5

Use the information you just obtained from Figure 15-3 to do the calculations for a child who weighs 35 lb and has a moderately severe infection.

1. What is the lower daily dosage range?   _____

2. What is the upper daily dosage range?   _____

3. If the medication is given in 4 divided dosages, what will the per dosage range be?   _____

4. If a dosage of 125 mg is ordered every 6 hours, will you need to question it?   _____

Answers 1. 350 mg/day **2.** 700 mg/day **3.** 87.5–175 mg per dose **4.** no; within normal range

▶▶▶ PROBLEMS 15.6

Refer to the dosage information in Figure 15-4 to answer the following questions about adult IV dosages.

1. What is the recommended daily dosage range for serious infections? _____

2. In how many divided doses should this daily dosage be given? _____

3. What is the maximum daily dosage? _____

4. Calculate the daily dosage range in g for a 176 lb adult. _____

5. If this dosage is to be given every 6 hours, what will this individual's dosage range be? _____

6. If a dosage of 2 g is ordered, what initial assessment would you make about it? _____

7. If a dosage of 10 g is ordered every 6 hours, what assessment would you make? _____

DOSAGE AND ADMINISTRATION

MEZLIN® (sterile mezlocillin sodium) may be administered intravenously or intramuscularly. For serious infections, the intravenous route of administration should be used. Intramuscular doses should not exceed 2g per injection.

The recommended adult dosage for serious infections is 200–300 mg/kg per day given in 4 to 6 divided doses. The usual dose is 3g given every 4 hours (18g/day) or 4g given every 6 hours (16g/day). For life-threatening infections, up to 350 mg/kg per day may be administered, but the total daily dosage should ordinarily not exceed 24g.

[See table below.]

For patients with life-threatening infections, 4g may be administered every 4 hours (24g/day).

Used with permission from Novartis AG.

▲ FIGURE 15-4

Answers 1. 200–300 mg/kg 2. 4–6 doses; every 6 or 4 hours 3. 24 g 4. 16–24 g 5. 4–6 g
6. The dosage is too low. 7. The dosage is too high.

▶▶▶ PROBLEMS 15.7

Refer to the dosage recommendations for the antineoplastic agent in Figure 15-5 to answer the following questions for treatment of testicular tumors in a patient weighing 240 lb.

1. What is the recommended daily dosage range in mcg/kg? _____

2. How often is this dosage to be given and for how long? _____ _____

3. What is the daily dosage range in mcg for this patient? In mg? (Calculate kg weight to the nearest tenth.) _____ _____

4. If a dosage of 3 mg IV is ordered every morning, does this need to be questioned? _____

MITHRACIN®　　　　　　　　　　　　℞
(plicamycin)
FOR INTRAVENOUS USE

DOSAGE
The daily dose of Mithracin is based on the patient's body
weight. If a patient has abnormal fluid retention such as
edema, hydrothorax or ascites, the patient's ideal weight
rather than actual body weight should be used to calculate
the dose.
Treatment of Testicular Tumors: In the treatment of patients with testicular tumors the recommended daily dose of
Mithracin (plicamycin) is 25 to 30 mcg (0.025–0.030 mg) per
kilogram of body weight. Therapy should be continued for a
period of 8 to 10 days unless significant side effects or toxicity
occur during therapy. A course of therapy consisting of more
than 10 daily doses is not recommended. Individual daily
doses should not exceed 30 mcg (0.030 mg) per kilogram of
body weight.

Used with permission of Bayer Corporation.

▲ **FIGURE 15-5**

Answers　1. 25–30 mcg/kg　**2.** Once a day; 8–10 days　**3.** 2728–3273 mcg/day; 2.7–3.3 mg/day
4. no; within normal range

▶▶▶　PROBLEMS 15.8

**Refer to the ceftriaxone literature in Figure 15-6 to answer the following questions
on pediatric dosages.**

1. What is the maximum daily dose of ceftriaxone for a child with a skin
   structure infection?　　　　　　　　　　　　　　　　　_____

2. What is the dosage range for skin structure infections?　　　_____

3. What is the initial dosage for meningitis?　　　　　　　　_____

4. What will the initial dosage be for a child weighing 12.6 kg who
   has meningitis? In mg? In g?　　　　　　　　　　　　　_____

5. What is the twice-daily dosage in mg for this child to
   follow the initial dose?　　　　　　　　　　　　　　　_____

6. What will the initial meningitis dosage be for a child
   weighing 19½ lb?　　　　　　　　　　　　　　　　　_____

7. How many days must ceftriaxone therapy be continued for
   meningitis after the initial dose?　　　　　　　　　　　_____

> **DOSAGE AND ADMINISTRATION**
>
> Ceftriaxone for injection may be administered intravenously or intramuscularly. However, the intent of this Pharmacy Bulk Package is for the preparation of solutions for intravenous infusion only. Ceftriaxone for injection should be administered intravenously by infusion over a period of 30 minutes.
>
> **Do not use diluents containing calcium, such as Ringer's solution or Hartmann's solution, to reconstitute ceftriaxone for injection. Particulate formation can result. Ceftriaxone and calcium-containing solutions, including continuous calcium-containing infusions such as parenteral nutrition, should not be mixed or co-administered to any patient irrespective of age, even via different infusion lines at different sites (see CONTRAINDICATIONS and WARNINGS).**
>
> **NEONATES**
>
> Hyperbilirubinemic neonates, especially prematures, should not be treated with ceftriaxone (see **CONTRAINDICATIONS**).
>
> **PEDIATRIC PATIENTS**
>
> For the treatment of skin and skin structure infections, the recommended total daily dose is 50 to 75 mg/kg given once a day (or in equally divided doses twice a day). The total daily dose should not exceed 2 grams.
>
> For the treatment of serious miscellaneous infections other than meningitis, the recommended total daily dose is 50 to 75 mg/kg, given in divided doses every 12 hours. The total daily dose should not exceed 2 grams.
>
> In the treatment of meningitis, it is recommended that the initial therapeutic dose be 100 mg/kg (not to exceed 4 grams). Thereafter, a total daily dose of 100 mg/kg/day (not to exceed 4 grams daily) is recommended. The daily dose may be administered once a day (or in equally divided doses every 12 hours). The usual duration of therapy is 7 to 14 days.
>
> **ADULTS**
>
> The usual adult daily dose is 1 to 2 grams given once a day (or in equally divided doses twice a day) depending on the type and severity of infection. The total daily dose should not exceed 4 grams.
>
> If *Chlamydia trachomatis* is a suspected pathogen, appropriate antichlamydial coverage should be added, because ceftriaxone sodium has no activity against this organism.
>
> For preoperative use (surgical prophylaxis), a single dose of 1 gram administered intravenously 1/2 to 2 hours before surgery is recommended.
>
> Generally, ceftriaxone for injection therapy should be continued for at least 2 days after the signs and symptoms of infection have disappeared. The usual duration of therapy is 4 to 14 days; in complicated infections, longer therapy may be required.
>
> When treating infections caused by *Streptococcus pyogenes*, therapy should be continued for at least 10 days.
>
> No dosage adjustment is necessary for patients with impairment of renal or hepatic function; however, blood levels should be monitored in patients with severe renal impairment (e.g. dialysis patients) and in patients with both renal and hepatic dysfunctions.

▲ **FIGURE 15-6**

Answers **1.** 2 g **2.** 50–75 mg/kg once a day or equally divided dosages twice a day **3.** 100 mg/kg not to exceed 4 g **4.** 1260 mg; 1.26 g **5.** 630 mg **6.** 887 mg (890 mg if rounded) **7.** 7–14 days

---

Summary

This concludes the chapter on calculation and assessment of dosages based on body weight. The important points to remember from this chapter are:

▽ Dosages are frequently ordered on the basis of weight, especially for children.

▽ Dosages may be recommended based on mcg or mg per kg or lb per day, usually administered in divided doses.

▽ Body weight may need to be converted from kg to lb or lb to kg to correlate with dosage recommendations.

▽ To convert lb to kg, divide by 2.2; to convert kg to lb, multiply by 2.2.

▽ Calculating dosage is a two-step procedure: first, calculate the total daily dosage for the weight; then, divide this by the number of doses to be administered.

▽ To check the accuracy of a prescriber's order, calculate the correct dosage and compare it with the dosage ordered.

▽ Dosage discrepancies are much more critical if the dosage range is low—for example, 2–5 mg, as opposed to high, for example 250–500 mg.

▼ Factors that make discrepancies particularly serious are age, low body weight, and severity of medical condition.

▼ If the drug label does not contain all the necessary information for safe administration, additional information should be obtained from drug package inserts, the *PDR*, drug formularies, or the hospital pharmacist.

Summary Self-Test

Read the dosage labels and literature provided to answer the questions.

1. A 43 lb child has an order for oral cefaclor. What is the daily dosage for this child? _____

2. What is the per dose dosage? _____

3. Is an order for 250 mg of cefaclor every 8 hours correct for this child? _____

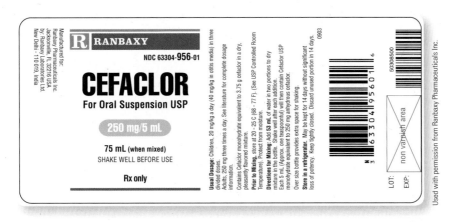

4. A 140 lb adult has an order for IV methylprednisolone. Calculate this patient's per dose dosage. _____

5. How often is this dosage to be given? _____

6. Children's dosages are smaller. What is the lowest mg/kg dosage recommended? _____

7. Calculate the lowest daily dosage for a child weighing 43 lb. _____

8. When given intravenously, what period of time is specified for the Solu-Medrol® administration? _____

SOLU–MEDROL®
brand of methylprednisolone sodium succinate sterile powder
(methylprednisolone sodium succinate for injection, USP)
For Intravenous or Intramuscular Administration

DOSAGE AND ADMINISTRATION

When high dose therapy is desired, the recommended dose of SOLU-MEDROL Sterile Powder (methylprednisolone sodium succinate) is 30 mg/kg administered intravenously over at least 30 minutes. This dose may be repeated every 4 to 6 hours for 48 hours.

Dosage may be reduced for infants and children but should be governed more by the severity of the condition and response of the patient than by age or size. It should not be less than 0.5 mg per kg every 24 hours.

Copyright Pfizer Inc. Reproduced with permission.

9. Refer to the penicillin V potassium oral solution label and identify the dosage strength in mg. _____

10. What is the dosage strength in units? _____

11. This medication is shipped in powdered form. How much diluent is needed for reconstitution? _____

12. What kind of diluent? _____

13. What dosage in mg/kg is specified for infants? _____

14. If an infant weighs 6.2 kg, what will the dosage range be? _____

15. What will the dosage range be for a 16 lb infant? _____

16. A 7.9 kg infant has an order for 125 mg every 8 hours. Calculate the per dose dosage based on this infant's body weight. Is the penicillin dosage ordered correct? _____

NDC 0000-0000-00

PENICILLIN V POTASSIUM

125 mg (200,000 units)   Rx only
For Oral Solution U.S.P.

per 5 mL when mixed as directed;
200 mL after mixing

Contains penicillin V potassium equivalent to 5 grams penicillin V in a dry mixture.

Each 5 mL teaspoon of prepared solution yields penicillin V potassium equivalent to 125 mg (200,000 units) penicillin V.

DIRECTIONS FOR PREPARATION

Use 117 mL of water to prepare 200 mL oral solution. Loosen powder then add water and shake vigorously.
Usual dosage: Adults and children — 1 to 2 teaspoons, given three or four times per day. Infants —15 to 56 mg/kg body weight daily, given in three to six divided doses. See insert for detailed information.
Store at room temperature in dry form.

Do Not Use If Caked

Lot:
Exp. Date:

CL Cengage Learning
For Educational Purposes Only

0000-0000-00

© Cengage Learning 2015.

17. Cefaclor oral suspension has been ordered for a child weighing 100 lb. Calculate the daily dose.   _____

18. What will the per dose dosage be?   _____

19. Would a 5 mL dosage every 8 hours be reasonable for this child?   _____

20. How is this oral cefaclor suspension to be reconstituted?   _____

21. What precautions did you learn about pouring and administering suspensions such as cefaclor?   _____

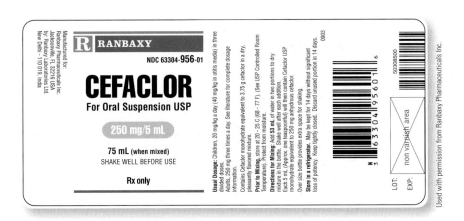

22. Refer to the acyclovir sodium injection insert to locate the adult and adolescent dosage in mg/kg.   _____

23. What will the dosage be per dose for an adult with mucosal herpes simplex weighing 61.4 kg?   _____

24. What would the dosage be for an adolescent with herpes simplex encephalitis weighing 180 lb?   _____

25. What mg/kg dosage is recommended for an infant with herpes simplex encephalitis?   _____

26. Read the literature to locate the time period recommended for intravenous infusion.   _____

27. There are bold print precautions regarding parenteral administration on this insert. What are they?   _____

ACYCLOVIR SODIUM

INJECTION

DOSAGE AND ADMINISTRATION:
CAUTION - AVOID RAPID OR BOLUS INTRAVENOUS INJECTION.
(see WARNINGS and PRECAUTIONS).

AVOID INTRAMUSCULAR OR SUBCUTANEOUS INJECTION
(see WARNINGS).
Initiate therapy as early as possible following onset of signs
and symptoms of herpes infections.
Do not exceed a dose equivalent to 20 mg/kg every 8 hours for
any patient.

DOSAGE IN HERPES SIMPLEX INFECTION:
MUCOSAL AND CUTANEOUS HERPES SIMPLEX (HSV-1 and HSV-2)
INFECTIONS IN IMMUNOCOMPROMISED PATIENTS:

Adults and Adolescents 12 years of age and older: 5 mg/kg
infused at a constant rate over 1 hour, every 8 hours for 7 days.

Children under 12 years of age: 10 mg/kg infused at a constant
rate over 1 hour, every 8 hours for 7 days.

DOSAGE IN SEVERE INITIAL CLINICAL EPISODES OF HERPES GENITALIS:

Adults and Adolescents 12 years of age and older: 5 mg/kg infused at a
constant rate over 1 hour, every 8 hours for 5 days.

DOSAGE IN HERPES SIMPLEX ENCEPHALITIS:
Adults and Adolescents 12 years of age and older: 10 mg/kg infused at a
constant rate over 1 hour, every 8 hours for 10 days.

Children 3 months to 12 years of age: 20 mg/kg infused at a constant rate
over 1 hour, every 8 hours for 10 days.

Administration
Further dilute the calculated dose in an appropriate intravenous solution at a
volume selected for administration during each 1 hour infusion. Infusion
concentrations of approximately 7 mg/mL or lower are recommended.
Clinical studies reveal that the average 70 kg adult received between 60 and
150 mL of fluid per dose. Higher concentrations (e.g.,10 mg/mL) may produce
phlebitis or inflammation at the injection site upon inadvertent extravasation. Standard, commercially available electrolyte and glucose solutions are
suitable for intravenous administration; biologic or colloidal fluids (e.g., blood
products, protein solutions, etc.) are not recommended.
Once diluted, each dose should be used within 24 hours.
Visually inspect for particulate matter and discoloration prior to
administration, whenever solution and container permit.

NDC 0000-0000-00

CL **Cengage Learning**
For Educational Purposes Only

Lot:
Exp. Date:

© Cengage Learning 2015.

---

28. A 198 lb adult is to be treated with IV ticarcillin disodium for
    bacterial septicemia. What is the daily dosage range in mg
    for this patient?   _____

29. If the drug is administered every 4 hours, what will the per dose
    be in g?   _____

30. Do you need to question a per dose dosage of 4 g of ticarcillin
    every 4 hours for this patient?   _____

TICARCILLIN DISODIUM

FOR INTRAMUSCULAR OR INTRAVENOUS ADMINISTRATION

DOSAGE AND ADMINISTRATION
In serious urinary tract and systemic infections, intravenous therapy in the higher doses should be used. Intramuscular injections
should not exceed 2 grams per injection.

Adults:

Bacterial septicemia	200 to 300 mg/kg/day by I.V. infusion in divided doses every four or six hours.
Respiratory tract infection	Usual dose is 3 grams every four hours (18 grams/day) or 4 grams every six hours
Skin and soft-tissue infection	(16 grams/day) depending on weight and the severity of the infection.
Intra-abdominal infection	
Infections of the female pelvis and genital tract	

Urinary tract infections	
Complicated:	Give 150 to 200 mg/kg/day by I.V. infusion every four to six hours in divided doses.
	Recommended dosage for average (70 kg) adult: 3 grams four times daily.
Uncomplicated:	Give 1 gram I.M. or direct I.V. every six hours.

NDC 0000-0000-00

CL **Cengage Learning**
For Educational Purposes Only

Lot:
Exp. Date:

© Cengage Learning 2015.

31. Refer to the VFEND® package insert information to locate the IV maintenance dosage in mg/kg every 12 hours (written with the abbreviation q12h, now slated for deletion) for invasive aspergillosis. _____

32. What would the daily IV dosage be for an individual weighing 92.7 kg? _____

33. What would the daily oral dosage be for this same 92.7 kg individual? _____

34. What will a single IV maintenance dosage be for the same 92.7 kg individual? _____

35. Locate the VFEND information on the maximum rate of administration for intravenous administration. _____

36. There is a bold type and capitalized warning for IV administration of VFEND on this insert. What is it? _____

VFEND® I.V.

(voriconazole) for Injection

VFEND® Tablets

(voriconazole)

VFEND® (voriconazole) **for Oral Suspension**

DESCRIPTION

VFEND® (voriconazole), a triazole antifungal agent, is available as a lyophilized powder for solution for intravenous infusion, film-coated tablets for oral administration, and as a powder for oral suspension.

DOSAGE AND ADMINISTRATION

Administration

VFEND Tablets or Oral Suspension should be taken at least one hour before, or one hour following, a meal.

VFEND I.V. for Injection requires reconstitution to 10 mg/mL and subsequent dilution to 5 mg/mL or less prior to administration as an infusion, at a maximum rate of 3 mg/kg per hour over 1–2 hours (see Intravenous Administration).

NOT FOR IV BOLUS INJECTION

Recommended Dosing Regimen

Infection	Loading dose	Maintenance Dose	
	IV	IV	Oral[a]
Invasive Aspergillosis	6 mg/kg q12h for the first 24 hours	4 mg/kg q12h	200 mg q12h
Candidemia in nonneutropenic patients and other deep tissue *Candida* infections	6 mg/kg q12h for the first 24 hours	3–4 mg/kg q12h[b]	200 mg q12h
Esophageal Candidiasis	c	c	200 mg q12h
Scedosporiosis and Fusariosis	6 mg/kg q12h for the first 24 hours	4 mg/kg q12h	200 mg q12h

37. Refer to the fluconazole injection insert to locate the first day dosage for a child with esophageal candidiasis. _____

38. What is the dosage recommendation for subsequent days? _____

39. How long must treatment for this condition be continued? _____

40. What will the first dose be for a child weighing 18.2 kg? _____

41. What will the subsequent dosage be for this same 18.2 kg child? _____

42. How often will this dosage be administered? _____

43. What is the maximum mg/kg dosage recommended if the child has a particularly severe infection? _____

44. What would the first dose of fluconazole be for a child weighing 72 lb? _____

FZC-P01

FLUCONAZOLE INJECTION

For Intravenous Infusion Only
Rx ONLY
DESCRIPTION

Fluconazole, the first of a new subclass of synthetic triazole antifungal agents, is available as a sterile solution for intravenous use in glass vials.

Dosage and Administration in Children:
The following dose equivalency scheme should generally provide equivalent exposure in pediatric and adult patients:

Pediatric Patients	Adults
3 mg/kg	100 mg
6 mg/kg	200 mg
12*mg/kg	400 mg

*Some older children may have clearances similar to that of adults. Absolute doses exceeding 600 mg/day are not recommended. Experience with fluconazole in neonates is limited to pharmacokinetic studies in premature newborns. (See **CLINICAL PHARMACOLOGY.**) Based on the prolonged half-life seen in premature newborns (gestational age 26 to 29 weeks), these children, in the first two weeks of life, should receive the same dosage (mg/kg) as in older children, but administered every 72 hours. After the first two weeks, these children should be dosed once daily. No information regarding fluconazole pharmacokinetics in full-term newborns is available.

Oropharyngeal candidiasis: The recommended dosage of fluconazole for oropharyngeal candidiasis in children is 6 mg/kg on the first day, followed by 3 mg/kg once daily. Treatment should be administered for at least 2 weeks to decrease the likelihood of relapse.

Esophageal candidiasis: For the treatment of esophageal candidiasis, the recommended dosage of fluconazole in children is 6 mg/kg on the first day, followed by 3 mg/kg once daily. Doses up to 12 mg/kg/day may be used based on medical judgment of the patient's response to therapy. Patients with esophageal candidiasis should be treated for a minimum of three weeks and for at least 2 weeks following the resolution of symptoms.

Systemic Candida infections: For the treatment of candidemia and disseminated *Candida* infections, daily doses of 6 to 12 mg/kg/day have been used in an open, noncomparative study of a small number of children.

Cryptococcal meningitis: For the treatment of acute cryptococcal meningitis, the recommended dosage is 12 mg/kg on the first day, followed by 6 mg/kg once daily. A dosage of 12 mg/kg once daily may be used, based on medical judgment of the patient's response to therapy. The recommended duration of treatment for initial therapy of cryptococcal meningitis is 10 to 12 weeks after the cerebrospinal fluid becomes culture negative. For suppression of relapse of cryptococcal meningitis in children with AIDS, the recommended dose of fluconazole is 6 mg/kg once daily.

Answers

1. 390 mg
2. 130 mg/dose
3. no, too high
4. 1908 mg/dose
5. every 4–6 hours for 48 hours
6. 0.5 mg/kg every 24 hours
7. 9.8 mg/day
8. at least 30 minutes
9. 125 mg/5 mL
10. 200,000 units/ 5 mL
11. 117 mL
12. water
13. 15–56 mg/kg
14. 93–347 mg
15. 110–409 mg/ daily
16. 40–147 mg/dose; the 125 ordered is correct
17. 910 mg/day
18. 303 mg/dose
19. yes
20. Add 53 mL water in two portions. Shake well after each addition until mixed.
21. Shake well to mix completely before pouring; administer immediately to prevent settling out.
22. 5 mg/kg
23. 307 mg
24. 818 mg
25. 20 mg/kg
26. 1 hour
27. No rapid or bolus injection; no intramuscular or subcutaneous injection
28. 18,000–27,000 mg daily
29. 3–4.5 g/dose
30. no
31. 4 mg/kg
32. 742 mg daily
33. 400 mg daily
34. 371 mg/dose
35. 3 mg/kg per hour over 1–2 hours
36. not for IV bolus injection
37. 6 mg/kg
38. 3 mg/kg
39. minimum of three weeks and at least two weeks following resolution of symptoms
40. 109 mg
41. 55 mg
42. once daily
43. 12 mg/kg/day
44. 196 mg

16

ADULT AND PEDIATRIC DOSAGES BASED ON BODY SURFACE AREA

OBJECTIVES

The learner will:

1. calculate BSA using formulas for weight and height.

2. use BSA to calculate dosages.

3. assess the accuracy of dosages prescribed on the basis of BSA.

Body surface area (BSA or SA) is a major factor in calculating dosages for a number of drugs, because many of the body's physiologic processes are more closely related to body surface than they are to weight. Body surface is used extensively to calculate dosages of antineoplastic agents for cancer chemotherapy, and for patients with severe burns. However, increasing numbers of other drugs are also calculated using BSA. **The nursing responsibility for checking dosages based on BSA varies widely in clinical facilities; therefore, this chapter covers all three essentials: calculation of BSA, calculation of dosages based on BSA, and assessment of physician orders based on BSA.**

Body surface is calculated in **square meters (m²)** using the patient's **weight and height** and a calculator that has **square root ($\sqrt{\ }$)** capabilities. Two formulas are used by physicians and pharmacists: one using kg and cm measurements, and another using lb (pound) and in (inch) measurements. We'll look at these separately.

CALCULATING BSA FROM kg AND cm

The safest way to calculate BSA is by using a time-tested formula with kilogram and centimeter measurements.

$$BSA = \sqrt{\frac{wt\,(kg) \times ht\,(cm)}{3600}}$$

EXAMPLE 1 Calculate the BSA of a man who weighs **104 kg** and whose height is **191 cm**. Express BSA to the nearest hundredth.

$$\sqrt{\frac{104\,(kg) \times 191\,(cm)}{3600}}$$

$$= \sqrt{5.517}$$

$$= 2.348 = \mathbf{2.35\ m^2}$$

Calculators vary in the way a square root must be obtained. Here is how the BSA was calculated in this example and throughout the chapter:

$$104. \times 191. \div 3600. = 5.517,\ \text{then immediately enter } \sqrt{}$$

Practice with your own calculator to determine how to calculate a square root. Be careful to **insert periods after all whole numbers** or you may obtain a wrong answer from preset decimal placement.

   The m² BSA is rounded to hundredths. Answers may vary slightly depending on how your calculator is set. Consider answers within 2–3 hundredths correct. Fractional weights and heights are also used in calculations. Refer to Examples 2 and 3.

EXAMPLE 2 Calculate the BSA of an adolescent who weighs **59.1 kg** and is **157.5 cm** in height. Express BSA to the nearest hundredth.

$$\sqrt{\frac{59.1\,(kg) \times 157.5\,(cm)}{3600}}$$

$$= \sqrt{2.585}$$

$$= 1.607 = \mathbf{1.61\ m^2}$$

EXAMPLE 3 A child is **96.2 cm** tall and weighs **15.17 kg**. What is his BSA in m² to the nearest hundredth?

$$\sqrt{\frac{15.17\,(kg) \times 96.2\,(cm)}{3600}}$$

$$= \sqrt{0.4053}$$

$$= 0.636 = \mathbf{0.63\ m^2}$$

▶▶▶ PROBLEMS 16.1

Calculate the BSA in m². Express answers to the nearest hundredth.

1. An adult weighing 59 kg whose height is 160 cm. _____

2. A child weighing 35.9 kg whose height is 63.5 cm. _____

3. A child weighing 7.7 kg whose height is 40 cm. _____

4. An adult weighing 92 kg whose height is 178 cm. _____

5. A child weighing 46 kg whose height is 102 cm. _____

Answers 1. 1.62 m² **2.** 0.8 m² **3.** 0.29 m² **4.** 2.13 m² **5.** 1.14 m²

CALCULATING BSA FROM lb AND in

The formula for calculating BSA from lb and in measurements is equally easy to use. **The only difference is the denominator, which is 3131.**

$$\text{BSA} = \sqrt{\frac{\text{wt (lb)} \times \text{ht (in)}}{3131}}$$

EXAMPLE 1 Calculate BSA to the nearest hundredth for a child who is **24 in** tall and weighs **34 lb.**

$$\sqrt{\frac{34\,(\text{lb}) \times 24\,(\text{in})}{3131}}$$

$$= \sqrt{0.260}$$

$$= 0.510 = \textbf{0.51 m}^2$$

EXAMPLE 2 Calculate BSA to the nearest hundredth for an adult who is **61.3 in** tall and weighs **142.7 lb.**

$$\sqrt{\frac{142.7\,(\text{lb}) \times 61.3\,(\text{in})}{3131}}$$

$$= \sqrt{2.793}$$

$$= 1.671 = \textbf{1.67 m}^2$$

EXAMPLE 3 A child weighs **105 lb** and is **51 in** tall. Calculate BSA to the nearest hundredth.

$$\sqrt{\frac{105\,(\text{lb}) \times 51\,(\text{in})}{3131}}$$

$$= \sqrt{1.710}$$

$$= 1.307 = \textbf{1.31 m}^2$$

▶▶▶ PROBLEMS 16.2

Determine the BSA. Express answers to the nearest hundredth.

1. A child weighing 92 lb who measures 35 in. _____

2. An adult who weighs 175 lb and who is 67 in tall. _____

3. An adult who is 70 in tall and weighs 194 lb. _____

4. A child who weighs 72.4 lb and is 40.5 in tall.   _____

5. A child who measures 26 in and weighs 36 lb.   _____

Answers 1. 1.01 m² **2.** 1.94 m² **3.** 2.08 m² **4.** 0.97 m² **5.** 0.55 m²

DOSAGE CALCULATION BASED ON BSA

Once you know the BSA in m², dosage calculation is straight multiplication.

EXAMPLE 1   Dosage recommended is **5 mg per m²**. The child has a BSA of **1.1 m²**.

$$1.1 (m^2) \times 5 \text{ mg} = \textbf{5.5 mg}$$

EXAMPLE 2   The recommended child's dosage is 25–50 mg/m². The child has a BSA of **0.76 m²**.

Lower dosage $0.76 (m^2) \times 25 \text{ mg} = 19 \text{ mg}$

Upper dosage $0.76 (m^2) \times 50 \text{ mg} = 38 \text{ mg}$

The dosage range is 19–38 mg.

▶▶▶ PROBLEMS 16.3

Determine the dosage for the following drugs. Express answers to the nearest whole number.

1. The recommended child's dosage is 5–10 mg/m².
   The BSA is 0.43 m².   _____

2. A child with a BSA of 0.81 m² is to receive a drug with a
   recommended dosage of 40 mg/m².   _____

3. Calculate the recommended dosage of 20 mg/m² for a
   child with a BSA of 0.51 m².   _____

4. An adult is to receive a drug with a recommended
   dosage of 20–40 units/m². The BSA is 1.93 m².   _____

5. The adult recommended dosage is 3–5 mg/m².
   Calculate dosage for 2.08 m².   _____

Answers 1. 2–4 mg **2.** 32 mg **3.** 10 mg **4.** 39–77 units **5.** 6–10 mg

ASSESSING ORDERS BASED ON BSA

In situations where you will have to check a dosage against m² recommendations, you will be referring to drug package inserts, medication protocols, or the *Physicians' Desk Reference* (*PDR*) to determine what the dosage should be.

EXAMPLE 1 Refer to the vinblastine information insert in Figure 16-1 and calculate the **first dose** for an adult whose BSA is **1.66 m²**. Calculations are to the nearest whole number.

Recommended first dose = 3.7 mg/m²

$1.66(m^2) \times 3.7\ mg = 6.14 = $ **6 mg**

EXAMPLE 2 A child with a BSA of 0.96 m² is to receive her **fourth dose** of vinblastine.

Recommended fourth dose = 6.25 mg/m²

$0.96(m^2) \times 6.25\ mg = $ **6 mg**

cetus oncology

STERILE VINBLASTINE SULFATE, USP

DOSAGE AND ADMINISTRATION
Caution: It is extremely important that the needle be properly positioned in the vein before this product is injected.

If leakage into surrounding tissue should occur during intravenous administration of vinblastine sulfate, it may cause considerable irritation. The injection should be discontinued immediately, and any remaining portion of the dose should then be introduced into another vein. Local injection of hyaluronidase and the application of moderate heat to the area of leakage help disperse the drug and are thought to minimize discomfort and the possibility of cellulitis.

There are variations in the depth of the leukopenic response which follows therapy with vinblastine sulfate. For this reason, it is recommended that the drug be given no more frequently than *once every 7 days*. It is wise to initiate therapy for adults by administering a single intravenous dose of 3.7 mg/M² of body surface area (bsa); the initial dose for children should be 2.5 mg/M². Thereafter, white-blood-cell counts should be made to determine the patient's sensitivity to vinblastine sulfate. A reduction of 50% in the dose of vinblastine is recommended for patients having a direct serum bilirubin value above 3 mg/100 mL. Since metabolism and excretion are primarily hepatic, no modification is recommended for patients with impaired renal function.

A simplified and conservative incremental approach to dosage *at weekly intervals* may be outlined as follows:

	Adults		Children	
First dose	3.7	mg/M² bsa	2.5	mg/M² bsa
Second dose	5.5	mg/M² bsa	3.75	mg/M² bsa
Third dose	7.4	mg/M² bsa	5	mg/M² bsa
Fourth dose	9.25	mg/M² bsa	6.25	mg/M² bsa
Fifth dose	11.1	mg/M² bsa	7.5	mg/M² bsa

The above-mentioned increases may be used until a maximum dose (not exceeding 18.5 mg/M² bsa for adults and 12.5 mg/M² bsa for children) is reached. The dose should not be increased after that dose which reduces the white-cell count to approximately 3000 cells/mm³. In some adults, 3.7 mg/M² bsa may produce this leukopenia; other adults may require more than 11.1mg/M² bsa; and, very rarely, as much as 18.5 mg/M² bsa may be necessary. For most adult patients, however, the weekly dosage will prove to be 5.5 to 7.4 mg/M² bsa.

▲ FIGURE 16-1

▶▶▶ PROBLEMS 16.4

Calculate the following dosages of vinblastine to the nearest whole number from the information available in Figure 16-1.

1. Calculate the dosage for an adult's third dose.
    The patient's BSA is 1.91 m². _____

2. Calculate the child's first dosage for a patient with
    a BSA of 1.2 m². _____

3. Calculate the adult's fifth dosage. The BSA is 1.53 m². _____

4. Calculate the child's second dosage for a BSA of 1.01 m². _____

5. Calculate the adult's second dose for a BSA of 2.12 m². _____

Answers **1.** 14 mg **2.** 3 mg **3.** 17 mg **4.** 4 mg **5.** 12 mg

▶▶▶ PROBLEMS 16.5

Refer to Figure 16-2 for BiCNU˙ to locate the following information. Express all dosages to the nearest whole number.

1. What is the dosage per m² if the drug is to be given
    in a single dose? _____

2. If the patient has a BSA of 1.91 m², what will the
    daily dosage range be? _____

3. If the order for this patient is a single dosage of 325 mg,
    is there any need to question it? _____

4. If the dosage ordered is 450 mg, is there any need to question it? _____

BiCNU ®
(carmustine for injection)

DOSAGE AND ADMINISTRATION
The recommended dose of BiCNU as a single agent in previously un-treated patients is 150 to 200 mg/m² intravenously every 6 weeks. This may be given as a single dose or divided into daily injections such as 75 to 100 mg/m² on 2 successive days. When BiCNU is used in combination with other myelosuppressive drugs or in pa-tients in whom bone marrow reserve is depleted, the doses should be adjusted accordingly.

▲ FIGURE 16-2

Answers **1.** 150–200 mg/m² **2.** 287–382 mg **3.** no **4.** yes, too high

PROBLEMS 16.6

Refer to the package insert for the antineoplastic medication bleomycin in Figure 16-3 to answer the following questions.

1. Locate the dosage information on Hodgkin's disease and identify the dosage per m^2.   _____

2. This insert also identifies the dosage per kg. What is this dosage?   _____

3. Calculate the unit dosage based on m^2 for an adult with a BSA of 1.73 m^2.   _____

4. How often is the dosage recommended?   _____

BEDFORD LABORATORIES™

BLEOMYCIN FOR INJECTION USP

BLE-P03

Rx ONLY

To reduce the development of drug-resistant bacteria and maintain the effectiveness of bleomycin and other antibacterial drugs, bleomycin should be used only to treat or prevent infections that are proven or strongly suspected to be caused by bacteria.

WARNING

It is recommended that bleomycin be administered under the supervision of a qualified physician experienced in the use of cancer chemotherapeutic agents. Appropriate management of therapy and complications is possible only when adequate diagnostic and treatment facilities are readily available.

Pulmonary fibrosis is the most severe toxicity associated with bleomycin. The most frequent presentation is pneumonitis occasionally progressing to pulmonary fibrosis. Its occurrence is higher in elderly patients and in those receiving greater than 400 units total dose, but pulmonary toxicity has been observed in young patients and those treated with low doses.

A severe idiosyncratic reaction consisting of hypotension, mental confusion, fever, chills, and wheezing has been reported in approximately 1% of lymphoma patients treated with bleomycin.

DOSAGE AND ADMINISTRATION

Because of the possibility of an anaphylactoid reaction, lymphoma patients should be treated with 2 units or less for the first two doses. If no acute reaction occurs, then the regular dosage schedule may be followed.

The following dose schedule is recommended:

Squamous cell carcinoma, non-Hodgkin's lymphoma, testicular carcinoma—0.25 to 0.50 units/kg (10 to 20 units/m²) given intravenously, intramuscularly, or subcutaneously weekly or twice weekly.

Hodgkin's Disease—0.25 to 0.50 units/kg (10 to 20 units/m²) given intravenously, intramuscularly, or subcutaneously weekly or twice weekly. After a 50% response, a maintenance dose of 1 unit daily or 5 units weekly intravenously or intramuscularly should be given.

Pulmonary toxicity of bleomycin appears to be dose related with a striking increase when the total dose is over 400 units. Total doses over 400 units should be given with great caution.

Note: When bleomycin for injection is used in combination with other antineoplastic agents, pulmonary toxicities may occur at lower doses.

Improvement of Hodgkin's Disease and testicular tumors is prompt and noted within 2 weeks. If no improvement is seen by this time, improvement is unlikely Squamous cell cancers respond more slowly, sometimes requiring as long as 3 weeks before any improvement is noted.

Malignant Pleural Effusion—60 units administered as a single dose bolus intrapleural injection (see **Administration: Intrapleural**).

▲ **FIGURE 16-3**

Answers   1. 10–20 units/m²   **2.** 0.25–0.5 units/kg   **3.** 17–35 units   **4.** weekly or twice weekly

▶▶▶ **PROBLEMS 16.7**

Refer to the mitomycin package insert information in Figure 16-4 to answer the following questions.

1. This preparation is a combination of two different drugs. It is shipped in powdered form. How much diluent must be added to prepare a mitomycin 40 mg and mannitol 80 mg dosage strength?   _____

2. What kind of diluent is specified?   _____

3. What dosage is required in m^2?   _____

4. What mitomycin dosage will be required for an individual with a BSA of 1.73? _____

5. How will this be administered? _____

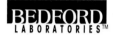

MITOMYCIN FOR INJECTION, USP
Rx ONLY.

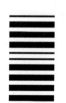

DOSAGE AND ADMINISTRATION

Mitomycin should be given intravenously only, using care to avoid extravasation of the compound. If extravasation occurs, cellulitis, ulceration, and slough may result.

Each vial contains either mitomycin 5 mg and mannitol 10 mg, or mitomycin 20 mg and mannitol 40 mg, or mitomycin 40 mg and mannitol 80 mg. To administer, add Sterile Water for Injection, 10 mL 40 mL, or 80 mL, respectively. Shake to dissolve. If product does not dissolve immediately, allow to stand at room temperature until solution is obtained.

After full hematological recovery (see guide to dosage adjustment) from any previous chemotherapy, the following dosage schedule may be used at 6- to 8-week intervals:

     20 mg/m² intravenously as a single dose via a functioning intravenous catheter.

Because of cumulative myelosuppression, patients should be fully reevaluated after each course of mitomycin, and the dose reduced if the patient has experienced any toxicities. Doses greater than 20 mg/m² have not been shown to be more effective and are more toxic than lower doses.

▲ **FIGURE 16-4**

Answers   **1.** 80 mL   **2.** sterile water for injection   **3.** mitomycin 20 mg/m²   **4.** 35 mg
5. intravenously as a single dose via a functioning intravenous catheter

Summary

This concludes the chapter on dosage calculation based on BSA. The important points to remember from this chapter are:

▼   The BSA in m² is calculated from a patient's weight and height.

▼   BSA is more important than weight alone in calculating some drug dosages because many physiologic processes are more closely related to surface area than they are to weight.

▼   BSA is calculated in square meters (m²) using a formula.

▼   Two formulas for calculation of BSA are available:

Using kg and cm: $\sqrt{\dfrac{\text{wt (kg)} \times \text{ht (cm)}}{3600}}$ Using lb and in: $\sqrt{\dfrac{\text{wt (lb)} \times \text{ht (in)}}{3131}}$

▼   After the BSA has been obtained, it can be used to calculate specific drug dosages and assess accuracy of physician orders.

Summary Self-Test

Use the formula method to calculate the following BSAs. Express m^2 to the nearest hundredth.

1. The weight is 58 lb and the height is 36 in. _____

2. An adult weighing 74 kg and measuring 160 cm. _____

3. A child who is 14.2 kg and measures 64 cm. _____

4. An adult weighing 69 kg whose height is 170 cm. _____

5. An adolescent who is 55 in and 103 lb. _____

6. A child who is 112 cm and weighs 25.3 kg. _____

7. An adult who weighs 55 kg and measures 157.5 cm. _____

8. An adult who weighs 65.4 kg and is 132 cm in height. _____

9. A child whose height is 58 in and whose weight is 26.5 lb. _____

10. A child whose height is 60 cm and weight is 13.6 kg. _____

Read the drug insert information provided in Figure 16-5 to answer the following questions. Calculate dosages to the nearest whole number.

11. Read the information on children's dosage to calculate the daily dosage for a 6-year-old child whose BSA is 0.78 m^2. _____

12. If a dosage of 4 mg is ordered for this 6-year-old child, would you question it? _____

13. What would the daily dosage be for a 4-year-old child whose BSA is 0.29 m^2? _____

14. What would the daily dosage be for a 5-year-old child with a BSA of 0.51 m^2? _____

Antibiotic

DOSAGE AND ADMINISTRATION

  DOSAGE SHOULD BE INDIVIDUALIZED ACCORDING TO THE NEEDS AND THE RESPONSE OF THE PATIENT.
  Each tablet contains 4 mg of antibiotic.

Pediatric Patients

Age 2 to 6 years
  The total daily dosage for pediatric patients may be calculated on the basis of body weight or body area using approximately 0.25 mg/kg/day or 8 mg per square meter of body surface (8 mg/m^2).
  The usual dose is 2 mg ($^1/_2$ tablet) two or three times a day, adjusted as necessary to the size and response of the patient. The dose is not to exceed 12 mg a day.

Age 7 to 14 years
  The usual dose is 4 mg (1 tablet) two or three times a day, adjusted as necessary to the size and response of the patient. The dose is not to exceed 16 mg a day.

Adults
  The total daily dose for adults should not exceed 0.5 mg/kg/day.
  The therapeutic range is 4 to 20 mg a day, with the majority of patients requiring 12 to 16 mg a day. An occasional patient may require as much as 32 mg a day for adequate relief. It is suggested that dosage be initiated with 4 mg (1 tablet) three times a day and adjusted according to the size and response of the patient.

© Cengage Learning 2015.

▲ **FIGURE 16-5**

Refer to Figure 16-6 to answer the following questions.

15. A patient is to be treated with the drug carboplatin for ovarian carcinoma. Her BSA is 1.61 m². What will her dosage be? _____

16. Another patient with ovarian cancer, who weighs 130 lb and measures 62 in, is to receive carboplatin. What is her BSA? _____

17. What dosage of carboplatin will she require? _____

18. Carboplatin is given in conjunction with cyclophosphamide. What is the recommended m² dosage for this drug? _____

19. Calculate the BSA of a third patient who is receiving therapy for ovarian cancer. She weighs 53.2 kg and measures 150.3 cm. _____

20. What will the companion dosage of cyclophosphamide be for this patient? _____

Manufactured by:
Ben Venue Laboratories, Inc.
Bedford, OH 44146

Manufactured for:
Bedford Laboratories™
Bedford, OH 44146

Patient Information
CARBOplatin for Injection

Read this entire leaflet carefully.
Keep it for future reference.

This information will help you learn more about CARBOplatin for Injection. It cannot, however, cover all the possible warnings or side effects relating to CARBOplatin, and it does not list all of the benefits and risks of CARBOplatin. Your doctor should always be your first choice for detailed information about your medical condition and your treatment. Be sure to ask your doctor about any questions you may have.

DOSAGE AND ADMINISTRATION
NOTE: Aluminum reacts with carboplatin causing precipitate formation and loss of potency, therefore, needles or intravenous sets containing aluminum parts that may come in contact with the drug must not be used for the preparation or administration of carboplatin.
Single Agent Therapy
Carboplatin for injection, as a single agent, has been shown to be effective in patients with recurrent ovarian carcinoma at a dosage of 360 mg/m² IV on day 1 every 4 weeks (alternatively see **Formula Dosing**). In general, however, single intermittent courses of carboplatin should not be repeated until the neutrophil count is at least 2000 and the platelet count is at least 100,000.
Combination Therapy with Cyclophosphamide
In the chemotherapy of advanced ovarian cancer, an effective combination for previously untreated patients consists of:
Carboplatin injection—300 mg/m² IV on day 1 every four weeks for six cycles (alternatively see **Formula Dosing**).
Cyclophosphamide—600 mg/m² IV on day 1 every four weeks for six cycles. For directions regarding the use and administration of cyclophosphamide please refer to its package insert. (See **CLINICAL STUDIES**.)

▲ FIGURE 16-6

Answers			
1. 0.82 m²	**6.** 0.89 m²	**11.** 6 mg per day	**16.** 1.6 m²
2. 1.81 m²	**7.** 1.55 m²	**12.** yes; too low	**17.** 576 mg
3. 0.50 m²	**8.** 1.55 m²	**13.** 2 mg per day	**18.** 600 mg/m²
4. 1.81 m²	**9.** 0.70 m²	**14.** 4 mg	**19.** 1.49 m²
5. 1.35 m²	**10.** 0.48 m²	**15.** 580 mg	**20.** 894 mg

SECTION

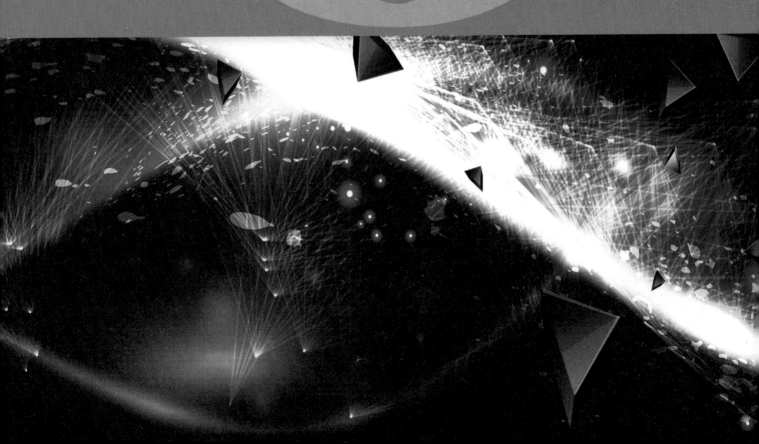

Intravenous Calculations

6

INTRODUCTION TO IV THERAPY

OBJECTIVES

The learner will:

1. differentiate among primary, secondary, peripheral, and central IV lines.

2. explain the function of IV drip chambers, roller and slide clamps, and on-line and indwelling injection ports.

3. differentiate between heparin flush and heparin admixture dosage strengths.

4. differentiate among volumetric pumps, syringe pumps, and PCAs.

5. identify the abbreviations used for IV fluid orders.

The calculations associated with IV therapy will be easier to understand if you have some general understanding of IV therapy. Intravenous fluid and medication administration is one of the most challenging of all nursing responsibilities. There are currently estimated to be over 200 different manufactured IV fluids, and at least as many additives are used with IV fluids, including medications, electrolytes, and nutrients. In addition, there are hundreds of different types of IV administration sets and components, and dozens of different models of electronic infusion devices (EIDs) to infuse and monitor IV fluids. This would appear to make the entire subject of IV therapy overwhelming, but it is not. This chapter presents the essentials in understandable segments and provides you with an excellent base of instruction upon which to build. Let's begin by looking at a basic sterile IV setup, which is referred to as a primary line.

KEY*point:* The choice of IV fluids and additives is a physician responsibility. The preparation of IVs containing additives is a pharmacist's, or specially designated and trained IV nurse practitioner's, responsibility. The staff nurse responsibility in almost all clinical settings will be to double-check for the correct solution, and set and regulate IV flow rates of the solutions ordered. Use of IV pumps is a hospital in-service education responsibility.

PRIMARY LINE

Refer to Figure 17-1, which shows a typical primary IV line connecting an IV fluid bag or bottle to the needle or cannula in a vein. The IV **tubing is connected to the IV solution bag** (using sterile technique), and the bag is hung on an IV stand.

KEY*point:* Close all roller clamps on the IV tubing before connecting it to the solution bag. This step prevents air bubbles from entering the tubing.

The **drip chamber**, Figure 17-1A, is then squeezed to **half-fill** it with fluid. This level is very important because **IV flow rates are set and**

monitored by counting the drops falling in this chamber. If the chamber is too full, the drops cannot be counted. On the other hand, if the outlet at the bottom of the chamber is not completely covered, air can enter the tubing during infusions and, subsequently, the vein and circulatory system. So, the half-full fluid level is extremely important.

 KEY*point:* The correct fluid level for IV drip chambers is half-full to allow drops to be counted and prevent air from entering the tubing.

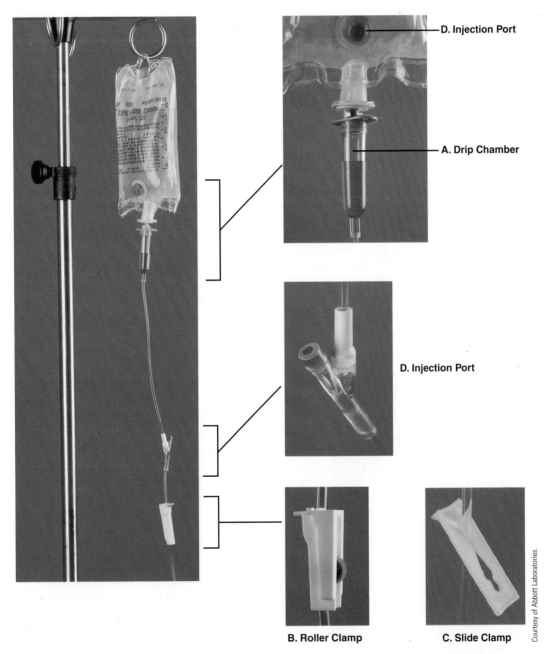

D. Injection Port

A. Drip Chamber

D. Injection Port

B. Roller Clamp

C. Slide Clamp

Courtesy of Abbott Laboratories.

▲ **FIGURE 17-1** IV tubing and solution bag.

Next, notice Figure 17-1B, the **roller clamp**. This is adjusted while the drops falling in the drip chamber are counted to **set the flow rate**. It provides an extremely accurate control of rate. A second type of clamp, Figure 17-1C, called a **slide clamp**, is present on all IV tubings. The **slide clamp** can be used to **temporarily stop an IV without disturbing the rate set** on the roller clamp.

Next, notice Figure 17-1D, the **injection port**. Rubber ports are located in several locations on the tubing, typically near the cannula end, drip chamber, and middle of the line, and also on most IV solution bags. **Ports allow injection of medication directly into the line or bag** or the **attachment to the primary line of secondary IV lines** containing compatible IV fluids or medications.

Intravenous fluids run by gravity flow. This necessitates that the IV solution bag be hung **above the patient's heart level** to exert sufficient pressure to infuse. Three feet above heart level is considered an average height.

KEY*point:* The higher an IV bag is hung, the greater the pressure and the faster the IV will infuse.

This pressure differential also means that if the flow rate is adjusted while the patient is lying in bed, it will slow down if he or she sits or stands, and, in fact, it changes slightly with each turn from side to side. For this reason, **monitoring IV flow rate is ongoing**, officially **done every hour**, but routinely checked **after each major position change**.

There are two additional terms relating to primary lines that you must know. If an arm or hand (or, less commonly, leg) vein is used for an infusion, it is referred to as a **peripheral line**. This is to distinguish it from a **central line**, which uses a special catheter whose tip is located centrally **in a deep chest vein**. Central lines may access the chest vein directly through the chest wall, via a neck vein, or through a peripheral vein in the arm or leg.

SECONDARY LINE

Secondary lines attach to the primary line at an injection port. They are used primarily **to infuse medications**, frequently on an intermittent basis; for example, every 6–8 hours. They may also be used to infuse other compatible IV fluids. Secondary lines are commonly referred to as **IV piggybacks**. They are abbreviated **IVPB**. Refer to Figure 17-2, which illustrates a primary and secondary line setup.

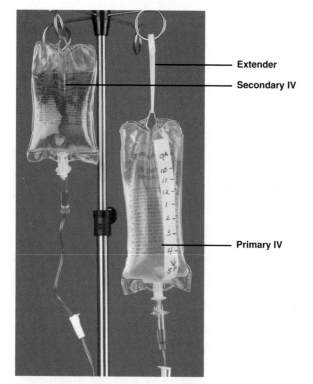

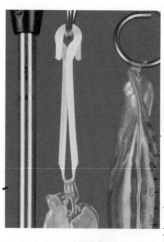

— Extender

— Secondary IV

— Primary IV

A. Extender

Courtesy of Abbott Laboratories.

▲ **FIGURE 17-2** Primary and secondary IV setup.

The IVPB is connected to a port located below the drip chamber on the primary line. Notice that **the IVPB bag is hanging higher than the primary**. This gives it greater pressure and causes it to **infuse first**. Each IVPB set includes a plastic or metal **extender**, in Figure 17-2 A, which is used to lower the primary solution bag to obtain this pressure differential. The flow rate for the IVPB is set by a separate roller clamp located on the secondary line. When the IVPB bag has emptied, the primary line will automatically resume its flow. Secondary medication bags are usually much smaller than primary bags. Fifty, 100, 150, 200, and 250 mL bags are frequently used.

Another type of secondary medication setup is provided by the Abbott Laboratories **ADD-Vantage System**® (Figure 17-3). In this system, a specially designed IV fluid bag that contains a **medication vial port** is used. The medication vial containing the ordered drug and dosage is inserted into the port, and the drug (frequently in powdered form) is mixed using IV fluid as the diluent, as illustrated in Figure 17-4. The vial contents are then displaced back into the solution bag and thoroughly mixed in the total solution before infusion. The vial remains in the solution bag port throughout the infusion, making it possible to cross-check the vial label for drug and dosage at any time.

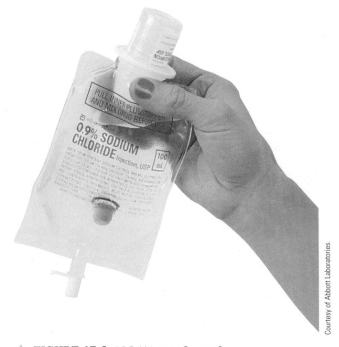

Courtesy of Abbott Laboratories.

▲ **FIGURE 17-3** ADD-Vantage System®.

If a drug is not available in either a prepackaged or ADD-Vantage format, it is often prepared and labeled by the hospital pharmacy. And, finally, an IV medication may be prepared, added to the appropriate IV fluid, thoroughly mixed, labeled and initialed, and administered by the nurse who initiates the infusion.

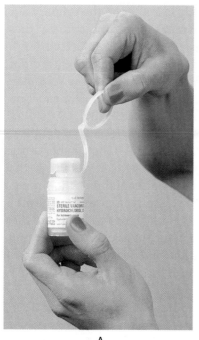

A

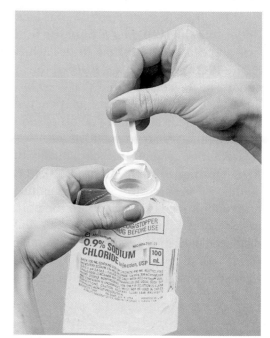

B

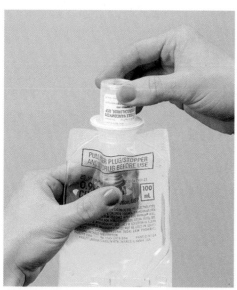

C

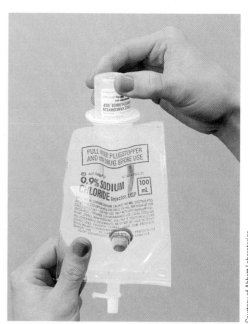

D

Courtesy of Abbott Laboratories.

▲ **FIGURE 17-4** ADD-Vantage® System **A**, The ADD-Vantage® medication vial is opened first. **B**, The medication vial port on the IV bag is opened. **C**, The vial top is inserted into the IV bag port and twisted to lock tightly in place. **D**, The vial stopper is removed "inside" the IV bag, and the medication and solution are thoroughly mixed before infusion.

VOLUME-CONTROLLED BURETTES

For greater accuracy in the measurement of **small-volume** IV medications and fluids, a **calibrated burette chamber** such as the one shown in Figure 17-5 may be used. The total capacity of burettes varies from 100 to 150 mL, calibrated in 1 mL increments. Many burettes are calibrated to deliver very small drops (microdrops), which also contributes to their accuracy. Burettes are most often referred to by their trade names; for example, Buretrols,® Solusets,® or Volutrols®. Burette chambers are most often connected to a secondary solution bag and used as a secondary line, but they can also be primary lines. When medication is ordered, it is injected into the burette through its injection port. The exact amount of IV fluid is then added as a diluent. After thorough mixing, the flow rate is set using a separate clamp on the burette line. Burettes are used extensively in pediatric and intensive care units, where medication dosages and fluid volumes are critical.

INDWELLING INFUSION PORTS/ INTERMITTENT LOCKS

When a continuous IV is not necessary, but intermittent IV medication administration is, an **infusion port adapter** (Figure 17-6) can be attached to an indwelling cannula in a vein. Infusion ports are frequently referred to as **heplocks** or **saline locks (or ports)**. This terminology evolved because the ports must be irrigated with 1–2 mL of sterile saline every 6–8 hours, or with a heparin lock flush solution (100 units/mL) to prevent clotting and blockage. To infuse medication, the port top is cleansed and the medication line is attached. When the infusion is complete, the line is disconnected until the next dosage is due. Ports are also used for **direct injection of medication using a syringe**, which is called an **IV push** or **bolus.**

Heparin anticoagulant therapy will be discussed in detail in a later chapter, where you will learn that heparin is most commonly diluted in large volume intravenous solutions for administration. **The heparin vial dosage strengths available for IV dilution range from 1000 to 50,000 units/mL**. Stop now, and think about the **enormous difference in dosage strengths between heparin flush solutions and intravenous admixture dosages: 10 to 100 units/mL for a flush; 1000 to 50,000 units/mL for IV admixes.**

These large differences in dosage strength demonstrate why **extreme caution is necessary in heparin flush dosage preparation.**

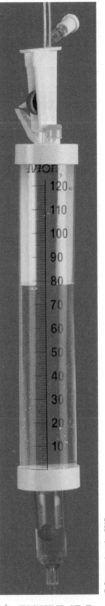

© Cengage Learning 2015.

▲ **FIGURE 17-5**
A calibrated burette chamber.

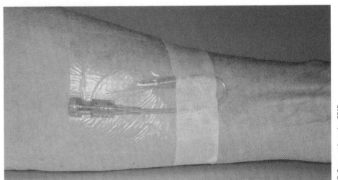

© Cengage Learning 2015.

▲ **FIGURE 17-6** An infusion port adapter.

HEPARIN FLUSH DOSAGE ALERT

Heparin flush solutions used to maintain patent (open) indwelling infusion ports come in **two dosage strengths: 10 units/mL and 100 units/mL.** Refer to the Heparin Lock Flush vial label in Figure 17-7 and identify its 10 units/mL strength.

In early 2008, errors in heparin flush dosages became national news when actor Dennis Quaid publicized the near-death of his newborn twins by not one, but two successive errors in flush dosages, which caused the newborns to almost hemorrhage to death.

Thanks to Mr. Quaid, this error was taken all the way to a Congressional hearing to publicize the danger. Similar heparin vial size and label colors were cited as contributing to the errors. But the fact remains that **these errors in dosage were caused by failure to correctly identify label dosage strengths,** not vial size or label color.

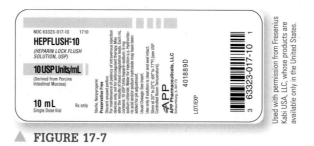

▲ FIGURE 17-7

KEY*point:* The average heparin flush dosage strength is 10 units and never exceeds 100 units.

▶▶▶ PROBLEMS 17.1

Answer the questions about IV administration sets as briefly as possible.

1. What is the correct fluid level for an IV drip chamber? _____

2. Which clamp is used to regulate IV flow rate? _____

3. When might a slide clamp be used? _____

4. What is a peripheral line? _____

5. What is a central line? _____

6. What is the common abbreviation for an intravenous piggyback? _____

7. Is the IVPB a primary or secondary line? _____

8. What must the height of a primary solution bag be when a secondary bag is infusing? _____

9. When is a saline lock used? _____

10. What are the two strengths of heparin flush solutions available? _____

Answers **1.** middle of chamber **2.** roller clamp **3.** stop the IV temporarily without disturbing the rate set on the roller clamp **4.** arm or leg vein **5.** IV catheter inserted into a deep chest vein **6.** IVPB **7.** secondary **8.** lower than secondary bag **9.** for intermittent infusions when a continuous IV is not necessary **10.** 10 units/mL and 100 units/mL

VOLUMETRIC PUMPS

Refer now to Figure 17-8 of the Alaris® SE Dual pump. Notice that the IV tubing with the AccuSlide® flow regulator has been inserted into the channels on the right and left. The center pumping mechanism maintains the desired flow rates.

All volumetric pumps look similar, and may physically resemble the Alaris SE pump, but the **functions of different models vary widely**. Some models continue to pump fluids even if an IV infiltrates, whereas others have a built-in pressure sensor that will sound an alarm if a resultant increased infusion resistance pressure occurs. Some models sound an alarm when the solution has completely infused; other models do not.

Because of the wide variation in pump models and their functions, caution is mandatory when they are used. It is estimated that a significant number of IV medication errors results from errors in pump programming.

KEY*point:* Hospital or clinical in-service education is required for the use of all infusion devices.

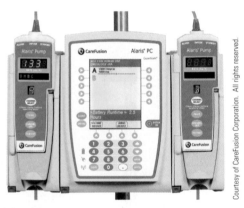

▲ **FIGURE 17-8** Alaris® Dual Pump.

Infusion devices are also widely used for IV medication administration, and their precautions in use apply less to the difficulty of the skill than in becoming familiar with the particular infusion model being used. A single hospital or clinic could realistically have a dozen different models in use, and it is an ongoing nursing responsibility to learn how to use each particular model.

KEY*point:* Double-checking of programming is mandatory in the use of infusion devices.

Because errors in infusion device programming are factors in IV medication errors, it is mandatory that all programming be double-checked. A new generation of sophisticated infusion safety systems has built-in libraries of usual drug dosages, offers customizable drug libraries for facility-specific needs, and is capable of alerting users to programming errors outside hospital-defined parameters. The Sigma Spectrum from Baxter shown in Figure 17-9 is one example. Another dose-specific pump is the Alaris System with Guardrails® Suite MX of safety software shown in Figure 17-10, a lightweight, modular platform that integrates infusion, patient monitoring, and clinical best-practice guidelines. As you can clearly see from the photograph, this is an infusion device that requires in-service instruction and certification to use.

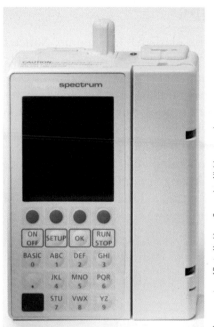

▲ **FIGURE 17-9** Sigma Spectrum Electronic Infusion device.

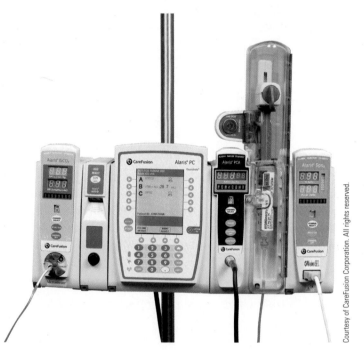

▲ **FIGURE 17-10**   Alaris® System from CareFusion featuring the Alaris PCA module, Auto-ID module and Alaris EtCO2 and SpO2 monitoring modules.

SYRINGE PUMPS

Syringe pumps, as their name implies, are devices that **use a syringe to administer medications or fluids** (Figure 17-11). Syringe pumps are particularly valuable when **drugs that cannot be mixed with other solutions or medications must be administered at a controlled rate over a short period of time**; for example, 5, 10, or 20 minutes. The drug is measured in the syringe, which is inserted into the device, and the medication is infused at the rate set.

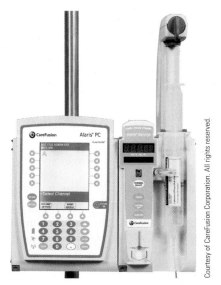

▲ **FIGURE 17-11** Alaris® System with syringe module.

PATIENT-CONTROLLED ANALGESIA (PCA) DEVICES

PCA devices allow a patient to **self-administer medication to control pain**. A prefilled syringe or medication bag containing pain medication is inserted into the device (Figure 17-12), and the **dosage and frequency of administration ordered are set**. The patient presses the control button as medication is needed, and the medication is administered and recorded by the PCA.

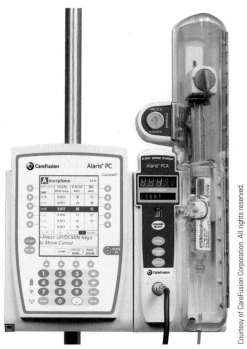

▲ **FIGURE 17-12** Alaris® Systems with CareFusion PCA Pump.

The device also keeps a record of the number of times a patient **attempts** to use it and thus provides a record of the effectiveness of the dosage prescribed. If a patient's pain is not being relieved, new orders must be obtained and the PCA reset to administer the new dosage.

 KEY*point:* All electronic devices must be monitored frequently to be sure they are functioning properly.

Is the IV infusing at the rate that was set? Is the patient who activates a PCA getting relief of pain? If not, is it possible the PCA itself is malfunctioning? Electronic devices have been in use for many years and are relatively trouble-free, but if the desired goal is not being obtained, in the absence of other obvious reasons, **the possibility of malfunction must always be considered**.

▶▶▶ PROBLEMS 17.2

Answer the questions about infusion devices as briefly as possible.

1. What is the function of a volumetric pump? _____
2. List two major precautions in the use of volumetric pumps. _____
3. When might a syringe pump be used? _____
4. What is a PCA? _____

Answers 1. to administer IVs at a controlled rate **2.** accurate programming; rate and site monitoring
3. to infuse small volumes of drugs that are not compatible with other drugs and/or fluids
4. patient-controlled analgesia device

INTRODUCTION TO IV FLUIDS

Intravenous fluids are prepared in plastic solution bags or glass bottles in volumes ranging from 50 mL (bags only) to 1000 mL. The 500 and 1000 mL sizes are the most commonly used. The bags and bottles are labeled with the **complete name** of the fluid they contain, and the fine print under the solution name identifies the exact amount of each component of the fluid. **Orders and charting**, however, are done **using abbreviations**.

 KEY*point:* In IV fluid abbreviations, D identifies dextrose; W identifies water; S identifies saline; NS identifies normal saline; and numbers identify percentage (%) strengths.

Solutions may be abbreviated in different ways; for example, D5W, 5%D/W, D5%W, or other combinations. But the **initials and percentage have the identical meaning regardless of the way they are abbreviated**. Normal saline solutions are frequently written with the 0.9, or % sign included; for example, D5 0.9NS, or D5 0.9%S. Solutions with different percentages of saline are also available: 0.45%, often written as ½ (0.45% is half of 0.9%), and 0.225%, sometimes written as ¼ (¼ of 0.9) are examples. Some typical orders might be abbreviated D5 ½S or D5 ¼NS.

Another commonly used solution is **Ringer's lactate**, a balanced electrolyte solution, which is also called Lactated Ringer's Solution. As you would now expect, this solution is abbreviated **RL**, **LR**, or **RLS**. Electrolytes may also be added to the basic fluids (DW and DS) just discussed. One electrolyte so commonly added that it must be mentioned is **potassium chloride**, which is abbreviated **KCl**. It is measured in milliequivalents (**mEq**).

▶▶▶ PROBLEMS 17.3

List the components and percentage strengths of the IV solutions.

1. D10NS   _____

2. D5NS   _____

3. D2.5 ½S   _____

4. D5 ¼S   _____

5. D20W   _____

6. D5NS 20 mEq KCl _____

7. D5RL   _____

Answers   1. 10% dextrose in 0.9% saline   **2.** 5% dextrose in normal (0.9%) saline   **3.** 2.5% dextrose in 0.45% saline   **4.** 5% dextrose in 0.225% saline   **5.** 20% dextrose in water   **6.** 5% dextrose in 0.9% saline with 20 mEq potassium chloride   **7.** 5% dextrose in Ringer's lactate solution

PERCENTAGES IN IV FLUIDS

You will recall that **percent means grams of drug per 100 mL of fluid**. This means that a 5% dextrose solution will have 5 g of dextrose in each 100 mL. A 500 mL bag of a 5% solution will contain 5 g × 5, or 25 g of dextrose, whereas 500 mL of a 10% solution contains 10 g × 5, or 50 g of dextrose. The fine print on IV labels always lists the name and amount of all ingredients.

The Ringer's lactate solution in Figure 17-13 illustrates this very well. Take a minute to read the components of this solution.

The point being made here is that **percentages make IV fluids significantly different from each other**. As with drugs, reading labels and making sure the IVs are administered as ordered is critically important.

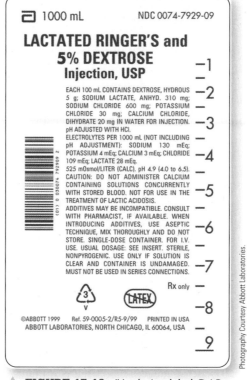

▲ **FIGURE 17-13**   IV solution label: D_5LR.

PARENTERAL NUTRITION

One of the options available for providing nutrition when a patient is unable to eat is to **administer a nutrient solution via a central vein**. This is referred to as parenteral nutrition. The solutions infused are generally of a high caloric content and contain varying percentages of glucose, amino acids, and/or fat emulsions. A number of abbreviations/descriptions are used for parenteral nutrients. Some of the more common are **total parenteral nutrition (TPN)**, **partial parenteral nutrition (PPN)**, **and hyper-alimentation (nutrition in excess of maintenance needs)**. There is a noticeable difference in fluids that contain lipids (fat, intralipids) in that they are **opaque-white** in appearance, similar to nonfat milk. These fluids are normally **infused slowly**, but **not usually over a period of more than 24 hours because they can spoil and support bacterial growth**. All precautions applicable to IVs in general apply equally to parenteral nutrients, with more care necessary for the IV site to prevent infection. Flow rate and infusion time calculations covered in subsequent chapters are also applicable for parenteral nutrition solutions.

Summary

This concludes your introduction to IV therapy. The important points to remember from this chapter are:

▼ Sterile technique is used to set up all IV solutions, tubings, and devices.

▼ The correct fluid level for an IV drip chamber is half full.

▼ Injection ports on an IV line are used to connect secondary lines and to infuse medications.

▼ A peripheral line refers to an IV infusing in a hand, arm, or leg vein.

▼ A central line refers to an IV infusing into a deep chest vein.

▼ IVs flow by gravity pressure, and the higher the solution bag, the faster the IV will infuse.

▼ The average height for an IV solution bag above the patient's heart level is 3 feet.

▼ Secondary solution bags must hang higher than the primary bag to infuse first.

▼ Volume-controlled burettes are used for very exact measurements of IV medications and fluids.

▼ Intermittent infusion locks or ports are used to infuse IV medications or fluids on an intermittent basis when a continuous IV is not necessary.

▼ Infusion locks or ports may be irrigated with sterile saline, or heparin flush solutions not to exceed 10–100 units/mL.

▼ Volumetric pumps are electronic devices that force fluids into a vein under pressure and control infusion rates.

▼ Syringe pumps are used to infuse medications that cannot be mixed with other fluids or medications.

▼ Patient-controlled analgesia (PCA) devices allow a patient to self-administer pain medication.

▼ In IV fluid abbreviations, D identifies dextrose, W identifies water, S identifies saline, NS identifies normal saline, RL or LR identify Ringer's lactate solution, and numbers identify percentage (%) strengths.

Summary Self-Test

You are to assist with some IV procedures. Answer the situational questions concerning these procedures.

1. A patient is admitted and an IV of 1000 mL D5RL is started.
   These initials identify what type of solution? _____
   This is referred to as what type of IV line? _____

2. All roller clamps on the IV tubing are closed before connection to the solution bag. Why? _____

3. The IV is started in the back of the patient's left hand. This makes it what type of line? _____

4. You are asked to check the fluid level in the drip chamber, and you observe that it is correct, which is … _____

5. You are then asked to adjust the flow rate. You will use what type of clamp to do this? _____

6. It is decided to use an electronic infusion control device to administer this IV. The device used is a… _____

7. An IV antibiotic is ordered for the patient. This is sent from the pharmacy already prepared in a small-volume IV solution bag. The setup used to infuse this medication is referred to as an IV… _____

8. How is this abbreviated? _____

9. In order for the antibiotic to infuse first, how must it be hung in relation to the original solution bag? _____

10. Some days later, the patient's IV is to be discontinued, but he is to continue to receive IV antibiotics. What is the site used for this intermittent administration called? _____

11. The patient had a PCA in use for one day. What do these initials mean? What does this device control? _____ _____

Answer these as briefly as possible.

12. A small-volume IV medication is to be diluted in 20 mL and infused. This can be most accurately measured using a _____.

13. These devices are calibrated in _____ increments.

14. When an IV medication is injected directly into the vein via a port, it is called an IV_____ or _____.

15. What heparin dosage strengths are used for IV port flush? _____

16. Ports may be irrigated with _____ mL of _____ to prevent blockage every _____ hours.

17. In IV fluid abbreviations, D5NS identifies what IV fluid? _____

Answers

1. 5% dextrose in Ringer's lactate; primary
2. to prevent air from entering the tubing
3. peripheral
4. half full
5. roller
6. volumetric pump
7. piggyback
8. IVPB
9. higher
10. intermittent infusion port; saline or heparin lock
11. patient-controlled analgesia; administration of pain medication
12. calibrated burette
13. 1 mL
14. push or bolus
15. 10 units/mL or 100 units/mL
16. 1–2; normal saline; 6–8
17. 5% dextrose in normal saline

18

IV FLOW RATE CALCULATION

This chapter presents a number of ways to calculate IV flow rates: ratio and proportion, dimensional analysis, and the formula and division factor method.

Intravenous fluids are ordered on the basis of **mL/hr** to be administered; for example, 125 mL/hr. With the widespread use of electronic infusion devices that can be **set to deliver a mL/hr rate**, simply setting the rate ordered on the device and making sure it is working properly is all that is required for many infusions.

The most common flow rate calculation is necessary **when an infusion device is not being used**. It involves **converting a mL/hr order to the gtt/min rate necessary to infuse it**; for example, **1000 mL to infuse at 125 mL/hr** or **3000 mL/24 hr**.

IV TUBING CALIBRATION

The size of IV drops is regulated by the type of IV set being used, which is **calibrated in number of gtt/mL**. Unfortunately, not all sets (or their drop size) are the same. Each clinical facility uses at least two sizes of infusion sets: a standard **macrodrip set calibrated at 10, 15, or 20 gtt/mL** that is used for routine adult IV administrations, and a **microdrip set calibrated at 60 gtt/mL** which is used when more exact measurements are needed; for example, to infuse medications or in critical care and pediatric infusions. Figure 18-1 gives a graphic representation of the various drop/gtt sizes.

 KEYpoint: IV administration sets are calibrated in gtt/mL.

The **gtt/mL calibration of each IV infusion set is clearly printed on each package**, and the first step in calculating flow rates is to identify the gtt/mL calibration of the set to be used for an infusion.

OBJECTIVES

The learner will:

1. identify the calibrations in gtt/mL on IV administration sets.

2. calculate flow rates using ratio and proportion.

3. calculate flow rates using dimensional analysis.

4. calculate flow rates using the formula and division factor method.

5. recalculate flow rates to correct off-schedule infusions.

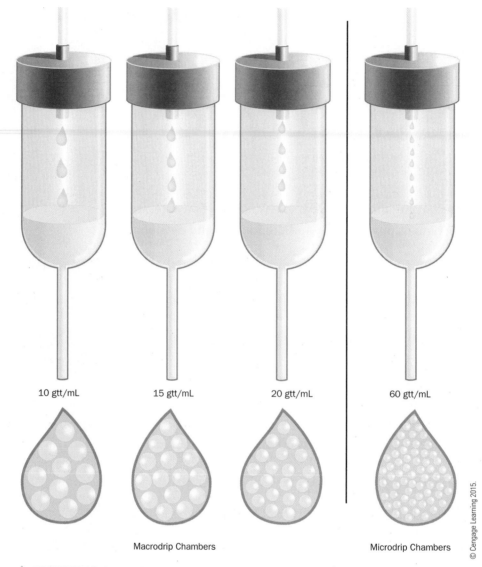

10 gtt/mL   15 gtt/mL   20 gtt/mL   60 gtt/mL

Macrodrip Chambers   Microdrip Chambers

© Cengage Learning 2015.

▲ **FIGURE 18-1** Comparative IV drop sizes.

▶▶▶ PROBLEMS 18.1

Identify the calibration in gtt/mL for each IV infusion set.

1. Figure 18-2 _____
2. Figure 18-3 _____

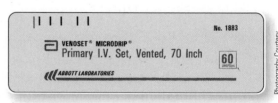

▲ **FIGURE 18-2**

Photography Courtesy
Abbott Laboratories.

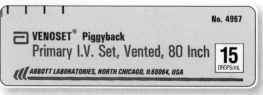

▲ **FIGURE 18-3**

Photography Courtesy
Abbott Laboratories.

3. Figure 18-4 _____

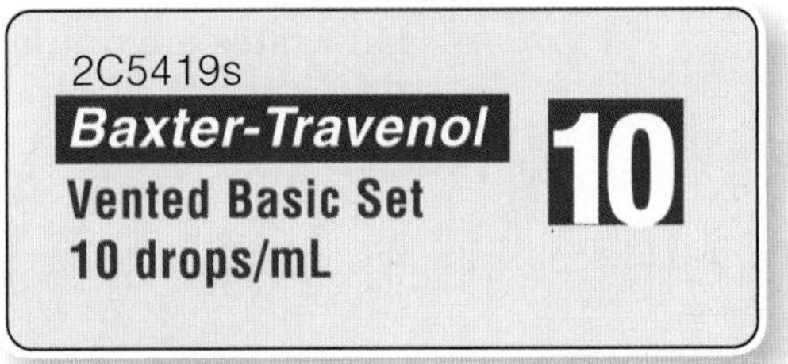

> 2C5419s
> **Baxter-Travenol**
> Vented Basic Set
> 10 drops/mL
>
> **10**

▲ **FIGURE 18-4**

Answers 1. 60 gtt/mL **2.** 15 gtt/mL **3.** 10 gtt/mL

USING RATIO AND PROPORTION TO CALCULATE gtt/min FLOW RATES

The flow rate in **gtt/min** is calculated from the **gtt/mL calibration of the IV set being used**, either 10, 15, 20, or 60 gtt/mL, and the **mL/hr ordered**.

EXAMPLE 1   An IV is ordered to infuse at a rate of **125 mL/hr** using a set calibrated at **10 gtt/mL**. Calculate the **gtt/min** flow rate.

You are calculating **gtt/min**. Start by converting **mL/hr** to **mL/min**. This is done by **dividing the 125 mL/hr rate by 60 min.**

- **Convert the 125 mL/hr ordered to mL/min.**

  125 mL ÷ 60 min = **2 mL/min**

- **Calculate the gtt/min rate for 2 mL/min. Enter the 10 gtt/mL set calibration as the first ratio in the proportion. The X gtt in 2 mL is entered next.**

$$\frac{10 \text{ gtt}}{1 \text{ mL}} = \frac{X \text{ gtt}}{2 \text{ mL}} = \textbf{20 gtt} \qquad \text{or} \quad 10 \text{ gtt} : 1 \text{ mL} = X \text{ gtt} : 2 \text{ mL}$$
$$X = \textbf{20 gtt}$$

To infuse an IV at 125 mL/hr using a set calibrated at 10 gtt/mL, set the drip rate at 20 gtt/min.

EXAMPLE 2   An IV of **150 mL** is to infuse in **1 hr** using a set calibrated at **15 gtt/mL**. Calculate the **gtt/min** flow rate.

- **Convert the 150 mL/hr to mL/min.**

  150 mL ÷ 60 min = **2.5 mL/min**

- **Calculate the gtt/min rate for 2.5 mL/min.**

$$\frac{15 \text{ gtt}}{1 \text{ mL}} = \frac{X \text{ gtt}}{2.5 \text{ mL}} = 37.5 = \textbf{38 gtt} \quad \text{or} \quad 15 \text{ gtt} : 1 \text{ mL} = X \text{ gtt} : 2.5 \text{ mL}$$
$$X = 37.5 = \textbf{38 gtt}$$

To infuse 150 mL/hr using a set calibrated at 15 gtt/mL, set the drip rate at 38 gtt/min.

KEY_point:_ Flow rates are routinely rounded to the nearest whole gtt.

Let's now look at some IVs ordered to infuse in more than 1 hour.

EXAMPLE 3 An IV of **2500 mL** is to infuse in **24 hr** using a **20 gtt/mL** calibrated set. Calculate the **gtt/min** flow rate.

- **Convert 2500 mL/24 hr to mL/hr.**

  2500 mL ÷ 24 hr = 104.1 = **104 mL/hr**

- **Convert the 104 mL/hr to mL/min.**

  104 mL ÷ 60 min = 1.73 = **1.7 mL/min**

- **Calculate the gtt/min rate for 1.7 mL/min.**

$$\frac{20 \text{ gtt}}{1 \text{ mL}} = \frac{X \text{ gtt}}{1.7 \text{ mL}} = \textbf{34 gtt} \quad \text{or} \quad 20 \text{ gtt} : 1 \text{ mL} = X \text{ gtt} : 1.7 \text{ mL}$$

$$X = \textbf{34 gtt}$$

To infuse an IV of 2500 mL in 24 hr using an IV set calibrated at 20 gtt/mL, set the flow rate at 34 gtt/min.

EXAMPLE 4 An IV of **1000 mL** is ordered to infuse in **5 hr** using a set calibrated at **15 gtt/mL**.

- **Convert 1000 mL/5 hr to mL/hr.**

  1000 mL ÷ 5 hr = **200 mL/hr**

- **Convert 200 mL/hr to mL/min.**

  200 mL ÷ 60 min = **3.3 mL/min**

- **Calculate the gtt/min rate for 3.3 mL/min.**

$$\frac{15 \text{ gtt}}{1 \text{ mL}} = \frac{X \text{ gtt}}{3.3 \text{ mL}} = 49.5 = \textbf{50 gtt} \quad \text{or} \quad 15 \text{ gtt} : 1 \text{ mL} = X \text{ gtt} : 3.3 \text{ mL}$$

$$X = 49.5 = \textbf{50 gtt}$$

To infuse 1000 mL in 5 hr using a set calibrated at 15 gtt/mL, set the rate at 50 gtt/min.

 KEY_point:_ Flow rate answers may vary by 1–2 gtt/min depending on how the numbers are rounded in calculations.

A 1–2 gtt/min variation is considered insignificant for most infusions, because flow rates fluctuate as the infusion limb is moved, or positional changes are made.

▶▶▶ PROBLEMS 18.2

Calculate gtt/min flow rates. Round to the nearest whole gtt.

1. An IV of 2000 mL is to infuse in 12 hr using a 10 gtt/mL set   _____

2. 3500 mL are ordered to infuse in 24 hr using a set calibrated at 20 gtt/mL   _____

3. Infuse 500 mL in 3 hr using a 15 gtt/mL set   _____

4. A volume of 1500 mL is to infuse in 5 hr using a 15 gtt/mL set   _____

5. 1750 mL are ordered to infuse in 9 hr using a 20 gtt/mL set   _____

6. An IV of 2500 mL is to infuse in 18 hr on a set calibrated at 10 gtt/mL   _____

7. A 3000 mL volume is to infuse in 24 hr on a set calibrated at 20 gtt/mL   _____

8. A volume of 2750 mL is to infuse in 22 hr on a 15 gtt/mL set   _____

9. An IV of 750 mL is ordered to infuse in 8 hr on a 10 gtt/mL set   _____

10. A volume of 1250 mL is to infuse in 12 hr using a 15 gtt/mL set   _____

Answers   **1.** 28 gtt/min   **2.** 49 gtt/min   **3.** 42 gtt/min   **4.** 75 gtt/min   **5.** 65 gtt/min   **6.** 23 gtt/min
7. 42 gtt/min   **8.** 31 gtt/min   **9.** 16 gtt/min   **10.** 26 gtt/min

NOTE: Continue with Using Dimensional Analysis to Calculate gtt/min Flow Rates or turn to *page 277 for the Formula and Division Factor Methods of Flow Rate Calculation.*

USING DIMENSIONAL ANALYSIS TO CALCULATE gtt/min FLOW RATES

The flow rate in **gtt/min** is calculated from the **calibration of the IV set being used**, either 10, 15, 20, or 60 gtt/mL, and the **mL/hr ordered**. You will immediately notice a difference from the previous DA calculations you have learned because **this calculation includes two values: gtt and min**. However, the DA calculation steps are identical.

EXAMPLE 1   Calculate a **gtt/min** flow rate to infuse **125 mL/hr** using a set calibrated at **10 gtt/mL**.

- Enter the **gtt/min** to be calculated as a **common fraction** followed by an equal sign.

$$\frac{gtt}{min} =$$

- **Begin ratio entries as if you were calculating only the gtt numerator**. Locate the ratio containing gtt—the 10 gtt/mL set calibration. Enter 10 gtt as the numerator to match the gtt numerator being calculated; 1 mL becomes the denominator.

$$\frac{gtt}{min} = \frac{10\ gtt}{1\ mL}$$

- Match the mL denominator with the 125 mL of the 125 mL/hr ordered; 1 hr becomes the denominator.

$$\frac{gtt}{min} = \frac{10\ gtt}{1\ mL} \times \frac{125\ mL}{1\ hr}$$

- Enter a **1 hr equals 60 min conversion ratio**, with 1 hr as the numerator and 60 min as the denominator. Notice that **the min being calculated falls automatically into place** as the final denominator to complete the equation.

$$\frac{gtt}{min} = \frac{10\ gtt}{1\ mL} \times \frac{125\ mL}{1\ hr} \times \frac{1\ hr}{60\ min}$$

- Cancel the mL/mL and hr/hr denominator/numerators to check for correct ratio entry. Do the math.

$$\frac{gtt}{min} = \frac{10\ gtt}{1\ \cancel{mL}} \times \frac{125\ \cancel{mL}}{1\ \cancel{hr}} \times \frac{1\ \cancel{hr}}{60\ min} = 20.8 = \textbf{21 gtt/min}$$

To infuse 125 mL/hr using a 10 gtt/mL infusion set, the flow rate is 21 gtt/min.

 KEY_point:_ Flow rates are rounded to the nearest whole gtt.

EXAMPLE 2   A **20 gtt/mL** set is used to infuse **90 mL/hr**. Calculate the **gtt/min** flow rate.

- Enter the gtt/min to be calculated followed by an equal sign.

$$\frac{gtt}{min} =$$

- Enter the 20 gtt/mL infusion set ratio with 20 gtt to match the gtt numerator being calculated; 1 mL becomes the denominator.

$$\frac{gtt}{min} = \frac{20\ gtt}{1\ mL}$$

- Match the mL denominator with the 90 mL of the mL/hr ordered; 1 hr is the new denominator.

$$\frac{gtt}{min} = \frac{20\ gtt}{1\ mL} \times \frac{90\ mL}{1\ hr}$$

- Enter a 1 hr equals 60 min conversion ratio, with 1 hr as the numerator and 60 min as the denominator, to complete the equation.

$$\frac{gtt}{min} = \frac{20\ gtt}{1\ mL} \times \frac{90\ mL}{1\ hr} \times \frac{1\ hr}{60\ min}$$

- Cancel the mL/mL and hr/hr denominator/numerators to check for correct ratio entry. Do the math.

$$\frac{gtt}{min} = \frac{20\ gtt}{1\ mL} \times \frac{90\ mL}{1\ hr} \times \frac{1\ hr}{60\ min} = 30\ gtt/min$$

To infuse 90 mL/hr using a set calibrated at 20 gtt/mL, the rate is 30 gtt/min.

EXAMPLE 3 Calculate the **gtt/min** rate to infuse **2500 mL** in **24 hr** using a **15 gtt/mL** infusion set.

- Enter the gtt/min to be calculated followed by an equal sign.

$$\frac{gtt}{min} =$$

- Enter the 15 gtt/mL infusion set ratio with 15 gtt to match the gtt numerator being calculated; 1 mL becomes the denominator.

$$\frac{gtt}{min} = \frac{15\ gtt}{1\ mL}$$

- Enter the 2500 mL/24 hr ordered with 2500 mL as the numerator to match the previous mL denominator. Enter 24 hr as the new denominator.

$$\frac{gtt}{min} = \frac{15\ gtt}{1\ mL} \times \frac{2500\ mL}{24\ hr}$$

- Enter a 1 hr equals 60 min conversion ratio, with 1 hr as the numerator and 60 min as the denominator, to complete the equation.

$$\frac{gtt}{min} = \frac{15\ gtt}{1\ mL} \times \frac{2500\ mL}{24\ hr} \times \frac{1\ hr}{60\ min}$$

- Cancel the mL/mL and hr/hr denominator/numerators to check for correct ratio entry. Do the math.

$$\frac{gtt}{min} = \frac{15\ gtt}{1\ mL} \times \frac{2500\ mL}{24\ hr} \times \frac{1\ hr}{60\ min} = 26.04 = \mathbf{26\ gtt/min}$$

To infuse 2500 mL in 24 hr using a 15 gtt/mL calibrated infusion set, the rate is 26 gtt/min.

EXAMPLE 4 Calculate the **gtt/min** rate to infuse **2000 mL** in **10 hr** using a **10 gtt/mL** IV infusion set.

- Enter the gtt/min to be calculated followed by an equal sign.

$$\frac{gtt}{min} =$$

- Enter the 10 gtt/mL infusion set ratio with 10 gtt as the numerator to match the gtt numerator being calculated; 1 mL becomes the denominator.

$$\frac{gtt}{min} = \frac{10\ gtt}{1\ mL}$$

- Enter the 2000 mL in 10 hr ordered with 2000 mL as the numerator to match the previous mL denominator; 10 hr is the next denominator to be matched.

$$\frac{gtt}{min} = \frac{10\ gtt}{1\ mL} \times \frac{2000\ mL}{10\ hr}$$

- Enter a 1 hr equals 60 min conversion ratio, with 1 hr as the numerator and 60 min as the denominator, to complete the equation.

$$\frac{gtt}{min} = \frac{10\ gtt}{1\ mL} \times \frac{2000\ mL}{10\ hr} \times \frac{1\ hr}{60\ min}$$

- Cancel the mL/mL and hr/hr denominator/numerators to check for correct ratio entry. Do the math.

$$\frac{gtt}{min} = \frac{10\ gtt}{1\ \cancel{mL}} \times \frac{2000\ \cancel{mL}}{10\ \cancel{hr}} \times \frac{1\ \cancel{hr}}{60\ min} = 33.3 = \mathbf{33\ gtt/min}$$

To infuse 2000 mL in 10 hr using a 10 gtt/mL calibrated infusion set, the rate is 33 gtt/min.

▶▶▶ PROBLEMS 18.3

Calculate gtt/min flow rates. Round to the nearest whole gtt.

1. An IV of 2000 mL is to infuse in 12 hr using a 10 gtt/mL set _____

2. 3500 mL are ordered to infuse in 24 hr using a set calibrated at 20 gtt/mL _____

3. Infuse 500 mL in 3 hr using a 15 gtt/mL set _____

4. A volume of 1500 mL is to infuse in 5 hr using a 15 gtt/mL set _____

5. 1750 mL are ordered to infuse in 9 hr using a 20 gtt/mL set _____

6. An IV of 2500 mL is to infuse in 18 hr on a set calibrated at 10 gtt/mL _____

7. A 3000 mL volume is to infuse in 24 hr on a set calibrated at 20 gtt/mL _____

8. A volume of 2750 mL is to infuse in 22 hr on a 15 gtt/mL set _____

9. An IV of 750 mL is ordered to infuse in 8 hr on a 10 gtt/mL set _____

10. A volume of 1250 mL is to infuse in 12 hr using a 15 gtt/mL set _____

Answers **1.** 28 gtt/min **2.** 49 gtt/min **3.** 42 gtt/min **4.** 75 gtt/min **5.** 65 gtt/min **6.** 23 gtt/min **7.** 42 gtt/min **8.** 31 gtt/min **9.** 16 gtt/min **10.** 26 gtt/min

FORMULA AND DIVISION FACTOR METHODS OF FLOW RATE CALCULATION

The **formula** and **division factor** methods are intrinsically related because **the division factor is derived from the formula method**. Let's start by looking at the formula method.

The formula method has a limitation in that it can **only be used if the flow rate is expressed as mL/hr (60 min) or less**; for example, 110 mL/60 min or 125 mL/60 min. It is especially suitable for small volume infusions to be completed in less than 60 min; for example, 30 mL in 20 min.

$$\text{Flow Rate} = \text{mL/hr} \; \frac{\text{Volume} \times \text{Set Calibration}}{\text{Time (60 min or less)}}$$

EXAMPLE 1 An IV is ordered to infuse at **125 mL/hr**. Calculate the **gtt/min** rate for a set calibrated at **10 gtt/mL**.

- **Convert the hr to 60 min.**

$$\frac{125 \,(\text{mL}) \times 10 \,(\text{gtt/mL})}{60 \,(\text{min})}$$

- **Calculate the gtt/min rate.**

$$\frac{125 \times 10}{60} = 20.8 = \textbf{21 gtt/min}$$

EXAMPLE 2 Administer an IV medication of **100 mL** in **40 min** using a set calibrated at **15 gtt/mL**.

$$\frac{100 \text{ mL} \times 15 \text{ gtt/mL}}{40 \text{ min}} = 37.5 = \textbf{38 gtt/min}$$

EXAMPLE 3 A **75 mL** volume of IV medication is ordered to infuse in **45 min**. The set is calibrated at **20 gtt/mL**.

$$\frac{75 \text{ mL} \times 20 \text{ gtt/mL}}{45 \text{ min}} = 33.3 = \textbf{33 gtt/min}$$

▶▶▶ PROBLEMS 18.4

Calculate the flow rate in gtt/min to the nearest whole drop using the formula method.

1. Administer an IV of 110 mL/hr using a set calibrated at 20 gtt/mL _____

2. An IV solution is ordered at 200 mL/hr using a set calibrated at 15 gtt/mL _____

3. A volume of 80 mL is to be infused in 20 min using a 10 gtt/mL set _____

4. An IV is ordered to infuse at 150 mL/hr using a 10 gtt/mL calibrated set _____

5. An IV rate of 90 mL/hr is ordered using a 15 gtt/mL calibrated set _____

6. An IV of 500 mL is to infuse at 120 mL/hr using a 20 gtt/mL calibrated set _____

7. A total of 90 mL is to infuse at 100 mL/hr using a 20 gtt/mL set   _____

8. A 15 gtt/mL set is used to infuse 120 mL at 80 mL/hr   _____

9. A rate of 60 mL/hr is ordered for a volume of 250 mL using a 10 gtt/mL set   _____

10. A medication volume of 50 mL is to infuse at 20 mL/hr using a 20 gtt/mL set   _____

Answers **1.** 37 gtt/min **2.** 50 gtt/min **3.** 40 gtt/min **4.** 25 gtt/min **5.** 23 gtt/min **6.** 40 gtt/min **7.** 33 gtt/min **8.** 20 gtt/min **9.** 10 gtt/min **10.** 7 gtt/min

When an IV is ordered to infuse in **more than 1 hour**, the formula method can still be used. However, it is necessary to add a preliminary step and determine the **mL/hr** the ordered volume will represent.

EXAMPLE 1   Calculate the gtt/min flow rate for an IV of **1000 mL** to infuse in **8 hr** on a set calibrated at **20 gtt/mL**.

- **Convert 1000 mL/8 hr to mL/hr.**

    1000 mL/8 hr = 1000 ÷ 8 = **125 mL/hr (60 min)**

- **Calculate the gtt/min flow rate.**

$$\frac{125 \, (\text{mL}) \times 20 \, (\text{gtt/mL})}{60 \, (\text{min})} = 41.6 = \textbf{42 gtt/min}$$

EXAMPLE 2   Calculate the gtt/min flow rate for a volume of **2500 mL** to infuse in **24 hr** on a set calibrated at **10 gtt/mL**.

- **Convert 2500 mL/24 hr to mL/hr.**

    2500 mL/24 hr = 2500 ÷ 24 = **104 mL/hr (60 min)**

- **Calculate the gtt/min flow rate.**

$$\frac{104 \, \text{mL} \times 10 \, \text{gtt/mL}}{60 \, \text{min}} = 17.3 = \textbf{17 gtt/min}$$

EXAMPLE 3   An IV of **1200 mL** is to infuse in **16 hr** on a set calibrated at **15 gtt/mL**.

1200 mL/16 hr = 1200 ÷ 16 = **75 mL/hr (60 min)**

$$\frac{75 \, \text{mL} \times 15 \, \text{gtt/mL}}{60 \, \text{min}} = 18.7 = \textbf{19 gtt/min}$$

▶▶▶ PROBLEMS 18.5

Calculate the gtt/min flow rate using the formula method.

1. A volume of 2000 mL to infuse in 24 hr on a set calibrated
   at 15 gtt/mL   _____

2. A volume of 300 mL to infuse in 6 hr on a 60 gtt/mL microdrip set   _____

3. A volume of 500 mL to infuse in 4 hr on a 15 gtt/mL calibrated set   _____

4. A 10 hr infusion of 1200 mL using a 20 gtt/mL set   _____

5. An infusion of 500 mL in 5 hr on a set calibrated at 10 gtt/mL   _____

6. A 2000 mL volume to infuse in 18 hr using a 20 gtt/mL set   _____

7. A 10 gtt/mL set to infuse 400 mL in 4 hr   _____

8. An 8 hr infusion of 1500 mL to use a set calibrated at 15 gtt/mL   _____

9. A volume of 250 mL to infuse in 2 hr using a 20 gtt/mL set   _____

10. A 5 hr infusion of 750 mL using a 10 gtt/mL set   _____

Answers 1. 21 gtt/min **2.** 50 gtt/min **3.** 31 gtt/min **4.** 40 gtt/min **5.** 17 gtt/min **6.** 37 gtt/min
7. 17 gtt/min **8.** 47 gtt/min **9.** 42 gtt/min **10.** 25 gtt/min

DIVISION FACTOR METHOD

The **division factor** is derived from the formula method, and it is invaluable for use in clinical facilities where **all the macrodrip infusion sets have the same calibration**—either 10, 15, or 20 gtt/mL. Once again, **this method can only be used if the rate is expressed in mL/hr (60 min)**. Let's start by looking at how the division factor is obtained.

$$\frac{mL \times gtt/mL}{60\ min} = gtt/min$$

EXAMPLE 1   Administer an IV at **125 mL/hr**. The set calibration is **10 gtt/mL**. Calculate the gtt/min rate. Express the hr rate as 60 min.

$$\frac{125\ (mL) \times \overset{1}{\cancel{10}}\ (gtt/mL)}{\underset{6}{\cancel{60}}\ (min)} = 20.8 = \textbf{21 gtt/min}$$

Look at the completed equation, and notice that because the time is restricted to 60 min, **the set calibration (10) will be divided into 60 (min) to obtain a constant number (6). This constant (6) is the division factor for a 10 gtt/mL calibrated set.**

 KEY *point:* The division factor can be obtained for any IV set by dividing 60 by the calibration of the set.

▶▶▶ PROBLEMS 18.6

Determine the division factor for these IV sets.

1. 20 gtt/mL _____

2. 15 gtt/mL _____

3. 60 gtt/mL _____

4. 10 gtt/mL _____

Answers **1.** 3 **2.** 4 **3.** 1 **4.** 6

Once the division factor is known, **the gtt/min rate can be calculated in one step by dividing the mL/hr rate by the division factor**. Look again at the example.

$$\frac{125\,(\text{mL}) \times \overset{1}{\cancel{10}}\,(\text{gtt/mL})}{\underset{6}{\cancel{60}}\,(\text{min})} = 20.8 = \textbf{21 gtt/min}$$

or 125 (mL/hr) ÷ **6** = 20.8 = **21 gtt/min**

The **125 mL/hr flow rate divided by the division factor 6 gives the same 21 gtt/min rate.**

 KEYpoint: The gtt/min flow rate can be calculated for mL/hr IV orders in one step by dividing the mL/hr to be infused by the division factor of the administration set.

EXAMPLE 1   Infuse an IV at **100 mL/hr** using a set calibrated at **10 gtt/mL**.

Determine the division factor: 60 ÷ 10 = **6**

Calculate the flow rate: 100 mL ÷ 6 = 16.6 = **17 gtt/min**

EXAMPLE 2   Infuse an IV at **125 mL/hr** using a set calibrated at **15 gtt/mL**.

60 ÷ 15 = 4   125 mL ÷ 4 = 31.2 = **31 gtt/min**

EXAMPLE 3   A set calibrated at **20 gtt/mL** is used to infuse **90 mL per hr**.

60 ÷ 20 = 3   90 mL ÷ 3 = **30 gtt/min**

▶▶▶ PROBLEMS 18.7

Calculate the flow rates in gtt/min using the division factor method.

1. A rate of 110 mL/hr via a set calibrated at 20 gtt/mL   _____

2. A set is calibrated at 15 gtt/mL. Infuse at 130 mL/hr   _____

3. To infuse 150 mL/hr using a 10 gtt/mL set   _____

4. A set calibrated at 20 gtt/mL to infuse 45 mL/hr   _____

5. A 75 mL/hr volume with a set calibrated at 15 gtt/mL   _____

6. A rate of 130 mL/hr using a 10 gtt/mL set   _____

7. A 200 mL rate using a 15 gtt/mL set   _____

8. A rate of 120 mL/hr using a 10 gtt/mL set   _____

9. A 100 mL/hr rate using a 20 gtt/mL set   _____

10. A rate of 125 mL/hr using a 15 gtt/mL set   _____

Answers   1. 37 gtt/min **2.** 33 gtt/min **3.** 25 gtt/min **4.** 15 gtt/min **5.** 19 gtt/min
6. 22 gtt/min **7.** 50 gtt/min **8.** 20 gtt/min **9.** 33 gtt/min **10.** 31 gtt/min

All the preceding examples and problems using the division factor were for **macrodrip** sets. Let's now look at what happens when a **microdrip** set calibrated at **60 gtt/mL** is used.

EXAMPLE 1   Infuse at **50 mL/hr** using a **60 gtt/mL** microdrip.

$$60 \div 60 = 1 \qquad 50 \text{ mL} \div 1 = \textbf{50 gtt/min}$$

Because the set calibration is 60 and the division factor is based on 60 min (1 hr), the division factor is 1. So, **for microdrip sets, the gtt/min flow rate will be identical to the mL/hr ordered**.

 KEYpoint: When a 60 gtt/mL microdrip set is used, the flow rate in gtt/min is identical to the volume in mL/hr to be infused.

▶▶▶ PROBLEMS 18.8

Calculate gtt/min rates for a microdrip.

1. 120 mL/hr   _____   6. 110 mL/hr   _____

2. 90 mL/hr   _____   7. 60 mL/hr   _____

3. 100 mL/hr   _____   8. 45 mL/hr   _____

4. 75 mL/hr   _____   9. 70 mL/hr   _____

5. 80 mL/hr   _____   10. 130 mL/hr   _____

Answers   1. 120 gtt/min **2.** 90 gtt/min **3.** 100 gtt/min **4.** 75 gtt/min **5.** 80 gtt/min
6. 110 gtt/min **7.** 60 gtt/min **8.** 45 gtt/min **9.** 70 gtt/min **10.** 130 gtt/min

The division factor can also be used to calculate the flow rate of **any volume that can be expressed in mL/hr**. Larger volumes can be divided, and smaller volumes can be multiplied and expressed in mL/hr. This does require the conversion step you used earlier.

EXAMPLE 1 $2400 \text{ mL}/24 \text{ hr} = 2400 \div 24 = \textbf{100 mL/hr}$

EXAMPLE 2 $1800 \text{ mL}/8 \text{ hr} = 1800 \div 8 = \textbf{225 mL/hr}$

EXAMPLE 3   10 mL/30 min = 10 × 2 (2 × 30 min) = **20 mL/hr**

EXAMPLE 4   15 mL/20 min = 15 × 3 (3 × 20 min) = **45 mL/hr**

REGULATING FLOW RATE

Manual flow rates are regulated by **counting the number of drops falling in the drip chamber**. The standard procedure for counting is to hold a watch next to the drip chamber and actually **count the number of drops falling**. The roller clamp is adjusted during the count until the required rate has been set. A 15 sec count is most commonly used because there is less chance of attention wandering during the count. This means that the ordered gtt/min (60 sec) rate must be divided by 4 to obtain the 15 sec drip count (60 sec ÷ 4 = 15 sec).

EXAMPLE 1   An IV is to run at a rate of **60 gtt/min**. What will the 15 sec count be?

60 gtt/min ÷ 4 = **15 gtt**

Adjust the rate to 15 gtt/15 sec.

EXAMPLE 2   A 70 **gtt/min** IV rate is ordered. What will the 15 sec count be?

70 gtt/min ÷ 4 = 17.5 = **18 gtt**

Adjust the rate to 18 gtt/15 sec.

EXAMPLE 3   Adjust an IV to a rate of **50 gtt/min** using a 15 sec count.

50 gtt/min ÷ 4 = 12.5 = **13 gtt**

Adjust the rate to 13 gtt/15 sec.

▶▶▶ PROBLEMS 18.9

Answer these questions about 15 sec drip rates.

1. The 15 sec count of an IV flow rate is 7 gtt. A 29 gtt/min rate is required. Is this rate correct?   _____

2. You are to regulate a newly started IV to deliver 67 gtt/min. Using a 15 sec count, how would you set the flow rate?   _____

3. An IV is to run at 48 gtt/min. What must the 15 sec drip rate be?   _____

4. How many gtt will you count in 15 sec if the rate is 55 gtt/min?   _____

5. An IV is to run at 84 gtt/min. What will the 15 sec rate be?   _____

6. What must the 15 sec count be to infuse 80 gtt/min?   _____

7. A 110 gtt/min rate is ordered. What must the 15 sec count be?   _____

8. A 100 gtt/min rate is ordered. What must the 15 sec count be?   _____

9. A rate of 90 gtt/min is ordered. Is a count of 15 gtt in 15 sec correct? _____

10. An IV is infusing at a rate of 30 gtt in 15 sec. A rate of 120 gtt/min was ordered. Is this rate correct? _____

Answers **1.** yes **2.** 17 gtt/15 sec **3.** 12 gtt/15 sec **4.** 14 gtt/15 sec **5.** 21 gtt/15 sec
6. 20 gtt/15 sec **7.** 28 gtt/15 sec **8.** 25 gtt/15 sec **9.** no, too slow **10.** yes

Individual clinical facilities and/or states/provinces may require a 30 or 60 sec (1 min) count. When a 60 sec count is required, particular care must be taken not to let your attention wander during the count, which can easily happen in this longer time frame. A 60 sec count will require a 1 min count, whereas a 30 sec count will require the gtt/min rate to be divided by 2 (60 sec ÷ 2 = 30 sec).

EXAMPLE 1   An IV is to be infused at 56 gtt/min. What is the 30 sec rate?

56 gtt/min ÷ 2 = 28 gtt

Adjust the rate to 28 gtt/30 sec.

EXAMPLE 2   A rate of 72 gtt/min has been ordered. What will the 30 sec count be?

72 gtt/min ÷ 2 = 36 gtt

Adjust the rate to 36 gtt/30 sec.

▶▶▶ PROBLEMS 18.10

Calculate a 30 sec flow rate count.

1. An IV to be run at a rate of 48 gtt/min _____
2. An IV ordered to infuse at 52 gtt/min _____
3. An IV to infuse at 120 gtt/min _____
4. An infusion rate of 90 gtt/min _____
5. An IV to infuse at 100 gtt/min _____

Answers **1.** 24 gtt/30 sec **2.** 26 gtt/30 sec **3.** 60 gtt/30 sec **4.** 45 gtt/30 sec **5.** 50 gtt/30 sec

CORRECTING OFF-SCHEDULE RATES

Because positional changes can alter the rate slightly, IVs occasionally infuse ahead of or behind schedule. When this occurs, the usual procedure is to **recalculate the flow rate using the volume and time remaining** and to **adjust the rate accordingly**. However, each situation must be individually evaluated, especially if the discrepancy is large. **If too much fluid has infused, immediately assess the individual's response** to the increased intake and take appropriate action. **If too little fluid has infused**, it will be necessary to **assess the individual's ability to tolerate an increased rate** because many medications and fluids have restrictions on the rate of administration. Both of these factors must be considered before rates can be increased to "catch up." In addition, **most clinical facilities will have specific policies to cover over- or underinfusion due to altered flow rates, and you will be responsible for knowing these.**

The following are some examples of how the rate can be recalculated. Because IVs are usually checked hourly, the focus will first be on recalculation using exact hours. Some recalculations have also been included using fractions of hours rounded to the nearest quarter hour: 15 min = 0.25 hr, 30 min = 0.5 hr, and 45 min = 0.75 hr. These equivalents are close enough for uncomplicated infusions because the exact time of completion is not totally predictable. IVs needing exact infusion would be monitored by electronic infusion devices.

EXAMPLE 1

An IV of **1000 mL** was ordered to infuse over **10 hr** at a rate of **25 gtt/min**. The set calibration is **15 gtt/mL**. After **5 hr**, a total of 650 mL have infused instead of the **500 mL** ordered. Recalculate the new gtt/min flow rate to complete the infusion on schedule.

Time remaining   10 hr – 5 hr = **5 hr**

Volume remaining   1000 mL – 650 mL = **350 mL**

350 mL ÷ 5 hr = **70 mL/hr**

Set calibration is **15 gtt/mL**.

70 ÷ 4 (division factor) = 17.5 = **18 gtt/min**

Slow the rate from 25 gtt/min to 18 gtt/min.

EXAMPLE 2

An IV of **800 mL** was to infuse over **8 hr** at **20 gtt/min**. After **4 hr 15 min** only **300 mL** have infused. Recalculate the **gtt/min** rate to complete on schedule. The set calibration is **15 gtt/mL**.

Time remaining   8 hr – 4.25 hr = **3.75 hr**

Volume remaining   800 mL – 300 mL = **500 mL**

500 mL ÷ 3.75 hr = 133.3 = **133 mL/hr**

Set calibration is **15 gtt/mL**.

133 ÷ 4 (division factor) = 33.2 = **33 gtt/min**

Increase the rate to 33 gtt/min.

EXAMPLE 3

An IV of **500 mL** is infusing at **28 gtt/min**. It was to complete in **3 hr**, but after **1½ hr**, only **175 mL** have infused. Recalculate the **gtt/min** rate to complete the infusion on schedule. Set calibration is **10 gtt/mL**.

Time remaining   3 hr – 1.5 hr = **1.5 hr**

Volume remaining   500 mL – 175 mL = **325 mL**

325 mL ÷ 1.5 hr = 216.6 = **217 mL/hr**

Set calibration is **10 gtt/mL**.

217 ÷ 6 (division factor) = 36.1 = **36 gtt/min**

Increase the rate to 36 gtt/min.

EXAMPLE 4 A volume of **250 mL** was to infuse **56 gtt/min** in **1½ hr** using a set calibrated at **20 gtt/mL**. After **30 min, 175 mL** have infused. Recalculate the flow rate.

Time remaining   1.5 hr – 30 min = **1 hr**

Volume remaining   250 mL – 175 mL = **75 mL**

Set calibration is **20 gtt/mL**.

75 ÷ 3 (division factor) = **25 gtt/min**

Decrease the rate to 25 gtt/min.

▶▶▶ PROBLEMS 18.11

Recalculate flow rates for infusions to complete on schedule.

1. An IV of 500 mL was ordered to infuse in 3 hr using a 15 gtt/mL set. With 1½ hr remaining, you discover that only 150 mL is left in the bag. At what rate will you need to reset the flow?   _____

2. An IV of 1000 mL was scheduled to run in 12 hr. After 4 hr, only 220 mL have infused. The set calibration is 20 gtt/mL. Recalculate the rate for the remaining solution.   _____

3. An IV of 1000 mL was ordered to infuse in 8 hr. With 3 hr of infusion time left, you discover that 600 mL have infused. The set delivers 20 gtt/mL. Recalculate the drip rate, and indicate how many drops you will count in 15 sec to set the new rate.   _____ _____

4. An IV of 750 mL was ordered to run in 6 hr with a set calibrated at 10 gtt/mL. After 2 hr, you notice that 300 mL have infused. Recalculate the flow rate, and indicate how many drops you will count in 15 sec to reset the rate.   _____ _____

5. An IV of 800 mL was started at 9 am to infuse in 4 hr. At 10 am, 150 mL have infused. The set is calibrated at 15 gtt/mL. Recalculate the flow rate in gtt/min.   _____

6. An IV of 600 mL was to infuse in 5 hr. After 2 hr, 400 mL have infused. Recalculate the gtt/min rate to complete on time. A 20 gtt/mL set is being used.   _____

7. A volume of 250 mL was to infuse in 2 hr. With 1 hr left, 70 mL have infused. Calculate a new gtt/min rate to complete on time using a 15 gtt/mL set.   _____

8. An infiltrated IV is restarted with a volume of 420 mL to complete in 3 hr. Calculate the gtt/min rate for a 20 gtt/mL set. What will the new 30 sec count be?   _____

9. After 1 hr 30 min, 350 mL of a 1000 mL IV has infused. It was ordered to complete in 4 hr using a set calibrated at 15 gtt/mL. Calculate the gtt/min rate to complete on time.   _____

10. A total of 300 mL of an ordered 1000 mL in 10 hr infusion
has completed in 4.5 hr. The set calibration is 15 gtt/mL.
What gtt/min rate is necessary to complete on time?
Calculate the 15 sec count to deliver this rate.   _____ _____

Answers **1.** 25 gtt/min **2.** 33 gtt/min **3.** 44 gtt/min; 11 gtt/15 sec **4.** 19 gtt/min; 4–5 gtt/15 sec
5. 54 gtt/min **6.** 22 gtt/min **7.** 45 gtt/min **8.** 47 gtt/min; 23–24 gtt/30 sec **9.** 65 gtt/min
10. 32 gtt/min; 8 gtt/15 sec

Summary

This concludes the chapter on IV flow rate calculation and monitoring. The important points to remember from this chapter are:

▽ IVs are ordered as mL/hr to be administered.

▽ Manual flow rates are counted in gtt/min.

▽ IV tubings are calibrated in gtt/mL.

▽ Macrodrip IV sets have a calibration of 10, 15, or 20 gtt/mL.

▽ Microdrip sets have a calibration of 60 gtt/mL.

▽ The formula for calculating flow rates is

$$\frac{\text{mL/hr Volume} \times \text{Set Calibration}}{\text{Time (60 min or less)}}$$

▽ The division factor method can be used to calculate flow rates only if the volume to be administered is specified in mL/hr (60 min).

▽ The division factor is obtained by dividing 60 by the set calibration.

▽ Flow rate by the division factor method is determined by dividing the mL/hr to be administered by the division factor.

▽ Because microdrip sets have a calibration of 60 gtt/mL, their division factor is 1, and the flow rate in gtt/min is the same as the mL/hr ordered.

▽ If an IV runs ahead of or behind schedule, a possible procedure is to use the time and mL remaining to calculate a new flow rate.

▽ If an IV is determined to have infused ahead of schedule, immediate assessment of the individual's tolerance to the excess fluid is required and appropriate action should be taken.

▽ If a rate must be increased to compensate for running behind schedule, the type of fluid being infused and the individual's ability to tolerate an increased rate must be assessed.

Summary Self-Test

Answer as briefly as possible.

1. Determine the division factor for the following IV sets.

   a. 60 gtt/mL

   b. 15 gtt/mL

   c. 20 gtt/mL

   d. 10 gtt/mL

2. How is the flow rate determined in the division factor method?

3. The division factor method can only be used if the volume to be administered is expressed in . . .

4. An IV is to infuse at 50 gtt/min. How will you set it using a 15 sec count?

5. You are to adjust an IV at a rate of 60 gtt/min. What will the 15 sec count be?

Calculate the flow rate in gtt/min.

6. An infusion of 2000 mL has been ordered to run 16 hr. The set calibration is 10 gtt/mL.

7. The order is for 500 mL in 8 hr. The set is calibrated at 15 gtt/mL.

8. Administer 150 mL in 3 hr. A microdrip is used.

9. 1500 mL has been ordered to infuse in 12 hr. Set calibration is 20 gtt/mL.

10. An IV medication of 30 mL is to be administered in 30 min using a 15 gtt/mL set.

11. Administer 100 mL in 1 hr using a 15 gtt/mL set.

12. Infuse 500 mL in 6 hr. Set calibration is 10 gtt/mL.

13. The order is to infuse a liter in 10 hr. At the end of 8 hr, you notice that there are 500 mL left. What would the new flow rate need to be to finish on schedule if the set calibration is 10 gtt/mL?

14. An IV was started at 9 am with orders to infuse 500 mL in 6 hr. At noon, the IV infiltrated with 350 mL left in the bag. At 1 pm, the IV was restarted. The set calibration is 20 gtt/mL. Calculate the new flow rate to deliver the infusion on time.

15. A 50 mL IV is to infuse in 15 min. The set calibration is 15 gtt/mL. After 5 min, the IV contains 40 mL. Calculate the flow rate to deliver the volume on time.

16. An IV of 1000 mL is ordered to run at 25 mL/hr using a microdrip set.

17. An infusion of 800 mL has been ordered to run in 5 hr. Set calibration is 10 gtt/mL.

18. Administer 1500 mL in 8 hr using a set calibrated at 20 gtt/mL.

19. The order is for 750 mL to run in 6 hr. Set calibration is 15 gtt/mL.

20. An IV of 1000 mL was ordered to run in 8 hr. After 4 hr, only 250 mL have infused. The set calibration is 20 gtt/mL. Recalculate the rate for the remaining solution to complete on time.   _____

21. The order is to infuse 50 mL in 1 hr. The set calibration is a microdrip.   _____

22. An IV of 500 mL is to infuse in 6 hr using a set calibrated at 10 gtt/mL.   _____

23. Infuse 120 mL in 1 hr. Set calibration is 10 gtt/mL.   _____

24. Administer 12 mL in 22 min using a microdrip set.   _____

25. A patient is to receive 3000 mL in 20 hr. Set is calibrated at 20 gtt/mL.   _____

26. Infuse 1 liter in 5 hr using a set calibration of 15 gtt/mL.   _____

27. A total of 1180 mL is to infuse in 12 hr using a set calibrated at 20 gtt/mL.   _____

28. A volume of 150 mL is to infuse in 30 min. At the end of 20 min, you discover that 100 mL have infused. The set calibration is 10 gtt/mL. Should the flow rate be adjusted? If so, what is the new rate?   _____ _____

29. The order is for 1000 mL in 5 hr. The set calibration is 20 gtt/mL.   _____

30. Infuse 15 mL in 14 min using a 20 gtt/mL set.   _____

31. The order is for 1000 mL in 10 hr using a 20 gtt/mL calibration.   _____

32. A microdrip is used to administer 12 mL in 17 min.   _____

33. Infuse 2750 mL in 20 hr using a 10 gtt/mL set.   _____

34. An IV of 1800 mL is to infuse in 15 hr using a 15 gtt/mL set.   _____

35. Infuse 600 mL in 6 hr with a 10 gtt/mL set.   _____

36. Administer 22 mL in 18 min using a microdrip set.   _____

37. An order of 1800 mL is to infuse in 10 hr. Set calibration is 20 gtt/mL.   _____

38. Infuse 8 mL in 9 min using a microdrip.   _____

39. Infuse 4000 mL in 20 hr. A 20 gtt/mL set is used.   _____

40. An IV of 500 mL that was to infuse in 2 hr is discovered to have only 150 mL left after 30 min. Recalculate the flow rate. Set calibration is 15 gtt/mL.   _____

Answers

1. a) 1 b) 4 c) 3 d) 6	11. 25 gtt/min	23. 20 gtt/min	34. 30 gtt/min
2. mL/hr ÷ division factor	12. 14 gtt/min	24. 33 gtt/min	35. 17 gtt/min
3. mL/hr (mL/60 min)	13. 42 gtt/min	25. 50 gtt/min	36. 73 gtt/min
4. 13 gtt/15 sec	14. 58 gtt/min	26. 50 gtt/min	37. 60 gtt/min
5. 15 gtt/15 sec	15. 60 gtt/min	27. 33 gtt/min	38. 53 gtt/min
6. 21 gtt/min	16. 25 gtt/min	28. no, rate is correct at 50 gtt/min	39. 67 gtt/min
7. 16 gtt/min	17. 27 gtt/min	29. 67 gtt/min	40. 25 gtt/min
8. 50 gtt/min	18. 63 gtt/min	30. 21 gtt/min	
9. 42 gtt/min	19. 31 gtt/min	31. 33 gtt/min	
10. 15 gtt/min	20. 63 gtt/min	32. 42 gtt/min	
	21. 50 gtt/min	33. 23 gtt/min	
	22. 14 gtt/min		

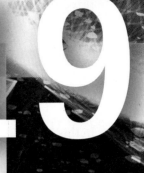

CALCULATING IV INFUSION AND COMPLETION TIMES

There are a number of reasons for calculating IV infusion and completion times: to know when an IV solution will complete so that additional solutions ordered can be prepared in advance and ready to hang; to discontinue an IV when it has completed; and to label an IV bag with start, progress, and completion times so that the infusion can be monitored and adjusted to keep it on schedule. Knowing the infusion time is also important because laboratory studies are sometimes made before, during, or after specified amounts of IV solutions have infused. The infusion time may be calculated in hours and/or minutes, depending on the type and amount of solution ordered.

OBJECTIVES

The learner will calculate:

1. infusion times.

2. completion times using international/military and standard time.

3. infusion time to label IV bag/bottle with start, progress, and completion times.

CALCULATING INFUSION TIME FROM mL/hr ORDERED

The infusion time is calculated for each bag/bottle to be hung and infused. The largest capacity IV solution bag or bottle is 1000 mL, but 500 mL, 250 mL, and 50 mL bags are also commonly used. Calculations for odd-numbered volumes remaining when an IV infiltrates are also routinely done. **Infusion time is calculated by dividing the volume being infused by the mL/hr rate ordered.**

Because most IVs take several hours to infuse, the unit of time being calculated most often includes hours (hr) and minutes (min).

 KEYpoint: IV infusion time is calculated by dividing the volume to be infused by the mL/hr flow rate.

EXAMPLE 1　Calculate the infusion time for an IV of **500 mL** to infuse at **50 mL/hr.**

Infusion Time = volume ÷ mL/hr rate

$$= 500 \text{ mL} \div 50 \text{ mL/hr} = \textbf{10 hr}$$

The infusion time for an IV of 500 mL infusing at 50 mL/hr is 10 hr.

EXAMPLE 2   The order is to infuse **1000 mL** at **75 mL/hr**. Calculate the infusion time.

1000 mL ÷ 75 mL/hr = **13.33 hr**

In this example, the 13 represents hr, whereas the **.33 represents the fraction of an additional hr**.

 KEY*point:* Fractional hr are converted to min by multiplying 60 min by the fraction obtained.

Calculate min by multiplying 60 min by the fractional .33 hr.

60 min/hr × .33 hr = 19.8 = **20 min**

The infusion time is 13 hr 20 min.

EXAMPLE 3   An IV of **1000 mL** is to infuse at **90 mL/hr**. Calculate the infusion time.

1000 mL ÷ 90 mL/hr = **11.11 hr**

Remember that .11 represents the fraction of an additional hr. Convert this to min by multiplying 60 min by .11

60 min/hr × .11 hr = 6.6 = **7 min**

The infusion time is 11 hr 7 min.

EXAMPLE 4   Calculate the infusion time for **750 mL** at a rate of **80 mL/hr**.

750 mL ÷ 80 mL/hr = **9.38 hr**

60 min/hr × .38 hr = 22.8 = **23 min**

The infusion time is 9 hr 23 min.

EXAMPLE 5   A rate of **75 mL/hr** is ordered for a volume of **500 mL**. Calculate the infusion time.

500 mL ÷ 75 mL/hr = **6.67 hr**

60 min/hr × .67 hr = 40.2 = **40 min**

The infusion time is 6 hr 40 min.

▶▶▶ PROBLEMS 19.1

Calculate the infusion times.

1. An IV of 900 mL to infuse at 80 mL/hr   _____

2. A volume of 250 mL to infuse at 30 mL/hr   _____

3. An infusion of 180 mL to run at 25 mL/hr   _____

4. A volume of 1000 mL ordered at 60 mL/hr   _____

5. An IV of 150 mL to infuse at 80 mL/hr _____

6. An infusion of 1000 mL at 125 mL/hr _____

7. A rate of 120 mL/hr for 500 mL _____

8. A volume of 800 mL at 60 mL/hr _____

9. An IV of 250 mL at 80 mL/hr _____

10. A rate of 135 mL/hr for 750 mL _____

Answers **1.** 11 hr 15 min **2.** 8 hr 20 min **3.** 7 hr 12 min **4.** 16 hr 40 min **5.** 1 hr 53 min
6. 8 hr **7.** 4 hr 10 min **8.** 13 hr 20 min **9.** 3 hr 8 min **10.** 5 hr 34 min
Note: Answers may vary due to rounding or calculator setting, so variations of 1–2 min may be considered correct.

CALCULATING INFUSION COMPLETION TIMES

The **completion time is the actual hour and/or minute an infusion bag or bottle will complete or empty**. Completion times are calculated in either **international/military time** using the 24-hour clock, or **standard time**, depending on individual clinical facility policy.

 KEY*point:* The completion time is calculated by adding the infusion time to the time the IV was started.

An example is the addition of an infusion time of 90 min to a 0515 international/ military or 5:15 am standard time when an IV was started.

INTERNATIONAL/MILITARY TIME CALCULATIONS

EXAMPLE 1 An IV started at **0400** is to complete in **2 hr 30 min**. Calculate the completion time.

■ **Add the 2 hr 30 min infusion time to the 0400 start time.**

```
   0400
+  230
───────
   0630
```

The completion time is 0630.

EXAMPLE 2 An IV started at **0750** is to complete in **5 hr 10 min**. Calculate the completion time.

■ **Add the 5 hr 10 min infusion time to the 0750 start time.**

```
   0750
+  510
───────
   1260
```

Change the 60 min to 1 hr and add to 1200 = 1300

The completion time is 1300.

EXAMPLE 3   An IV started at **2250** is to complete in **4 hr 20 min**. Calculate the completion time.

- **Add the infusion time to the start time.**

$$\begin{array}{r} 2250 \\ +\ 420 \\ \hline 2670 \end{array}$$

Change the 70 min to 1 hr 10 min = 2710

Deduct 24 hr from 2710 = 0310

The completion time is 0310.

▶▶▶ PROBLEMS 19.2

Calculate the international/military completion times.

1. An IV started at 0415 to infuse in 1 hr 30 min. _____
2. An infusion started at 1735 to complete in 2 hr 40 min. _____
3. An IV to complete in 1 hr 14 min that was started at 0025. _____
4. An IV started at 2300 to complete in 3 hr 40 min. _____
5. An infusion time of 6 hr 20 min for an infusion started at 0325. _____
6. An IV started at 0445 to complete in 3 hr 20 min. _____
7. A medication infusion started at 0740 to complete in 90 min. _____
8. An IV medication started at 1247 to complete in 45 min. _____
9. An IV started at 1430 to complete in 4 hr. _____
10. An IV started at 1605 to complete in 3 hr 30 min. _____

Answers **1.** 0545 **2.** 2015 **3.** 0139 **4.** 0240 **5.** 0945 **6.** 0805 **7.** 0910 **8.** 1332 **9.** 1830 **10.** 1935

STANDARD TIME CALCULATIONS

EXAMPLE 1   An IV medication will infuse in **20 minutes**. It is now **6:14 pm**. When will it complete?

- **Add the 20 minutes infusion time to the 6:14 pm start time.**

6:14 pm + **20 min** = **6:34 pm**

The completion time will be at 6:34 pm.

EXAMPLE 2   An IV is to infuse in **2 hr 33 min**. It is now **4:43 pm**. When will it complete?

- **Add the 2 hr 33 min infusion time to the 4:43 start time.**

$$\begin{array}{r} 4:43\ pm \\ +\ 2:33 \\ \hline 6:76 \end{array}$$

Change the 76 min to 1 hr 16 min to make the completion time 7:16 pm.

The infusion will complete at 7:16 pm.

EXAMPLE 3   An IV infusion time is **13 hr 20 min**. What is its completion time if it was started at **10:45 am**?

■ **Add the 13 hr 20 min infusion time to the 10:45 am start time.**

$$
\begin{array}{r}
10:45 \text{ am} \\
+\,13:20 \\
\hline
23:65
\end{array}
$$

Change the 65 min to 1 hr 5 min = 24:05. Subtract 12 hr.

The completion time will be 12:05 am.

EXAMPLE 4   A IV with an infusion time of **10 hr 7 min** is started at **9:42 am**. When will it complete?

■ **Add the 10 hr 7 min infusion time to the 9:42 am start time.**

$$
\begin{array}{r}
9:42 \text{ am} \\
+\,10:07 \\
\hline
19:49
\end{array}
$$

Subtract 12 hr to make the completion time 7:49 pm.

The completion time will be 7:49 pm.

EXAMPLE 5   An IV with an infusion time of **12 hr 30 min** is started at **2:10 am**. When will it complete?

■ **Add the 12 hr 30 min infusion time to the 2:10 am start time.**

$$
\begin{array}{r}
2:10 \text{ am} \\
+\,12:30 \\
\hline
14:40
\end{array}
$$

Subtract 12 hr to make the time 2:40 pm.

The completion time will be 2:40 pm.

▶▶▶ PROBLEMS 19.3

Calculate IV completion using standard time.

1. An IV started at 4:40 am that has an infusion time of 9 hr 42 min.   _____

2. An IV medication started at 7:30 am that has an infusion time of 45 min.   _____

3. An IV with an infusion time of 7 hr 7 min that was restarted at 10:42 am.   _____

4. An IV with a restart time of 9:07 pm that has an infusion time of 6 hr 27 min.   _____

5. An IV with an infusion time of 3 hr 30 min was started at 11:49 pm.

6. An IV started at 2:43 pm to infuse in 40 min.

7. An IV medication started at 10:15 am to complete in 90 min.

8. An infusion started at 7:05 pm to complete in 8 hr.

9. An IV started at 5:47 am to complete in 5 hr.

10. An IV started at 4:20 am to complete in 12 hr.

Answers 1. 2:22 pm **2.** 8:15 am **3.** 5:49 pm **4.** 3:34 am **5.** 3:19 am **6.** 3:23 pm **7.** 11:45 am
8. 3:05 am **9.** 10:47 am **10.** 4:20 pm

LABELING SOLUTION BAGS WITH INFUSION AND COMPLETION TIMES

IV bags/bottles are calibrated so that the amount of fluid remaining can be checked at any time. In the majority of clinical facilities, it is routine to label bags when they are hung with start, progress, and finish times to provide a visual reference of the status of the infusion. Commercially prepared labels are available for this purpose; however, you can prepare one using any tape available.

Refer to Figure 19-1, where you can see close up the calibrations on a 1000 mL bag. Notice that each 50 mL is calibrated but that only the 100 mL calibrations are numbered: 1, 2, 3 (for 100, 200, 300), etc. Also, notice that the calibrations on the IV bag are not all the same width. They are somewhat wider at the bottom because gravity and the pressure of the solution force more fluid to the bottom of the bag.

The tape on the IV solution bag in Figure 19-1 is for an 8 hr infusion, from 9 am to 5 pm. The 9A represents the start time of 9 am, and the 5P at the bottom represents the completion time of 5 pm. An 8 hr infusion time for 1000 mL means that 125 mL are to be infused per hour (1000 mL ÷ 8 hr = 125 mL/hr). Each 125 mL is labeled on the calibrated scale along with the hour the IV should be at this level. This tape allows for constant visual monitoring of the IV. Regardless of your clinical responsibility, develop the habit of reading infusion time labeling, particularly if you have been giving personal care that involves movement or repositioning of the patient.

Let's look at an example of how you could label an IV that is just being started.

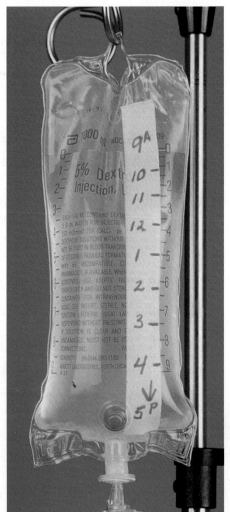

▲ **FIGURE 19-1**

EXAMPLE 1 An IV of **1000 mL** has been ordered to run at **150 mL/hr**. It was started at **1:40 pm.** Tape the bag with start, progress, and completion times.

Add the tape to the bag/bottle so that it is near but does not cover the calibrations. Enter the start time as 1:40 pm at the 1000 mL level. Next, mark each 150 mL from top to bottom with the successive hours the IV will run.

1000 mL − 150 mL = 850 mL	Label 850 mL for 2:40 pm
850 mL − 150 mL = 700 mL	Label 700 mL for 3:40 pm
700 mL − 150 mL = 550 mL	Label 550 mL for 4:40 pm
550 mL − 150 mL = 400 mL	Label 400 mL for 5:40 pm
400 mL − 150 mL = 250 mL	Label 250 mL for 6:40 pm
250 mL − 150 mL = 100 mL	Label 100 mL for 7:40 pm

Calculate the infusion time for the remaining 100 mL.

$$100 \text{ mL} \div 150 \text{ mL/hr} = 0.66 = \textbf{0.67 hr}$$

$$60 \text{ min/hr} \times 0.67 \text{ hr} = 40.2 = \textbf{40 min}$$

$$7\text{:}40 \text{ pm} + \textbf{40 min} = \textbf{8:20 pm}$$

The completion time is 8:20 pm.

EXAMPLE 2 An infiltrated IV with **625 mL** remaining is restarted at **5:30 pm** to run at **150 mL/hr**. Relabel the bag with the new start, progress, and completion times.

Label the 625 mL level with the 5:30 pm restart time.

625 mL − 150 mL = 475 mL	Label 475 mL for 6:30 pm
475 mL − 150 mL = 325 mL	Label 325 mL for 7:30 pm
325 mL − 150 mL = 175 mL	Label 175 mL for 8:30 pm
175 mL − 150 mL = 25 mL	Label 25 mL for 9:30 pm

Calculate the infusion time for the remaining 25 mL.

$$25 \text{ mL} \div 150 \text{ mL/hr} = 0.166 = \textbf{0.17 hr}$$

$$60 \text{ min/hr} \times 0.17 \text{ hr} = 10.2 = \textbf{10 min}$$

$$9\text{:}30 \text{ pm} + \textbf{10 min} = \textbf{9:40 pm}$$

The completion time is 9:40 pm.

EXAMPLE 3 An infiltrated IV with **340 mL** remaining is restarted at **4:15 am** to run at **70 mL/hr**. Relabel the bag with the new start, progress, and completion times.

Label the 340 mL level with the 4:15 am restart time.

340 mL − 70 mL = 270 mL	Label 270 mL for 5:15 am
270 mL − 70 mL = 200 mL	Label 200 mL for 6:15 am
200 mL − 70 mL = 130 mL	Label 130 mL for 7:15 am
130 mL − 70 mL = 60 mL	Label 60 mL for 8:15 am

Calculate the infusion time for the remaining 60 mL.

60 mL ÷ 70 mL/hr = 0.857 = **0.86 hr**

60 min/hr × 0.86 hr = 51.6 = **52 min**

8:15 am + **52 min** = **9:07 am**

The completion time is 9:07 am.

▶▶▶ PROBLEMS 19.4

Calculate the infusion and completion times. Label the IV bags provided with start, progress, and completion times. Have your instructor check your labeling.

1. The IV in Figure 19-2 of 1000 mL was started at 0710 to run at 75 mL/hr.

   Infusion time _____   Completion time _____

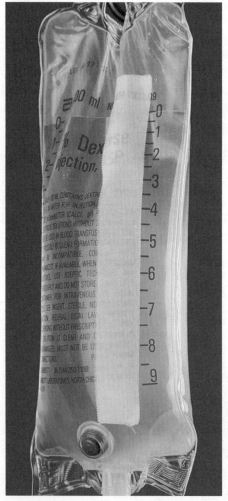

Photography Courtesy Abbott Laboratories.

▲ **FIGURE 19-2**

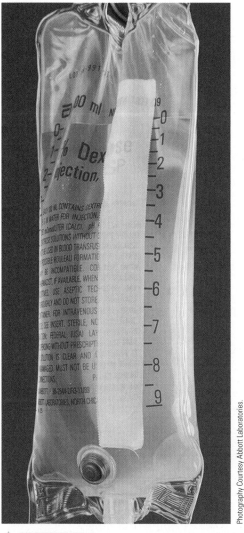

▲ FIGURE 19-3

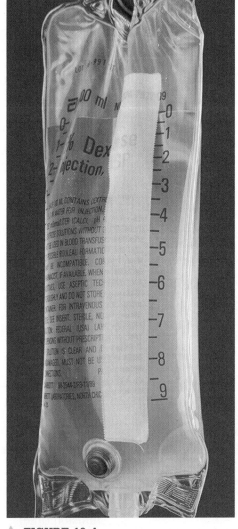

▲ FIGURE 19-4

Photography Courtesy Abbott Laboratories.

Photography Courtesy Abbott Laboratories.

2. The 1000 mL IV in Figure 19-3 has an ordered rate of 125 mL/hr. It was started at 6:30 pm.

   Infusion time_____   Completion time_____

3. The IV in Figure 19-4 of 1000 mL has an ordered rate of 80 mL/hr. It was started at 5:40 am.

   Infusion time_____   Completion time_____

Answers 1. 13 hr 20 min; 2030 **2.** 8 hr; 2:30 am **3.** 12 hr 30 min; 6:10 pm

Summary

This concludes the chapter on calculation of infusion and completion times and labeling of IV bags/bottles with start, progress, and completion times. The important points to remember from this chapter are:

▼ The infusion time is the time required for an IV to infuse completely.

▼ The infusion time is calculated by dividing the total volume to infuse by the mL/hr rate ordered.

▼ The completion time is calculated by adding the infusion time to the start time.

▼ When the min calculated are 60 or more, an additional hr is added to the completion time and 60 min are subtracted from the total min.

▼ Calculating completion times provides an opportunity to plan ahead and have the next solution ordered ready to hang or to discontinue an IV when it has completed.

▼ Most clinical facilities label IV solution bags/bottles with start, progress, and finish times to provide a visual record of the infusion status.

Summary Self-Test

Calculate the infusion and completion times.

1. The order is for 50 mL to infuse at 50 mL/hr. The infusion was started at 10:10 am.

   Infusion time_____   Completion time_____

2. An infusion of 950 mL is ordered at 80 mL/hr. It was started at 8:02 am.

   Infusion time_____   Completion time_____

3. A total of 280 mL remain in an IV bag. The flow rate is 70 mL/hr. It is now 11:03 am.

   Infusion time_____   Completion time_____

4. The order is to infuse 500 mL at 90 mL/hr. The IV was started at 2:40 pm.

   Infusion time_____   Completion time_____

5. An infiltrated IV with 850 mL remaining is restarted at 10 am at a rate of 150 mL/hr.

   Infusion time_____   Completion time_____

6. At 4:04 am, an IV of 500 mL is started at a rate of 50 mL/hr.

   Infusion time_____   Completion time_____

7. An IV medication with a volume of 150 mL is started at 1:45 pm to infuse at 60 mL/hr.

   Infusion time_____   Completion time_____

8. An IV of 520 mL is restarted at 0420 at a rate of 125 mL/hr.

   Infusion time_____   Completion time_____

9. It is 12:00 pm, and an IV of 900 mL is to infuse at a rate of 100 mL/hr.

   Infusion time_____   Completion time_____

10. An IV of 1000 mL is started at 0550 to infuse at 130 mL/hr.

    Infusion time_____   Completion time_____

11. An infusion of 250 mL is started at 11:20 am to infuse at a rate of 20 mL/hr.

    Infusion time_____   Completion time_____

12. The flow rate ordered for 1 L is 80 mL/hr. It was started at 8:07 pm.

    Infusion time_____   Completion time_____

13. A 250 mL volume is started at 3:40 pm to be infused at 90 mL/hr.

    Infusion time_____   Completion time_____

14. A medication volume of 100 mL is started at 4:00 pm to infuse at 42 mL/hr.

        Infusion time_____   Completion time_____

15. At 11:00 pm, 200 mL remain in an IV. The rate is 120 mL/hr.

        Infusion time_____   Completion time_____

16. An infusion of 350 mL is to run at 150 mL/hr. It is now 9:47 am.

        Infusion time_____   Completion time_____

17. An IV medication of 25 mL is started at 8:17 am to run at 25 mL/hr.

        Infusion time_____   Completion time_____

18. An IV of 425 mL is restarted at 0814 to infuse at 90 mL/hr.

        Infusion time_____   Completion time_____

19. At 10:30 pm, there are 180 mL left in an IV that is infusing at 25 mL/hr.

        Infusion time_____   Completion time_____

20. At 1400, 500 mL is started to run at a rate of 60 mL/hr.

        Infusion time_____   Completion time_____

21. An infusion of 250 mL is started at 3:04 am to run at 100 mL/hr.

        Infusion time_____   Completion time_____

22. With 525 mL remaining, a rate change to 108 mL/hr is ordered. It is 2:10 am.

        Infusion time_____   Completion time_____

23. A liter is started at 8:42 am at a rate of 120 mL/hr.

        Infusion time_____   Completion time_____

24. An infusion of 1000 mL is to run at 200 mL/hr. It is started at 6:40 pm.

        Infusion time_____   Completion time_____

25. An IV medication of 100 mL is started at 7:50 am to run at 150 mL/hr.

        Infusion time_____   Completion time_____

26. A volume of 500 mL is started at 4:04 pm at a rate of 75 mL/hr.

        Infusion time_____   Completion time_____

27. An IV of 950 mL is restarted at 2:10 am at 100 mL/hr.

        Infusion time_____   Completion time_____

28. An IV medication of 30 mL is started at 0915 at a rate of 60 mL/hr.

        Infusion time_____   Completion time_____

29. A medication volume of 90 mL was started at 6:15 am to be infused at 90 mL/hr.

        Infusion time_____   Completion time_____

30. A rate of 80 mL/hr is set at 4:20 pm to infuse a medication with a volume of 100 mL.

        Infusion time_____   Completion time_____

31. A volume of 750 mL is started at 0303 at a rate of 96 mL/hr.

        Infusion time_____   Completion time_____

Label the following solution bags for the times and rates indicated. Have your instructor check your labeling.

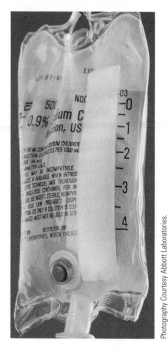

Photography Courtesy Abbott Laboratories.

32.
Started: 10:47 am
Rate: 80 mL/hr

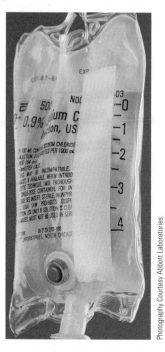

Photography Courtesy Abbott Laboratories.

33.
Started: 1315
Rate: 100 mL/hr

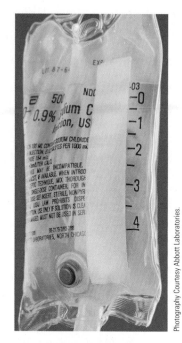

Photography Courtesy Abbott Laboratories.

34.
Started: 2:10 pm
Rate: 90 mL/hr

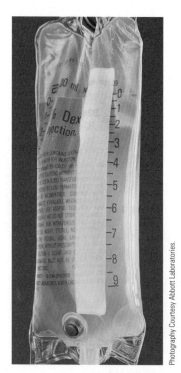

Photography Courtesy Abbott Laboratories.

35.
Started: 0440
Rate: 75 mL/hr

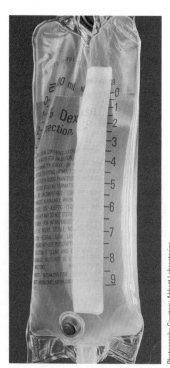

Photography Courtesy Abbott Laboratories.

36.
Started: 0730
Rate: 50 mL/hr

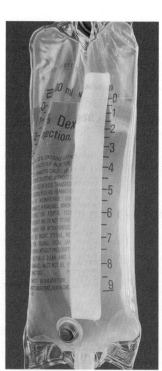

Photography Courtesy Abbott Laboratories.

37.
Started: 6:20 pm
Rate: 25 mL/hr

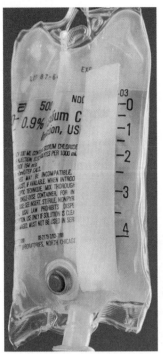

Photography Courtesy Abbott Laboratories.

38.
Started: 3:03 am
Rate: 50 mL/hr

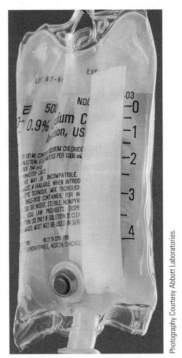

Photography Courtesy Abbott Laboratories.

39.
Started: 0744
Rate: 125 mL/hr

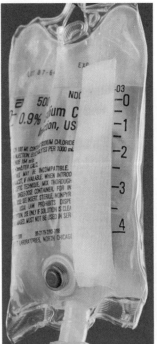

Photography Courtesy Abbott Laboratories.

40.
Started: 2140
Rate: 100 mL/hr

Answers

1. 1 hr; 11:10 am
2. 11 hr 53 min; 7:55 pm
3. 4 hr; 3:03 pm
4. 5 hr 34 min; 8:14 pm
5. 5 hr 40 min; 3:40 pm
6. 10 hr; 2:04 pm
7. 2 hr 30 min; 4:15 pm
8. 4 hr 10 min; 0830
9. 9 hr; 9 pm
10. 7 hr 41 min; 1331
11. 12 hr 30 min; 11:50 pm

12. 12 hr 30 min; 8:37 am
13. 2 hr 46 min; 6:26 pm
14. 2 hr 23 min; 6:23 pm
15. 1 hr 40 min; 12:40 am
16. 2 hr 20 min; 12:07 pm
17. 1 hr; 9:17 am
18. 4 hr 43 min; 1257
19. 7 hr 12 min; 5:42 am
20. 8 hr 20 min; 2220
21. 2 hr 30 min; 5:34 am
22. 4 hr 52 min; 7:02 am
23. 8 hr 20 min; 5:02 pm

24. 5 hr; 11:40 pm
25. 40 min; 8:30 am
26. 6 hr 40 min; 10:44 pm
27. 9 hr 30 min; 11:40 am
28. 30 min; 0945
29. 1 hr; 7:15 am
30. 1 hr 15 min; 5:35 pm
31. 7 hr 49 min; 1052
32–40. Verify your answers with your instructor.

Note: Answers may vary slightly due to rounding.

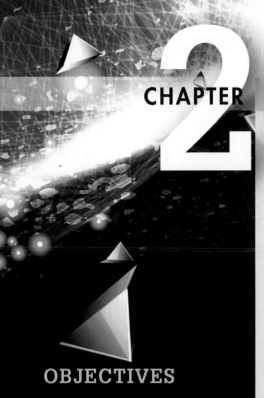

CHAPTER

20 IV MEDICATION AND TITRATION CALCULATIONS

Many IV drugs are used in critical and life-threatening situations to alter or maintain vital physiologic functions; for example heart rate, cardiac output, blood pressure, and respiration. In general, these drugs have a very rapid action and short duration. They are frequently administered diluted in 250–500 mL of IV solution, most commonly D5W.

Intravenous medications may be ordered by dosage (mcg/mg/units per min/hr) or based on body weight (mcg/mg/units per kg per min/hr). They may also be ordered to infuse within a specific dosage range—for example, 1–3 mcg/min—to elicit a measurable physiologic response; an example would be to maintain a systolic BP above 100 mm Hg. This adjustment of rate is called **titration**, and dosage increments are made within the ordered range until the desired response has been established. IV drugs require close and continuous monitoring, and an electronic infusion device (EID), either a volumetric pump or a syringe pump, is used for their administration. If an EID is not used, a microdrip set calibrated at 60 gtt/mL or a dosage controlled Soluset/Buretrol/Volutrol burette is used.

All calculations in this chapter are for an EID or microdrip, and the mL/hr and gtt/min rates are therefore interchangeable. Calculations include converting ordered dosages to the flow rates necessary to administer them, and using flow rates to calculate the dosage infusing at any given moment. Body weight is often a critical factor in IV dosages, and its use in calculations will also be covered. A number of EIDs display, and can be set to deliver, dosage and flow rate equivalents, but you must know how to do these calculations in case you encounter a situation in which you will have to do one. IV drugs that alter a basic physiologic function generally have narrow margins of safety, and accuracy is imperative in their calculation. Double-checking of math is both mandatory and routine. As a general rule, dosages are calculated to the nearest tenth and flow rates are rounded to the nearest mL or gtt.

KEY*point:* All calculations assume the use of an EID or microdrip infusion set; therefore, the mL/hr and gtt/min rates are identical and interchangeable.

 If you prefer to use Dimensional Analysis for these calculations, turn to page 310. To use Ratio and Proportion, continue on this page.

USING RATIO AND PROPORTION TO CALCULATE mL/hr RATE FOR DOSAGE ORDERED

One common calculation is to determine the mL/hr flow rate for a specific drug dosage ordered. Let's start by looking at some examples of these.

EXAMPLE 1 A dosage of **125 mg/100 mL** is to infuse at a rate of **20 mg/hr**. Calculate the **mL/hr** flow rate.

- Use the 125 mg/100 mL solution strength to calculate the mL/hr rate for 20 mg/hr.

$$\frac{125 \text{ mg}}{100 \text{ mL}} = \frac{20 \text{ mg}}{X \text{ mL}} = \textbf{16 mL/hr} \quad \text{or} \quad 125 \text{ mg} : 100 \text{ mL} = 20 \text{ mg} : X \text{ mL}$$
$$125X = 100 \times 20$$
$$X = \textbf{16 mL/hr}$$

To infuse 20 mg/hr, set the flow rate at 16 mL/hr.

EXAMPLE 2 A maintenance dose of **2 mcg/min** has been ordered using an **8 mg in 250 mL** solution. Calculate the **mL/hr** flow rate.

- **Convert 2 mcg/min to mcg per hr.**

  2 mcg/min × 60 min/hr = **120 mcg/hr**

- **Convert 120 mcg to mg to match the 8 mg in 250 mL solution strength.**

  120 mcg = **0.12 mg**

- **Calculate the mL/hr rate.**

$$\frac{8 \text{ mg}}{250 \text{ mL}} = \frac{0.12 \text{ mg}}{X \text{ mL}} = \textbf{4 mL/hr} \quad \text{or} \quad 8 \text{ mg} : 250 \text{ mL} = 0.12 \text{ mg} : X \text{ mL}$$
$$8X = 250 \times 0.12$$
$$X = 3.75 = \textbf{4 mL/hr}$$

To infuse 2 mcg/min, set the flow rate at 4 mL/hr.

 KEY*point:* Metric conversions may be made in either direction: solution strength to dosage ordered or dosage ordered to solution strength.

EXAMPLE 3 A **50 mg in 250 mL** strength solution is used to infuse a dosage of **200 mcg/min**. Calculate the flow rate in **mL/hr**.

- **Convert the mcg/min to mcg/hr.**

  200 mcg/min × 60 min/hr = **12,000 mcg/hr**

- **Convert 12,000 mcg to mg to match the mg solution strength.**

  12,000 mcg = **12 mg**

- **Calculate the mL/hr flow rate.**

$$\frac{50 \text{ mg}}{250 \text{ mL}} = \frac{12 \text{ mg}}{X \text{ mL}} = \textbf{60 mL/hr} \quad \text{or} \quad 50 \text{ mg} : 250 \text{ mL} = 12 \text{ mg} : X \text{ mL}$$

$$50X = 250 \times 12$$

$$X = \textbf{60 mL/hr}$$

To infuse 200 mcg/min, set the flow rate at 60 mL/hr.

EXAMPLE 4   A rate of **3 mcg/min** is ordered using a **1 mg/250 mL** solution. Calculate the **mL/hr** flow rate.

- **Convert the dosage per min to dosage per hr.**

  3 mcg/min × 60 min/hr = **180 mcg/hr**

- **Convert 180 mcg to mg to match the mg solution strength.**

  180 mcg = **0.18 mg**

- **Calculate the mL/hr flow rate.**

$$\frac{1 \text{ mg}}{250 \text{ mL}} = \frac{0.18 \text{ mg}}{X \text{ mL}} = \textbf{45 mL/hr} \quad \text{or} \quad 1 \text{ mg} : 250 \text{ mL} = 0.18 \text{ mg} : X \text{ mL}$$

$$X = 250 \times 0.18$$

$$X = \textbf{45 mL/hr}$$

To infuse 3 mcg/min, set the flow rate at 45 mL/hr.

▶▶▶ PROBLEMS 20.1

Calculate these mL/hr flow rates.

1. A 20 mg/hr rate is ordered using a 100 mg/100 mL solution strength. _____

2. An IV medication is ordered at the rate of 3 mcg/min. The solution strength is 8 mg in 250 mL. _____

3. A solution strength of 2 g in 500 mL is used to administer a dosage of 2 mg/min. _____

4. A rate of 2 mcg/min is ordered. The solution strength is 1 mg/250 mL. _____

5. A rate of 25 mg/hr is ordered. The solution strength is 125 mg/100 mL. _____

6. A 50 mg/200 mL solution strength is ordered at a rate of 6 mg/hr. _____

7. A solution strength of 75 mg/250 mL is to infuse at 10 mg/hr.   _____

8. A 500 mL/1 g solution is to infuse at 1 mg/min.   _____

9. A 100 mg/250 mL solution is to infuse at 8 mg/hr.   _____

10. A 1 g/250 mL solution is to infuse at 150 mg/hr.   _____

Answers 1. 20 mL/hr **2.** 6 mL/hr **3.** 30 mL/hr **4.** 30 mL/hr **5.** 20 mL/hr **6.** 24 mL/hr **7.** 33 mL/hr
8. 30 mL/hr **9.** 20 mL/hr **10.** 38 mL/hr

USING RATIO AND PROPORTION TO CALCULATE mL/hr RATE FOR DOSAGE PER kg ORDERED

Many drug dosages are calculated based on body weight; for example, 5 mg/kg/hr. **Body weight, to the nearest tenth kg**, is used for these calculations. **A preliminary step of calculating dosage based on weight** is necessary before the flow rate can be calculated. **Fractional dosage answers are expressed to the nearest tenth and mL/hr rates to the nearest whole mL**.

EXAMPLE 1   A drug is ordered at the rate of **3 mcg/kg/min** for a body weight of **95.9 kg**. The solution strength is **400 mg** in **250 mL**. Calculate the **mL/hr** flow rate.

- **Calculate the dosage per min for 95.9 kg.**

  3 mcg/kg/min × 95.9 kg = **287.7 mcg/min**

- **Convert 287.7 mcg/min to mcg/hr.**

  287.7 mcg/min × 60 min/hr = **17,262 mcg/hr**

- **Convert 17,262 mcg to mg.**

  17,262 mcg/hr ÷ 1000 mcg/mg = 17.26 = **17.3 mg/hr**

- **Calculate the flow rate.**

$$\frac{400 \text{ mg}}{250 \text{ mL}} = \frac{17.3 \text{ mg}}{X \text{ mL}} \quad \text{or} \quad 400 \text{ mg} : 250 \text{ mL} = 17.3 \text{ mg} : X \text{ mL}$$
$$400X = 250 \times 17.3$$
$$= 10.8 = \textbf{11 mL/hr} \qquad\qquad X = 10.8 = \textbf{11 mL/hr}$$

To infuse 3 mcg/kg/min, set the flow rate at 11 mL/hr.

EXAMPLE 2   A **2.5 g in 250 mL** solution is ordered at a rate of **100 mcg/kg/min** for a body weight of **104.6 kg**. Calculate the **mL/hr** flow rate.

- **Calculate the dosage per min for 104.6 kg.**

  100 mcg/kg/min × 104.6 kg = **10,460 mcg/min**

- **Convert 10,460 mcg to mg.**

  10,460 mcg/min ÷ 1000 mcg/mg = 10.46 = **10.5 mg/min**

- **Convert 10.5 mg/min to mg/hr.**

  10.5 mg/min × 60 min/hr = **630 mg/hr**

- **Calculate the flow rate.**

$$\frac{2500 \text{ mg}}{250 \text{ mL}} = \frac{630 \text{ mg}}{X \text{ mL}} = \textbf{63 mL/hr} \quad \text{or} \quad 2500 \text{ mg} : 250 \text{ mL} = 630 \text{ mg} : X \text{ mL}$$

$$2500X = 250 \times 630$$

$$X = \textbf{63 mL/hr}$$

To infuse 100 mcg/kg/min, set the rate at 63 mL/hr.

EXAMPLE 3 ▶ An IV medication has been ordered at **4 mcg/kg/min** using a solution of **50 mg** in **250 mL.** The body weight is **107.3 kg.** Calculate the **mL/hr** flow rate.

- **Calculate the dosage per min.**

  4 mcg/kg/min × 107.3 kg = **429.2 mcg/min**

- **Convert mcg/min to mcg/hr.**

  429.2 mcg/min × 60 min/hr = **25,752 mcg/hr**

- **Convert mcg to mg.**

  25,752 mcg/hr ÷ 1000 mcg/mg = 25.75 = **25.8 mg/hr**

- **Calculate the flow rate.**

$$\frac{50 \text{ mg}}{250 \text{ mL}} = \frac{25.8 \text{ mg}}{X \text{ mL}} = \textbf{129 mL/hr} \quad \text{or} \quad 50 \text{ mg} : 250 \text{ mL} = 25.8 \text{ mg} : X \text{ mL}$$

$$50X = 250 \times 25.8$$

$$X = \textbf{129 mL/hr}$$

To infuse 4 mcg/kg/min, set the rate at 129 mL/hr.

▶▶▶ PROBLEMS 20.2

Calculate the dosage per min to the tenths, and the mL/hr flow rates.

	Dosage per min	mL/hr
1. A dosage of 3 mcg/kg/min has been ordered for an 87.4 kg adult. The solution has a strength of 50 mg in 250 mL.	_____	_____
2. A dosage has been ordered at 4 mcg/kg/min using a 400 mg/250 mL solution. The body weight is 92.4 kg.	_____	_____
3. A dosage of 2.5 mcg/kg/min has been ordered. The solution is 500 mg/250 mL. The body weight is 80.7 kg.	_____	_____
4. A dosage of 150 mcg/kg/min has been ordered for a body weight of 92.1 kg. The solution strength is 2.5 g/250 mL.	_____	_____

5. A 5 mcg/kg/min dosage is ordered for a body weight of 80.3 kg. The solution strength is 1 g/100 mL.   _____ _____

6. A dosage of 2 mcg/kg/min has been ordered for an adult weighing 78.2 kg. The strength of the solution is 40 mg/200 mL.   _____ _____

7. A dosage of 6 mcg/kg/min has been ordered for an adult weighing 88.7 kg. A solution strength of 100 mg/500 mL is to be infused.   _____ _____

8. The body weight is 91.2 kg and a 1.5 mcg/kg/min rate is ordered using a 0.3 g/250 mL solution.   _____ _____

9. A 2 mcg/kg/min infusion is ordered for a 90.3 kg adult. The solution to be used has a strength of 0.5 g/250 mL.   _____ _____

10. A 20 mcg/kg/min dosage is ordered for a body weight of 81.7 kg. The solution available is 1 g/500 mL.   _____ _____

Answers 1. 262.2 mcg/min; 79 mL/hr **2.** 369.6 mcg/min; 14 mL/hr **3.** 201.8 mcg/min; 6 mL/hr **4.** 13,815 mcg/min; 83 mL/hr **5.** 401.5 mcg/min; 2 mL/hr **6.** 156.4 mcg/min; 47 mL/hr **7.** 532.2 mcg/min; 160 mL/hr **8.** 136.8 mcg/min; 7 mL/hr **9.** 180.6 mcg/min; 5 mL/hr **10.** 1634 mcg/min; 49 mL/hr

USING RATIO AND PROPORTION TO CALCULATE INFUSION TITRATIONS

Titration refers to the adjustment of dosage within a specific range to obtain a measurable physiologic response; for example, 2–4 mcg/min to maintain systolic BP >100. The dosage is increased or decreased within the ordered range until the desired response is obtained. The **lowest dosage is set first** and adjusted upward and downward as necessary. The **upper dosage is never exceeded** unless a new order is obtained.

EIDs are used for administration. Flow rates are calculated in mL/hr for the lowest and highest dosage ordered and adjusted within this range to elicit the desired physiologic response. Let's look at some examples.

EXAMPLE 1   A dosage of **2–4 mcg/min** has been ordered to maintain systolic BP > 100 mm. The solution being titrated has **8 mg** in **250 mL**. Calculate the flow rate for the **2–4 mcg range**.

Calculate the **lower** 2 mcg/min flow rate first.

- **Convert 2 mcg/min to mcg/hr.**

  2 mcg/min × 60 min/hr = **120 mcg/hr**

- **Convert 120 mcg/hr to mg/hr.**

  120 mcg/hr = **0.12 mg/hr**

- **Calculate the 0.12 mg/hr flow rate.**

$$\frac{8 \text{ mg}}{250 \text{ mL}} = \frac{0.12 \text{ mg}}{X \text{ mL}} \quad \text{or} \quad 8 \text{ mg} : 250 \text{ mL} = 0.12 \text{ mg} : X \text{ mL}$$

$$= 3.75 = \textbf{4 mL/hr} \qquad\qquad 8X = 250 \times 0.12$$

$$X = 3.75 = \textbf{4 mL/hr}$$

The flow rate for the lower 2 mcg/min dosage is 4 mL/hr.

The **upper** 4 mcg/min flow rate is exactly double the 2 mcg/min rate, so it can be calculated by multiplying the 4 mL/hr rate by 2.

4 mL/hr $\times$ 2 = **8 mL/hr**

The flow rate for the upper 4 mcg/min dosage is 8 mL/hr.
The flow rate range to titrate a dosage of 2–4 mcg/min is 4–8 mL/hr.

EXAMPLE 2 ▸ A drug is to be titrated between **415 and 830 mcg/min**. The solution concentration is **100 mg** in **40 mL**. Calculate the **mL/hr** flow rate range.

Calculate the **lower** 415 mcg/min flow rate first.

- **Convert 415 mcg/min to mcg/hr.**

  415 mcg/min $\times$ 60 min/hr = **24,900 mcg/hr**

- **Convert 24,900 mcg/hr to mg/hr.**

  24,900 mcg/hr $\div$ 1000 mcg/mg = **24.9 mg/hr**

- **Calculate the 24.9 mg/hr flow rate.**

$$\frac{100 \text{ mg}}{40 \text{ mL}} = \frac{24.9 \text{ mg}}{X \text{ mL}} \qquad \text{or} \quad 100 \text{ mg} : 40 \text{ mL} = 24.9 \text{ mg} : X \text{ mL}$$

$$100X = 40 \times 24.9$$

$$= 9.96 = \textbf{10 mL/hr} \qquad\qquad X = 9.96 = \textbf{10 mL/hr}$$

The **upper** 830 mcg/min dosage is exactly double the lower 415 mcg/min dosage, so the flow rate will be double 10 mL/hr.

10 mL/hr $\times$ 2 = **20 mL/hr**

The flow rate to titrate a dosage of 415–830 mcg/min is 10–20 mL/hr.

EXAMPLE 3 ▸ An adult weighing **103.1 kg** has orders for a titration between **0.3** and **3 mcg/kg/min**. The solution concentration is **50 mg in 250 mL**.

Calculate the dosage for 103.1 kg.

- **Calculate the lower 0.3 mcg/kg dosage per min.**

  0.3 mcg/kg/min $\times$ 103.1 kg = 30.93 = **30.9 mcg/min**

- **Calculate the upper 3 mcg/kg dosage per min.**

  3 mcg/kg/min $\times$ 103.1 kg = **309.3 mcg/min**

The dosage range for 103.1 kg is 30.9 to 309.3 mcg/min.

Calculate the flow rate for the lower 30.9 mcg/min dosage.

- **Convert 30.9 mcg/min to mcg/hr.**

  30.9 mcg/min $\times$ 60 min/hr = **1854 mcg/hr**

- **Convert 1854 mcg/hr to mg/hr.**

  1854 mcg/hr $\div$ 1000 mcg/mg = 1.85 = **1.9 mg/hr**

- Calculate the 1.9 mg/hr flow rate.

$$\frac{50 \text{ mg}}{250 \text{ mL}} = \frac{1.9 \text{ mg}}{X \text{ mL}} \qquad \text{or} \quad 50 \text{ mg} : 250 \text{ mL} = 1.9 \text{ mg} : X \text{ mL}$$
$$= 9.5 = \textbf{10 mL/hr} \qquad\qquad 50X = 250 \times 1.9$$
$$X = 9.5 = \textbf{10 mL/hr}$$

Calculate the flow rate for the upper 309.3 mcg/min dosage.

- **Convert 309.3 mcg/min to mcg/hr.**

  309.3 mcg/min $\times$ 60 min/hr = **18,558 mcg/hr**

- **Convert 18,558 mcg/hr to mg/hr.**

  18,558 mcg/hr $\div$ 1000 mcg/mg = 18.55 = **18.6 mg/hr**

- **Calculate the 18.6 mg/hr flow rate.**

$$\frac{50 \text{ mg}}{250 \text{ mL}} = \frac{18.6 \text{ mg}}{X \text{ mL}} = \textbf{93 mL/hr} \quad \text{or} \quad 50 \text{ mg} : 250 \text{ mL} = 18.6 \text{ mg} : X \text{ mL}$$
$$50X = 250 \times 18.6$$
$$X = \textbf{93 mL/hr}$$

To deliver 0.3–3 mcg/kg/min for a 103.1 kg adult, the flow rate must be titrated between 10 and 93 mL/hr.

▶▶▶ PROBLEMS 20.3

Calculate these mL/hr flow rate ranges. Express answers to the nearest whole mL/hr.

1. A 2 g in 500 mL solution is ordered to titrate at 1–2 mg/min.   _____

2. A drug is ordered to titrate between 1 and 3 mcg/min.
   The solution strength is 1 mg per 250 mL.   _____

3. The dosage range being titrated is 5–8 mcg/kg/min.
   The adult weighs 103.7 kg, and the solution strength
   is 100 mg in 40 mL.   _____

4. A drug is to titrate between 50 and 100 mcg/kg/min.
   The adult weighs 78.7 kg, and the solution strength
   is 2500 mg in 250 mL.   _____

5. An adult weighing 73.2 kg has a solution of 500 mg in 250 mL
   ordered to titrate between 3 and 10 mcg/kg/min.   _____

6. A dosage of 4–6 mg/min has been ordered using a solution
   strength of 2.5 g/400 mL.   _____

SECTION 6

7. A dosage of 2–4 mcg/min has been ordered using a solution strength of 2 mg/250 mL.

    _____

8. The body weight is 99.9 kg, and a range of 5–9 mcg/kg/min is ordered. A 120 mg/50 mL solution is to be used.

    _____

9. A range of 30–70 mcg/kg/min infusion is ordered for an 84.3 kg adult. The solution to be used has a strength of 2 g/250 mL.

    _____

10. A 75–125 mcg/kg/min dosage is ordered for a body weight of 81.2 kg. The solution available is 2.5 g/250 mL.

    _____

Answers **1.** 15–30 mL/hr **2.** 15–45 mL/hr **3.** 12–20 mL/hr **4.** 24–47 mL/hr **5.** 7–22 mL/hr **6.** 38–58 mL/hr **7.** 15–30 mL/hr **8.** 12–22 mL/hr **9.** 19–44 mL/hr **10.** 37–61 mL/hr

 If you chose the Ratio and Proportion method, turn to the Summary Self-Test on page 319. If you chose the Dimensional Analysis method, continue with the DA instructional section that follows.

USING DIMENSIONAL ANALYSIS TO CALCULATE mL/hr RATE FOR DOSAGE ORDERED

One common IV critical care calculation is to determine the mL/hr flow rate for a specific drug dosage ordered. Let's start by looking at some examples of these.

EXAMPLE 1 A cardiac medication with a strength of **125 mg/100 mL** is to infuse at a rate of **20 mg/hr**. Calculate the **mL/hr** flow rate.

$$\frac{mL}{hr} = \frac{100\,mL}{125\,mg} \times \frac{20\,mg}{1\,hr}$$

$$= \frac{100\,mL}{125\,mg} \times \frac{20\,mg}{1\,hr}$$

$$= 16\,\textbf{mL/hr}$$

To infuse 20 mg/hr, set the flow rate at 16 mL/hr.

EXAMPLE 2 A dosage of **2 mcg/min** has been ordered using an **8 mg in 250 mL** solution. Calculate the **mL/hr** flow rate.

This equation will need a 60 min = 1 hr and a 1 mg = 1000 mcg conversion.

$$\frac{mL}{hr} = \frac{250\,mL}{8\,mg} \times \frac{1\,mg}{1000\,mcg} \times \frac{2\,mcg}{1\,min} \times \frac{60\,min}{1\,hr}$$

$$= \frac{250\,mL}{8\,mg} \times \frac{1\,mg}{1000\,mcg} \times \frac{2\,mcg}{1\,min} \times \frac{60\,min}{1\,hr}$$

$$= 3.75 = 4\,\textbf{mL/hr}$$

To infuse 2 mcg/min, set the flow rate at 4 mL/hr.

EXAMPLE 3 A medication with a strength of **50 mg in 250 mL** is used to infuse a dosage of **200 mcg/min**. Calculate the flow rate in **mL/hr**.

This equation will need a 60 min = 1 hr and 1 mg = 1000 mcg conversion.

$$\frac{mL}{hr} = \frac{250\,mL}{50\,mg} \times \frac{1\,mg}{1000\,mcg} \times \frac{200\,mcg}{1\,min} \times \frac{60\,min}{1\,hr}$$

$$= \frac{250\,mL}{50\,\cancel{mg}} \times \frac{1\,\cancel{mg}}{1000\,\cancel{mcg}} \times \frac{200\,\cancel{mcg}}{1\,\cancel{min}} \times \frac{60\,\cancel{min}}{1\,hr}$$

$$= \textbf{60 mL/hr}$$

To infuse 200 mcg/min, set the flow rate at 60 mL/hr.

▶▶▶ PROBLEMS 20.4

Calculate these mL/hr flow rates. Express answers to the nearest whole mL/hr.

1. A 20 mg/hr dosage is ordered using a 100 mg/100 mL solution. _____

2. A medication is ordered at the rate of 3 mcg/min.
   The solution strength is 8 mg in 250 mL. _____

3. A solution of 2 g medication in 500 mL is used to
   administer a dosage of 2 mg/min. _____

4. A 2 mcg/min infusion is ordered. The solution strength
   is 1 mg/250 mL. _____

5. An initial dose of a drug is ordered at 25 mg/hr. The
   solution strength is 125 mg/100 mL. _____

6. A 100 mg/250 mL solution strength is ordered at a
   rate of 15 mg/hr. _____

7. A solution strength of 10 mg/250 mL is to infuse at 5 mcg/min. _____

8. A 500 mL/1.5 g solution is to infuse at 3 mg/min. _____

9. A 10 mg/250 mL solution is to infuse at 20 mcg/min. _____

10. A 250 mg/100 mL solution is to infuse at 30 mg/hr. _____

Answers   1. 20 mL/hr   **2.** 6 mL/hr   **3.** 30 mL/hr   **4.** 30 mL/hr   **5.** 20 mL/hr   **6.** 38 mL/hr
7. 8 mL/hr   **8.** 60 mL/hr   **9.** 30 mL/hr   **10.** 12 mL/hr

USING DIMENSIONAL ANALYSIS TO CALCULATE mL/hr RATE FOR DOSAGE PER kg ORDERED

Many IV medication infusions are calculated based on body weight; for example, 95.9 mcg/kg/hr. **Body weight to the nearest tenth kg** is used for the calculations. There are two ways the flow rate can be calculated. The first method requires two steps.

Two-Step Flow Rate Calculation

The dosage for the body weight is calculated to the nearest tenth, then used to determine the flow rate.

EXAMPLE 1 ▮ Medication is ordered at the rate of **3 mcg/kg/min** for an adult weighing **95.9 kg**. The solution strength is **400 mg** in **250 mL**. Calculate the flow rate.

- **Calculate the 3 mcg/min dosage for 95.9 kg.**

$$3 \text{ mcg/kg/min} \times 95.9 \text{ kg} = \textbf{287.7 mcg/min}$$

- **Calculate the mL/hr flow rate for 287.7 mcg/min.**

$$\frac{\text{mL}}{\text{hr}} = \frac{250 \text{ mL}}{400 \text{ mg}} \times \frac{1 \text{ mg}}{1000 \text{ mcg}} \times \frac{287.7 \text{ mcg}}{1 \text{ min}} \times \frac{60 \text{ min}}{1 \text{ hr}}$$

$$= \frac{250 \text{ mL}}{400 \text{ mg}} \times \frac{1 \text{ mg}}{1000 \text{ mcg}} \times \frac{287.7 \text{ mcg}}{1 \text{ min}} \times \frac{60 \text{ min}}{1 \text{ hr}}$$

$$= 10.79 = \textbf{11 mL/hr}$$

To infuse 3 mcg/kg/min, set the flow rate at 11 mL/hr.

EXAMPLE 2 ▮ A solution strength of **2.5 g in 250 mL** has been ordered at a rate of **100 mcg/kg/min** for an adult weighing **104.6 kg**. Calculate the flow rate.

- **Calculate the dosage for 104.6 kg.**

$$100 \text{ mcg/kg/min} \times 104.6 \text{ kg} = 10{,}460 \text{ mcg/min} = \textbf{10.5 mg/min}$$

- **Calculate the flow rate for 10.5 mg/min.**

$$\frac{\text{mL}}{\text{hr}} = \frac{250 \text{ mL}}{2.5 \text{ g}} \times \frac{1 \text{ g}}{1000 \text{ mg}} \times \frac{10.5 \text{ mg}}{1 \text{ min}} \times \frac{60 \text{ min}}{1 \text{ hr}}$$

$$= \frac{250 \text{ mL}}{2.5 \text{ g}} \times \frac{1 \text{ g}}{1000 \text{ mg}} \times \frac{10.5 \text{ mg}}{1 \text{ min}} \times \frac{60 \text{ min}}{1 \text{ hr}}$$

$$= 63 = \textbf{63 mL/hr}$$

To infuse 100 mcg/kg/min, set the flow rate at 63 mL/hr.

EXAMPLE 3 ▮ A medication has been ordered at **4 mcg/kg/min** from a solution of **50 mg in 250 mL**. The body weight is **107.3 kg**.

- **Calculate the dosage for 107.3 kg.**

$$4 \text{ mcg/kg/min} \times 107.3 \text{ kg} = \textbf{429.2 mcg/min}$$

- **Calculate the flow rate for 429.2 mcg/min.**

$$\frac{\text{mL}}{\text{hr}} = \frac{250 \text{ mL}}{50 \text{ mg}} \times \frac{1 \text{ mg}}{1000 \text{ mcg}} \times \frac{429.2 \text{ mcg}}{1 \text{ min}} \times \frac{60 \text{ min}}{1 \text{ hr}}$$

$$= \frac{250 \text{ mL}}{50 \text{ mg}} \times \frac{1 \text{ mg}}{1000 \text{ mcg}} \times \frac{429.2 \text{ mcg}}{1 \text{ min}} \times \frac{60 \text{ min}}{1 \text{ hr}}$$

$$= 128.7 = \textbf{129 mL/hr}$$

To infuse 4 mcg/kg/min, set the flow rate at 129 mL/hr.

▶▶▶ PROBLEMS 20.5

Calculate the mcg/min and mL/hr flow rates.

	mcg/min	mL/hr
1. A 3 mcg/kg/min dosage has been ordered for an adult weighing 87.4 kg. The solution being used has a strength of 50 mg in 250 mL.	_____	_____
2. IV medication has been ordered to infuse at 4 mcg/kg/min using a 400 mg/250 mL solution. The body weight is 92.4 kg.	_____	_____
3. A 2.5 mcg/kg/min dosage has been ordered. The solution strength is 0.5 g/250 mL. The body weight is 80.7 kg.	_____	_____
4. A rate of 150 mcg/kg/min has been ordered for a 92.1 kg body weight. The solution strength is 2.5 g in 250 mL.	_____	_____
5. A 5 mcg/kg/min infusion has been ordered for a body weight of 80.3 kg. The solution to be used has 1 g in 500 mL.	_____	_____
6. A 2 mcg/kg/min dosage has been ordered for an adult weighing 79.9 kg. The solution strength available is 50 mg/250 mL.	_____	_____
7. A dosage of 3 mcg/kg/min has been ordered using a 350 mg/250 mL solution strength. The body weight is 86.9 kg.	_____	_____
8. An adult weighing 84.3 kg has a dosage of 3 mcg/kg/min ordered. The solution to be used is 0.75 g/300 mL.	_____	_____
9. A 4.5 mcg/kg/min dosage is ordered for an 84.9 kg adult. The solution strength is 1.2 g/500 mL.	_____	_____
10. A 6 mcg/kg/min dosage is ordered for an adult weighing 85.8 kg. The solution strength is 800 mg/500 mL.	_____	_____

Answers **1.** 262.2 mcg/min; 79 mL/hr **2.** 369.6 mcg/min; 14 mL/hr **3.** 201.8 mcg/min; 6 mL/hr **4.** 13,815 mcg/min; 83 mL/hr **5.** 401.5 mcg/min; 12 mL/hr **6.** 159.8 mcg/min; 48 mL/hr **7.** 260.7 mcg/min; 11 mL/hr **8.** 252.9 mcg/min; 6 mL/hr **9.** 382.1 mcg/min; 10 mL/hr **10.** 514.8 mcg/min; 19 mL/hr

One-Step mL/hr Flow Rate Calculation

The one-step method of flow rate calculation requires very careful entry of ratios and equally careful cancellation of measurement units to verify accuracy in ratio entry. Let's look at the entire equation step by step. Express flow rates to the nearest mL.

EXAMPLE 1 ▸ Medication is ordered at the rate of **3 mcg/kg/min** for an adult weighing **95.9 kg**. The solution strength is **400 mg** in **250 mL**. Calculate the flow rate.

The first two ratios entered are the same as in the two-step method.

$$\frac{mL}{hr} = \frac{250\ mL}{400\ mg} \times \frac{1\ mg}{1000\ mcg}$$

The denominator to be matched next is mcg. This is provided by the 3 mcg/ kg/ min dosage. Enter this with 3 mcg as the numerator; two measures, kg and min, become the new denominators.

$$\frac{mL}{hr} = \frac{250\ mL}{400\ mg} \times \frac{1\ mg}{1000\ mcg} \times \frac{3\ mcg}{kg/min}$$

Both kg and min must be matched in the next numerators. Either can be entered first, but min is the best choice because a conversion ratio is needed to change min to the hr being calculated. Enter the 60 min = 1 hr conversion, with 60 min as the numerator, to match the previous min denominator.

$$\frac{mL}{hr} = \frac{250\ mL}{400\ mg} \times \frac{1\ mg}{1000\ mcg} \times \frac{3\ mcg}{kg/min} \times \frac{60\ min}{1\ hr}$$

Only one measure remains to be entered: the 95.9 kg body weight. Enter this as the final numerator to match the remaining kg denominator. This completes the equation.

$$\frac{mL}{hr} = \frac{250\ mL}{400\ mg} \times \frac{1\ mg}{1000\ mcg} \times \frac{3\ mcg}{kg/min} \times \frac{60\ min}{1\ hr} \times \frac{95.9\ kg}{}$$

Cancel the alternate denominator/numerator measures. Only mL and hr remain in the equation. Do the math.

$$\frac{mL}{hr} = \frac{250\ mL}{400\ \cancel{mg}} \times \frac{1\ \cancel{mg}}{1000\ \cancel{mcg}} \times \frac{3\ \cancel{mcg}}{\cancel{kg}/\cancel{min}} \times \frac{60\ \cancel{min}}{1\ hr} \times \frac{95.9\ \cancel{kg}}{}$$

$$= 10.79 = \mathbf{11\ mL/hr}$$

The 11 mL/hr answer is identical to the 11 mL/hr answer obtained in the two-step calculation previously demonstrated.

EXAMPLE 2 ▸ A dosage of **2.5 g in 250 mL** has been ordered at a rate of **100 mcg/ kg/min** for an adult weighing **104.6 kg**. Calculate the flow rate.

Enter the mL/hr being calculated. The first mL numerator is provided by the 250 mL containing 2.5 g medication. Enter it now.

$$\frac{mL}{hr} = \frac{250\ mL}{2.5\ g}$$

The dosage ordered is in mcg, so g to mg and mg to mcg conversion ratios are needed. Enter these now.

$$\frac{mL}{hr} = \frac{250\ mL}{2.5\ g} \times \frac{1\ g}{1000\ mg} \times \frac{1\ mg}{1000\ mcg}$$

Enter the 100 mcg/kg/min dosage next, with mcg as the numerator to match the previous mcg denominator.

$$\frac{mL}{hr} = \frac{250\ mL}{2.5\ g} \times \frac{1\ g}{1000\ mg} \times \frac{1\ mg}{1000\ mcg} \times \frac{100\ mcg}{kg/min}$$

Enter the min/hr conversion ratio.

$$\frac{mL}{hr} = \frac{250\ mL}{2.5\ g} \times \frac{1\ g}{1000\ mg} \times \frac{1\ mg}{1000\ mcg} \times \frac{100\ mcg}{kg/min} \times \frac{60\ min}{1\ hr}$$

Enter the 104.6 kg body weight to complete the equation.

$$\frac{mL}{hr} = \frac{250\ mL}{2.5\ g} \times \frac{1\ g}{1000\ mg} \times \frac{1\ mg}{1000\ mcg} \times \frac{100\ mcg}{kg/min} \times \frac{60\ min}{1\ hr} \times \frac{104.6\ kg}{}$$

Cancel the alternate denominator/numerator entries to double-check the accuracy of ratio entry. Do the math.

$$\frac{mL}{hr} = \frac{250\ mL}{2.5\ \cancel{g}} \times \frac{1\ \cancel{g}}{1000\ \cancel{mg}} \times \frac{1\ \cancel{mg}}{1000\ \cancel{mcg}} \times \frac{100\ \cancel{mcg}}{\cancel{kg}/\cancel{min}} \times \frac{60\ \cancel{min}}{1\ hr} \times \frac{104.6\ \cancel{kg}}{}$$

$$= 62.76 = \textbf{63 mL/hr}$$

The 63 mL/hr answer is identical to the 63 mL/hr answer obtained in the two-step calculation.

EXAMPLE 3   A medication has been ordered at 4 mcg/kg/min from a solution of **50 mg** in **250 mL**. The body weight is **107.3 kg**.

$$\frac{mL}{hr} = \frac{250\ mL}{50\ mg}$$

$$\frac{mL}{hr} = \frac{250\ mL}{50\ mg} \times \frac{1\ mg}{1000\ mcg}$$

$$\frac{mL}{hr} = \frac{250\ mL}{50\ mg} \times \frac{1\ mg}{1000\ mcg} \times \frac{4\ mcg}{kg/min}$$

$$\frac{mL}{hr} = \frac{250\ mL}{50\ mg} \times \frac{1\ mg}{1000\ mcg} \times \frac{4\ mcg}{kg/min} \times \frac{60\ min}{1\ hr}$$

$$\frac{mL}{hr} = \frac{250\ mL}{50\ mg} \times \frac{1\ mg}{1000\ mcg} \times \frac{4\ mcg}{kg/min} \times \frac{60\ min}{1\ hr} \times \frac{107.3\ kg}{}$$

$$= 128.76 = \textbf{129 mL/hr}$$

The 129 mL/hr answer is identical to the 129 mL/hr rate calculated in the two-step method.

SECTION 6

▶▶▶ PROBLEMS 20.6

Calculate these mL/hr flow rates. Express answers to the nearest whole mL/hr.

1. A 3.5 mcg/kg/min dosage has been ordered for an adult weighing 90.3 kg. The solution being used has a strength of 40 mg in 150 mL. _____

2. IV medication has been ordered to infuse at 3 mcg/kg/min using a 250 mg/250 mL solution. The body weight is 87.3 kg. _____

3. A 4 mcg/kg/min dosage has been ordered. The solution strength is 600 mg/250 mL. The weight is 90.3 kg. _____

4. A rate of 200 mcg/kg/min has been ordered for an 83.3 kg weight. The solution strength is 3.5 g in 250 mL. _____

5. A 4.5 mcg/kg/min infusion has been ordered for a 79.9 kg body weight. The solution to be used has 1.5 g in 200 mL. _____

6. A 4 mcg/kg/min dosage has been ordered for an adult weighing 83.8 kg. The solution strength available is 50 mg/150 mL. _____

7. A dosage of 5 mcg/kg/min has been ordered using a 300 mg/250 mL solution strength. The body weight is 86.6 kg. _____

8. An adult weighing 91.4 kg has a dosage of 4 mcg/kg/min ordered. The solution to be used is 700 mg/500 mL. _____

9. A 175 mcg/kg/min dosage is ordered for an 84.9 kg adult. The solution strength is 4 g/250 mL. _____

10. A 5 mcg/kg/min dosage is ordered for an adult weighing 78.9 kg. The solution strength is 2 g/250 mL. _____

Answers **1.** 71 mL/hr **2.** 16 mL/hr **3.** 9 mL/hr **4.** 71 mL/hr **5.** 3 mL/hr **6.** 60 mL/hr **7.** 22 mL/hr **8.** 16 mL/hr **9.** 56 mL/hr **10.** 3 mL/hr

USING DIMENSIONAL ANALYSIS TO CALCULATE INFUSION TITRATIONS

Titration refers to the **adjustment of dosage within a specific range to obtain a measurable physiologic response**; for example, a drug at 2–4 mcg/min to maintain systolic BP > 100. The dosage is increased or decreased within the ordered range until the desired response is obtained. The **lowest dosage is set first and adjusted upward and downward as necessary**. The **upper dosage is never exceeded** unless a new order is obtained.

Volumetric or syringe pumps are used for administration. Flow rates are calculated in mL/hr for the lowest and highest dosage ordered and adjusted within this range to elicit the desired physiologic response. Let's look at some examples.

EXAMPLE 1 ▸ A **2–4 mcg/min** dosage has been ordered. The solution being titrated has **8 mg** in **250 mL**. Calculate the flow rate of medication for the **2–4 mcg range**.

Calculate the lower 2 mcg/min flow rate first.

$$\frac{mL}{hr} = \frac{250\ mL}{8\ mg} \times \frac{1\ mg}{1000\ mcg} \times \frac{2\ mcg}{1\ min} \times \frac{60\ min}{1\ hr}$$

$$= \frac{250\ mL}{8\ \cancel{mg}} \times \frac{1\ \cancel{mg}}{1000\ \cancel{mcg}} \times \frac{2\ \cancel{mcg}}{1\ \cancel{min}} \times \frac{60\ \cancel{min}}{1\ hr}$$

$$= 3.75 = \mathbf{4\ mL/\ hr}$$

The upper 4 mcg/min flow rate is exactly double the 2 mcg/min rate.

$$4\ mL/hr \times 2 = \mathbf{8\ mL/hr}$$

A dosage of 2–4 mcg/min is delivered by a flow rate of 4–8 mL/hr.

EXAMPLE 2   A medication is to be titrated between **415–830 mcg/min**. The solution concentration is **100 mg** in **40 mL**. Calculate the **mL/hr** flow rate range.

Calculate the flow rate for the lower 415 mcg/min dosage.

$$\frac{mL}{hr} = \frac{40\ mL}{100\ mg} \times \frac{1\ mg}{1000\ mcg} \times \frac{415\ mcg}{1\ min} \times \frac{60\ min}{1\ hr}$$

$$= \frac{40\ mL}{100\ \cancel{mg}} \times \frac{1\ \cancel{mg}}{1000\ \cancel{mcg}} \times \frac{415\ \cancel{mcg}}{1\ \cancel{min}} \times \frac{60\ \cancel{min}}{1\ hr}$$

$$= 9.96 = \mathbf{10\ mL/hr}$$

The 830 mcg dosage is exactly double 415 mcg.

$$10\ mL/hr \times 2 = \mathbf{20\ mL/hr}$$

A dosage of 415–830 mcg/min requires a flow rate of 10–20 mL/hr.

EXAMPLE 3   An adult weighing **103.1 kg** has dosage orders for **0.3–3 mcg/kg/min**. The solution concentration is **50 mg** in **250 mL**.

Calculate the dosage range for 103.1 kg.

> **Lower dosage:** 0.3 mcg/kg/min × 103.1 kg = 30.93 = **30.9 mcg/min**
>
> **Upper dosage:** 3 mcg/kg/min × 103.1 kg = **309.3 mcg/min**

The dosage range for this 103.1 kg adult is 30.9–309.3 mcg/min.

Calculate the flow rate for the lower 30.9 mcg/min dosage.

$$\frac{mL}{hr} = \frac{250\ mL}{50\ mg} \times \frac{1\ mg}{1000\ mcg} \times \frac{30.9\ mcg}{1\ min} \times \frac{60\ min}{1\ hr}$$

$$= \frac{250\ mL}{50\ \cancel{mg}} \times \frac{1\ \cancel{mg}}{1000\ \cancel{mcg}} \times \frac{30.9\ \cancel{mcg}}{1\ \cancel{min}} \times \frac{60\ \cancel{min}}{1\ hr}$$

$$= 9.2 = \mathbf{9\ mL/hr}$$

Calculate the flow rate for the upper 309.3 mcg/min dosage.

$$\frac{mL}{hr} = \frac{250\ mL}{50\ mg} \times \frac{1\ mg}{1000\ mcg} \times \frac{309.3\ mcg}{1\ min} \times \frac{60\ min}{1\ hr}$$

$$= \frac{250\ mL}{50\ mg} \times \frac{1\ mg}{1000\ mcg} \times \frac{309.3\ mcg}{1\ min} \times \frac{60\ min}{1\ hr}$$

$$= 92.7 = \textbf{93 mL/hr}$$

To deliver 0.3–3 mcg/kg/min, the flow rate must be titrated from 9–93 mL/hr.

▶▶▶ PROBLEMS 20.7

Calculate these mL/hr flow rate ranges. Express answers to the nearest whole mL/hr.

1. A 2 g in 500 mL solution is ordered to titrate at 1–2 mg/min. _____

2. A drug is ordered to titrate between 1–3 mcg/min. The solution strength is 1 mg per 250 mL. _____

3. The dosage range is 5–8 mcg/kg/min. The body weight is 103.7 kg, and the solution strength is 100 mg in 40 mL. _____

4. A drug is to titrate between 50–100 mcg/kg/min. The body weight is 78.7 kg, and the solution strength is 2500 mg in 250 mL. _____

5. An adult weighing 73.2 kg has a solution of 500 mg medication in 250 mL ordered to titrate between 3–10 mcg/kg/min. _____

6. A 2–3 mg/min dosage has been ordered. The solution strength available is 1.5 g/400 mL. _____

7. A dosage of 6–7 mcg/min has been ordered using a 5 mg/500 mL solution strength. _____

8. An adult weighing 101.6 kg has a dosage of 4–7 mcg/kg/min ordered. The solution to be used is 75 mg/50 mL. _____

9. A 30–70 mcg/kg/min dosage is ordered for an 80.4 kg adult. The solution strength is 3 g/250 mL. _____

10. A 4–8 mcg/kg/min dosage is ordered for an adult weighing 72.1 kg. The solution strength is 400 mg/250 mL. _____

Answers 1. 15–30 mL/hr 2. 15–45 mL/hr 3. 12–20 mL/hr 4. 24–47 mL/hr 5. 7–22 mL/hr
6. 32–48 mL/hr 7. 36–42 mL/hr 8. 16–28 mL/hr 9. 12–28 mL/hr 10. 11–22 mL/hr

---

Summary

This concludes the chapter on titration of IV medications. The important points to remember about these medications are:

▼ They have a rapid action and short duration.

▼ They have a narrow margin of safety, and continuous monitoring is required in their use.

▼ They are frequency titrated within a specific dosage/flow rate to elicit a measurable physiologic response.

▼ When titrated, they are initiated at the lowest dosage ordered and increased or decreased slowly to obtain the desired response.

▼ They are infused using an EID or 60 gtt/mL microdrip set.

▼ The mL/hr flow rate for EIDs and the gtt/min microdrip rate are identical and interchangeable.

Summary Self-Test

Calculate dosages to the nearest tenth and flow rates to the nearest whole number using the calculations method, Ratio and Proportion or Dimensional Analysis, that you choose.

1. A 6 mcg/kg/min dosage is ordered for an adult weighing 75.4 kg. The solution available is 500 mg in 250 mL.

    mcg/min dosage _____   mL/hr flow rate _____

2. The order is to infuse a solution of 50 mg in 250 mL at 0.8 mcg/kg/min. Calculate the dosage and flow rate for a 65.9 kg adult.

    mcg/min dosage _____   mL/hr flow rate _____

3. A solution of 250 mg in 500 mL is to infuse between 0.5 and 0.7 mg/kg/hr. The adult weighs 82.4 kg.

    mg/hr dosage range _____   mL/hr flow rate range _____

4. A solution of 400 mg in 250 mL is infusing at 20 mL/hr.

    mcg/min dosage _____

5. A 1–6 mg/min dosage is ordered. The solution strength is 2 g/500 mL.

    mL/hr flow rate range _____

6. An infusion of 2 g in 500 mL is ordered at 60 mL/hr.

    mg/min dosage _____   mg/hr dosage _____

7. The solution available is 25 mg in 50 mL. The order is to infuse at 8 mg/hr.

    mL/hr flow rate _____

8. A solution of 100 mg in 40 mL is ordered to infuse at 5 mcg/kg/min for an adult weighing 77.1 kg.

    mL/hr flow rate _____

9. A drug is ordered at 4 mcg/min. The solution available is 1 mg in 250 mL.

    mL/hr flow rate _____

10. An adult weighing 80 kg has an infusion ordered at 8 mcg/kg/min. The solution strength is 800 mg in 500 mL.

    mcg/min dosage _____   mL/hr flow rate _____

11. A dosage of 400 mg is added to 250 mL and infused at 45 mL/hr. Calculate the mcg/min and mg/hr infusing.

    mcg/min dosage _____   mg/hr dosage _____

12. An adult has orders for a dosage of 1 mg/min. The solution strength is 250 mg in 250 mL.

mL/hr flow rate _____

13. An adult weighing 77.9 kg is to receive 80 mcg/kg/min. The solution strength is 2.5 g in 250 mL.

mcg/min dosage _____   mL/hr flow rate _____

14. A dosage of 4 mcg/min has been ordered using an 8 mg in 250 mL solution.

mL/hr flow rate _____

15. An adult who weighs 81.7 kg has orders for 8–10 mcg/kg/min. The solution strength is 400 mg in 250 mL.

mcg/min dosage range _____

16. A 6 mcg/kg/min dosage has been ordered for a 90.7 kg adult. The solution strength is 50 mg in 250 mL.

mcg/min dosage _____   mL/hr flow rate _____

17. A dosage of 5 mcg/kg/min is ordered. The solution available is 400 mg in 250 mL. The adult weighs 70.7 kg.

mcg/min dosage _____   mL/hr flow rate _____

18. A 3 mg/min dosage is ordered. The solution strength is 2 g in 500 mL.

mL/hr flow rate _____

19. A solution of 50 mg/250 mL is infusing at 15 mL/hr.

mcg/min infusing _____

20. A 2 g in 500 mL solution is to infuse at a rate of 2 mg/min.

mL/hr flow rate _____

21. An adult whose weight is 102.4 kg is to receive a dosage of 2 mg/kg/hr. The solution strength is 1 g in 500 mL.

mg/hr dosage _____   mL/hr flow rate _____

22. A solution strength of 1 g in 100 mL is to infuse at a rate of 15 mcg/kg/min. The body weight is 94.4 kg.

mcg/min dosage _____   mL/hr flow rate _____

23. An adult is receiving 4 mL/hr of a solution that contains 8 mg in 250 mL.

mcg/min infusing _____

24. A drug is ordered to titrate between 5 and 10 mcg/kg/min. The body weight is 97.1 kg, and the solution strength is 100 mg/40 mL.

mcg/min range _____   mL/hr flow rate range _____

25. A 500 mg in 250 mL solution is ordered for a 101.2 kg adult to titrate between 3 and 10 mcg/kg/min. _____

mcg/min dosage range _____   mL/hr flow rate range _____

26. An infusion of 500 mg in 250 mL is infusing at a rate of 14 mL/hr.

mcg/min infusing _____

27. A 5–10 mcg/kg/min dosage is to be titrated for an adult patient weighing 79.6 kg. The solution strength is 100 mg in 40 mL.

mcg/min dosage range _____   mL/hr flow rate range _____

28. A 400 mg in 250 mL solution is to be titrated at 2–20 mcg/kg/min. The body weight is 62.3 kg.

        mcg/min dosage range _____   mL/hr flow rate range _____

29. A drug has been ordered for an adult weighing 84.9 kg to titrate at 2.5–10 mcg/kg/min. The solution strength is 500 mg in 250 mL.

        mcg/min dosage range _____   mL/hr flow rate range _____

30. A drug is ordered at a rate of 1–4 mg/min. The solution strength is 2 g in 500 mL.

        mL/hr flow rate range _____

31. A 10 mcg/min dosage is ordered using an 8 mg/250 mL solution.

        mL/hr flow rate _____

32. A 2 g in 500 mL dosage is to infuse at 3 mg/min.

        mL/hr flow rate _____

33. A 250 mL solution with 1 mg of medication is to be infused at 5 mcg/min.

        mL/hr flow rate _____

34. A 4 mcg/min dosage is ordered. The solution is 250 mL with 8 mg of medication.

        mL/hr flow rate _____

35. A 2 g in 500 mL solution is ordered to infuse at a rate of 6 mg/min.

        mL/hr flow rate _____

36. A 2 g in 500 mL solution is ordered to infuse at 4 mg/min.

        mL/hr flow rate _____

37. A 12 mcg/min dosage using an 8 mg in 250 mL of solution is ordered.

        mL/hr flow rate _____

38. A 40 mg/hr dosage is ordered, and a 100 mg in 100 mL solution is ordered.

        mL/hr flow rate _____

39. The order is to infuse 4 mcg/min from a 250 mL solution containing 1 mg of medication.

        mL/hr flow rate _____

40. Infuse 10 mg/hr from a 125 mg/100 mL solution.

        mL/hr flow rate _____

Answers

1. 452.4 mcg/min; 14 mL/hr
2. 52.7 mcg/min; 16 mL/hr
3. 41.2–57.7 mg/hr; 82–115 mL/hr
4. 533.3 mcg/min
5. 15–90 mL/hr
6. 4 mg/min; 240 mg/hr
7. 16 mL/hr
8. 9 mL/hr
9. 60 mL/hr
10. 640 mcg/min; 24 mL/hr
11. 1200 mcg/min; 72 mg/hr
12. 60 mL/hr
13. 6232 mcg/min; 37 mL/hr
14. 8 mL/hr

15. 653.6–817 mcg/min
16. 544.2 mcg/min; 163 mL/hr
17. 353.5 mcg/min; 13 mL/hr
18. 45 mL/hr
19. 50 mcg/min
20. 30 mL/hr
21. 204.8 mg/hr; 102 mL/hr
22. 1416 mcg/min; 9 mL/hr
23. 2.1 mcg/min
24. 485.5–971 mcg/min; 12–23 mL/hr
25. 303.6–1012 mcg/min; 9–30 mL/hr
26. 466.7 mcg/min
27. 398–796 mcg/min; 10–19 mL/hr

28. 124.6–1246 mcg/min; 5–47 mL/hr
29. 212.3–849 mcg/min; 6–25 mL/hr
30. 15–60 mL/hr
31. 19 mL/hr
32. 45 mL/hr
33. 75 mL/hr
34. 8 mL/hr
35. 90 mL/hr
36. 60 mL/hr
37. 23 mL/hr
38. 40 mL/hr
39. 60 mL/hr
40. 8 mL/hr

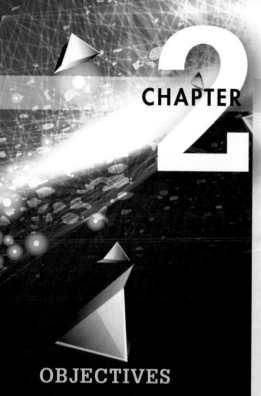

HEPARIN INFUSION CALCULATIONS

OBJECTIVES

The learner will calculate:

1. heparin dosages.

2. mL/hr flow rates for an EID.

3. gtt/min flow rates for microdrip and macrodrip sets.

4. hourly dosage infusing from mL/hr rate.

Heparin is a powerful anticoagulant drug that inhibits new blood clot formation or the extension of already-existing clots. Heparin dosages are expressed in USP units and may be given subcutaneously, mixed in IV solutions, or by IV push or bolus. Heparin is so commonly given, often postoperatively to prevent clot formation from venous stasis, that it is actually prepared in ready-to-hang IV bags; frequent checks of coagulation times during heparin therapy is essential. Heparin dosages are ordered based on clotting time and/or on an individual's body weight in kg. Subcutaneous heparin injections are given deeply at a 45° angle, to discourage medication leakage through the injection track, and subsequent bruising.

There is no essential difference in the calculations you have already practiced for critical care dosages and those for heparin dosages, except that heparin dosages for subcutaneous injection are measured using a TB syringe. However, heparin's action is so critical that it does deserve to be addressed separately. In this chapter, you will be introduced to labels of a variety of heparin dosages, practice measuring heparin dosages for addition to IV solutions, and calculate units per hour infusing from mL/hr flow rates.

HEPARIN IV AND VIAL LABELS

Let's start by taking a look at the heparin IV solution bag in Figure 21-1. This is an example of a premixed IV solution mentioned earlier. Notice the gray "Heparin Sodium 1000 units in 0.9% Sodium Chloride Injection" labeling on this 500 mL bag and the additional red labeling below. The red labeling draws particular attention to the fact that these bags contain heparin and make the bags instantly recognizable. They serve as an important safety factor in solution identification.

If a commercially prepared IV heparin dosage strength that you require is not available, you may be required to prepare the solution yourself from **a number of available vial dosage strengths**. Let's stop and look at several vial labels now so that you can refresh your memory with some typical calculations.

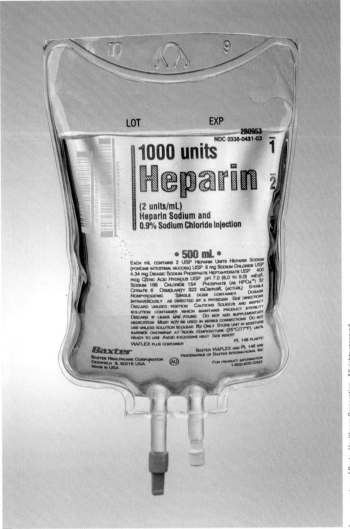

▲ **FIGURE 21-1**

▶▶▶ PROBLEMS 21.1

Read the heparin labels provided to determine how many mL of heparin will be necessary to prepare the solutions indicated.

1. Refer to the label in Figure 21-2 to determine how many mL will be required to add 20,000 units to an IV solution. _____

2. Refer to the label in Figure 21-3 to determine how many mL will be required to add 20,000 units to an IV solution. _____

3. Refer to the label in Figure 21-4 to determine how many mL of heparin will be required to add 25,000 units to an IV solution. _____

4. Refer to the label in Figure 21-5 to determine how many mL will be required to add 10,000 units to an IV solution. _____

Answers **1.** 4 mL **2.** 2 mL **3.** 12.5 mL **4.** 10 mL

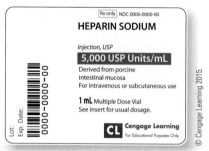

▲ FIGURE 21-2

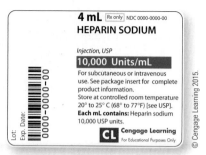

▲ FIGURE 21-3

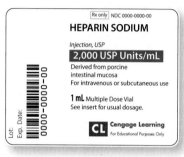

▲ FIGURE 21-4

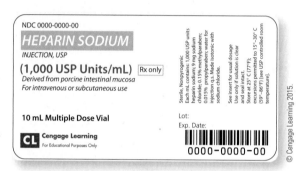

▲ FIGURE 21-5

CALCULATING mL/hr IV FLOW RATE FROM units/hr ORDERED

Because heparin is most frequently ordered in units/hr to be administered—for example, 1000 units/hr—and infused using an EID, a common calculation will be the mL/hr flow rate. Let's look at these calculations first, keeping in mind that **the mL/hr flow rate for an EID is identical to the gtt/min rate for a microdrip.**

CALCULATION USING RATIO AND PROPORTION

EXAMPLE 1

The order is to infuse heparin at **1000 units/hr** from a solution of **20,000 units in 500 mL** of D5W.

$$\frac{20{,}000 \text{ units}}{500 \text{ mL}} = \frac{1000 \text{ units}}{X \text{ mL}} = \textbf{25 mL/hr}$$

or

$$20{,}000 \text{ units} : 500 \text{ mL} = 1000 \text{ units} : X \text{ mL}$$

$$20{,}000X = 500 \times 1000$$

$$X = \textbf{25 mL/hr}$$

The flow rate to infuse 1000 units/hr from a solution of 20,000 units in 500 mL is 25 mL/hr.

EXAMPLE 2 The order is for heparin **800 units/hr**. The solution available is **40,000 units in 1000 mL** of D5W.

$$\frac{40,000 \text{ units}}{1000 \text{ mL}} = \frac{800 \text{ units}}{X \text{ mL}} = \textbf{20 mL/hr}$$

or

$$40,000 \text{ units} : 1000 \text{ mL} = 800 \text{ units} : X \text{ mL}$$

$$40,000X = 1000 \times 800$$

$$X = \textbf{20 mL/hr}$$

The flow rate to infuse 800 units/hr from a solution of 40,000 units in 1000 mL is 20 mL/hr.

EXAMPLE 3 The order is to infuse heparin **1100 units/hr** from a solution of **60,000 units in 1 L** of D5W.

$$\frac{60,000 \text{ units}}{1000 \text{ mL}} = \frac{1100 \text{ units}}{X \text{ mL}}$$

$$= 18.3 = \textbf{18 mL/hr}$$

or

$$60,000 \text{ units} : 1000 \text{ mL} = 1100 \text{ units} : X \text{ mL}$$

$$60,000X = 1000 \times 1100$$

$$X = 18.3 = \textbf{18 mL/hr}$$

The flow rate to infuse 1100 units/hr from a solution of 60,000 units in 1 L is 18 mL/hr.

CALCULATION USING DIMENSIONAL ANALYSIS

EXAMPLE 1 The order is to infuse heparin **1000 units/hr** from a solution of **20,000 units in 500 mL** D5W. Calculate the **mL/hr** flow rate.

Enter the mL/hr being calculated first. Locate the ratio containing mL, the 20,000 units/500 mL strength, and enter this as the starting ratio with mL as the numerator, to match the mL numerator of the units being calculated; 20,000 units becomes the denominator.

$$\frac{\text{mL}}{\text{hr}} = \frac{500 \text{ mL}}{20,000 \text{ units}}$$

The starting ratio denominator, units, must be matched in the next numerator. Enter the 1000 units/hr rate ordered, with units as the numerator. This completes the equation.

$$\frac{\text{mL}}{\text{hr}} = \frac{500 \text{ mL}}{20,000 \text{ units}} \times \frac{1000 \text{ units}}{1 \text{ hr}}$$

Cancel alternate denominator/numerator units in the equation to double-check that the ratios have been entered correctly. Only mL and hr should remain. Do the math.

$$\frac{mL}{hr} = \frac{500\ mL}{20{,}000\ units} \times \frac{1000\ units}{1\ hr} = \mathbf{25\ mL/hr}$$

A rate of 25 mL/hr is required to infuse 1000 units/hr from a solution strength of 20,000 units in 500 mL.

EXAMPLE 2 The order is for heparin **800 units/hr.** The solution available is **40,000 units in 1000 mL** D5W. Calculate the **mL/hr** flow rate.

Enter the mL/hr being calculated. Enter the 1000 mL/40,000 units ratio, with mL as the numerator.

$$\frac{mL}{hr} = \frac{1000\ mL}{40{,}000\ units}$$

Enter the next ratio, 800 units/hr, with 800 units as the numerator to match the starting ratio denominator.

$$\frac{mL}{hr} = \frac{1000\ mL}{40{,}000\ units} \times \frac{800\ units}{1\ hr}$$

Cancel to double-check for correct ratio entry, and do the math.

$$\frac{mL}{hr} = \frac{1000\ mL}{40{,}000\ units} \times \frac{800\ units}{1\ hr} = \mathbf{20\ mL/hr}$$

A rate of 20 mL/hr is required to infuse 800 units/hr from a solution strength of 40,000 units in 1000 mL.

EXAMPLE 3 The order is to infuse heparin **1100 units/hr** from a solution strength of **60,000 units in 1 L** D5W. Calculate the **mL/hr** flow rate.

$$\frac{mL}{hr} = \frac{1000\ mL}{60{,}000\ units} \times \frac{1100\ units}{1\ hr}$$

$$\frac{mL}{hr} = \frac{1000\ mL}{60{,}000\ units} \times \frac{1100\ units}{1\ hr} = 18.33 = \mathbf{18\ mL/hr}$$

A rate of 18 mL/hr will be required to infuse 1100 units per hour from a solution strength of 60,000 units in 1 L.

▶▶▶ PROBLEMS 21.2

Calculate these mL/hr flow rates using the calculation method you prefer.

1. The order is to infuse 1000 units heparin per hour from an available solution strength of 25,000 units in 500 mL D5W.   _____

2. Heparin has been ordered at 2500 units per hour. The solution strength is 50,000 units in 1000 mL D5W.   _____

3. The order is to infuse 1100 units per hour from a 15,000 units in 1 L D5W solution. _____

4. An adult has orders for 50,000 units of heparin in 1000 mL D5W to infuse at a rate of 2000 units per hour. _____

5. Administer 1500 units per hour of heparin from an available strength of 40,000 units in 1 L. _____

Answers **1.** 20 mL/hr **2.** 50 mL/hr **3.** 73 mL/hr **4.** 40 mL/hr **5.** 38 mL/hr

CALCULATING units/hr INFUSING FROM mL/hr FLOW RATE

On occasion it may be necessary to calculate the units/hr of heparin infusing from the mL/hr flow rate. This is done using the units/mL solution strength and mL/hr rate of infusion.

CALCULATION USING RATIO AND PROPORTION

EXAMPLE 1 An IV of **1000 mL** containing **40,000 units** of heparin is running at **30 mL/hr**. Calculate the **units/hr** infusing.

$$\frac{1000\ mL}{40,000\ units} = \frac{30\ mL}{X\ units} = \textbf{1200 units/hr}$$

or

1000 mL : 40,000 units = 30 mL : X units

$$X = \textbf{1200 units/hr}$$

A 1000 mL solution containing 40,000 units heparin running at 30 mL/hr is infusing 1200 units/hr.

EXAMPLE 2 A solution of **1 L** of D5W with **20,000 units** heparin is running at **80 mL/hr**. Calculate the **units/hr** infusing.

$$\frac{1000\ mL}{20,000\ units} = \frac{80\ mL}{X\ units} = \textbf{1600 units/hr}$$

or

1000 mL : 20,000 units = 80 mL : X units

$$X = \textbf{1600 units/hr}$$

A 1 L (1000 mL) solution containing 20,000 units heparin running at 80 mL/hr is infusing 1600 units/hr.

EXAMPLE 3 An IV of D5W **500 mL** containing **10,000 units** heparin is running at **40 mL/hr**. Calculate the **units/hr** infusing.

$$\frac{500\ mL}{10,000\ units} = \frac{40\ mL}{X\ units} = \textbf{800 units/hr}$$

or

$$500 \text{ mL} : 10{,}000 \text{ units} = 40 \text{ mL} : X \text{ units}$$

$$X = \textbf{800 units/hr}$$

A 500 mL solution containing 10,000 units heparin running at 40 mL/hr is infusing 800 units/hr.

CALCULATION USING DIMENSIONAL ANALYSIS

EXAMPLE 1   An IV of **1000 mL** containing **40,000 units** of heparin is running at **30 mL/hr**. Calculate the **units/hr** infusing.

$$\frac{\text{units}}{\text{hr}} = \frac{40{,}000 \text{ units}}{1000 \text{ mL}} \times \frac{30 \text{ mL}}{1 \text{ hr}}$$

$$\frac{\text{units}}{\text{hr}} = \frac{40{,}000 \text{ units}}{1000 \text{ mL}} \times \frac{30 \text{ mL}}{1 \text{ hr}} = \textbf{1200 units/hr}$$

A 1000 mL solution containing 40,000 units heparin running at 30 mL/hr is infusing 1200 units/hr.

EXAMPLE 2   A solution of **1 L** of D5W with **20,000 units** heparin is running at **80 mL/hr**. Calculate the **units/hr** infusing.

$$\frac{\text{units}}{\text{hr}} = \frac{20{,}000 \text{ units}}{1000 \text{ mL}} \times \frac{80 \text{ mL}}{1 \text{ hr}}$$

$$\frac{\text{units}}{\text{hr}} = \frac{20{,}000 \text{ units}}{1000 \text{ mL}} \times \frac{80 \text{ mL}}{1 \text{ hr}} = \textbf{1600 units/hr}$$

A 1 L (1000 mL) solution containing 20,000 units heparin running at 80 mL/hr is infusing 1600 units/hr.

EXAMPLE 3   An IV of D5W **500 mL** containing **10,000 units** heparin is running at **40 mL/hr**. Calculate the **units/hr** infusing.

$$\frac{\text{units}}{\text{hr}} = \frac{10{,}000 \text{ units}}{500 \text{ mL}} \times \frac{40 \text{ mL}}{1 \text{ hr}}$$

$$\frac{\text{units}}{\text{hr}} = \frac{10{,}000 \text{ units}}{500 \text{ mL}} \times \frac{40 \text{ mL}}{1 \text{ hr}} = \textbf{800 units/hr}$$

A 500 mL solution containing 10,000 units heparin running at 40 mL/hr is infusing 800 units/hr.

▶▶▶ PROBLEMS 21.3

Use your calculation method of choice to determine the units/hr of heparin infusing in the following IV administrations.

1. An IV of 750 mL containing 30,000 units heparin running at 25 mL/hr _____

2. A solution of 20,000 units in 500 mL running at 30 mL/hr _____

3. A 1 L volume of D5W containing heparin 30,000 units running at 40 mL/hr _____

4. An IV of 1 L DNS containing 20,000 units heparin running at 30 mL/hr _____

5. A 25,000 units heparin in 500 mL solution running at 30 mL/hr _____

6. An IV of 1000 mL containing 40,000 units heparin running at 25 mL/hr _____

7. A 1000 mL solution with 45,000 units heparin running at 25 mL/hr _____

8. A solution of 1000 mL containing 25,000 units heparin running at 30 mL/hr _____

9. A 1 L solution with 35,000 units heparin running at 45 mL/hr _____

10. A 20,000 units in 500 mL solution running at 20 mL/hr _____

Answers **1.** 1000 units/hr **2.** 1200 units/hr **3.** 1200 units/hr **4.** 600 units/hr **5.** 1500 units/hr **6.** 1000 units/hr **7.** 1125 units/hr **8.** 750 units/hr **9.** 1575 units/hr **10.** 800 units/hr

Summary

This concludes the chapter on heparin administration. The important points to remember are:

▼ Heparin is a potent anticoagulant that is frequently added to IV solutions.

▼ It is measured in USP units.

▼ Heparin therapy requires a frequent check of coagulation times.

▼ Subcutaneous heparin injections are given deeply at a 45° angle, to discourage medication leakage through the injection track, and subsequent bruising.

▼ IV heparin may be ordered by mL/hr flow rate or by units/hr to infuse.

▼ An EID or microdrip is used for heparin infusion.

▼ Commercially prepared IV heparin solutions are available in several strengths.

▼ Additional IV solution strengths may require the preparation of heparin from available vial strengths.

▼ Frequent blood tests for clotting time are required to monitor dosage.

Summary Self-Test

Calculate these mL/hr heparin flow rates using the calculation method of your choice.

1. An adult is to receive heparin 1000 units/hr. The IV solution available has 25,000 units in 1 L D5W, and a pump will be used.   _____

2. A solution of 35,000 units heparin in 1 L D5W is to infuse via volumetric pump at 1200 units/hr.   _____

3. The order is for 1000 units heparin per hour. The solution strength is 20,000 units in 500 mL D5NS.   _____

4. The order is for 1250 units/hr heparin from a solution strength of 15,000 units in 500 mL D5W. A pump is used to monitor the infusion.   _____

5. A solution of 10,000 units heparin in 500 mL D5W is ordered to infuse at 1000 units/hr.   _____

6. An IV of 1000 mL D5W with 40,000 units heparin is to infuse at 1200 units/hr via a pump.   _____

7. The order is to infuse 500 mL D5W with 25,000 units heparin at 1500 units/hr.   _____

8. 500 mL D5W with 30,000 units of heparin is to infuse via a pump at 1500 units/hr.   _____

9. The order is to infuse 1 L D5W with 45,000 units of heparin at 1875 units/hr.   _____

10. A rate of 500 units/hr is ordered using a 250 mL with 10,000 units IV solution.   _____

11. A solution of 40,000 units in 1000 mL is to be used to infuse 1500 units/hr.   _____

12. A rate of 1500 units/hr is ordered using a 30,000 units in 500 mL solution.   _____

13. Heparin 750 units/hr is ordered using an IV solution of 500 mL containing 5000 units heparin.   _____

14. An IV solution of 10,000 units in 1000 mL heparin is to infuse 500 units/hr.   _____

15. Heparin 1500 units per hour is to be infused using a solution strength of 15,000 units in 500 mL.   _____

Answers		
1. 40 mL/hr	**6.** 30 mL/hr	**12.** 25 mL/hr
2. 34 mL/hr	**7.** 30 mL/hr	**13.** 75 mL/hr
3. 25 mL/hr	**8.** 25 mL/hr	**14.** 50 mL/hr
4. 41.6 or 42 mL/hr	**9.** 41.6 or 42 mL/hr	**15.** 50 mL/hr
5. 50 mL/hr	**10.** 12.5 or 13 mL/hr	
	11. 37.5 or 38 mL/hr	

SECTION

Pediatric Medication Calculations

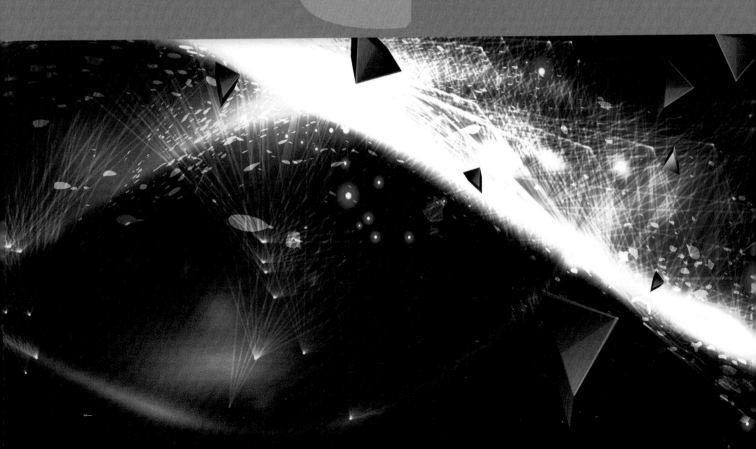

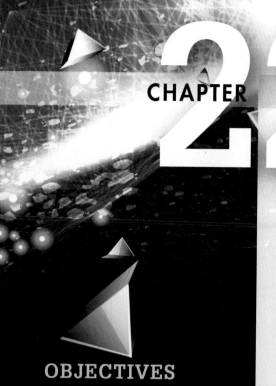

22 PEDIATRIC ORAL AND PARENTERAL MEDICATIONS

OBJECTIVES

The learner will:

1. explain how suspensions are measured and administered.

2. calculate pediatric oral dosages.

3. list the precautions of IM and subcutaneous injection in infants and children.

4. calculate pediatric IM and subcutaneous dosages.

Two differences between adult and pediatric dosages will be immediately apparent: **Most oral drugs are prepared as liquids** because infants and small children cannot be expected to swallow tablets easily, if at all, and **dosages are dramatically smaller.** The oral route is used whenever possible, but when a child cannot swallow or the drug is ineffective given orally, drugs will be administered by a parenteral route.

Both the subcutaneous and intramuscular routes may be used depending on the type of drug to be administered. However, the smaller size of infants and children limits the use of both routes, as does the nature of the drug being used. For example, many antibiotics are administered intravenously rather than intramuscularly.

ORAL MEDICATIONS

Most oral pediatric drugs are prepared as liquids to facilitate ease in swallowing. If the child is old enough to cooperate, these dosages may be measured in a medication cup. Solutions are also frequently measured using oral syringes, such as the ones shown in Figure 22-1. Notice that oral syringes have the same metric calibrations as hypodermic syringes, but they may also include household measures; for example, tsp. **Oral syringes have different-sized tips** to prevent use with hypodermic needles. On some oral syringes, the **tip is positioned off center (termed *eccentric*)**, to further distinguish them from hypodermic syringes, or they may be **amber-colored**, as in Figure 22-1.

If oral syringes are not available, hypodermic syringes **(without the needle)** can also be used for dosage measurement. In addition to accuracy, syringes provide an excellent method of administering oral liquid drugs to infants and small children. Some oral liquid preparations incorporate a calibrated medication dropper as an integral part of the medication bottle. These may be **calibrated in mL** like the dropper shown in Figure 22-2 or in **actual dosage;** for example, 25 mg or 50 mg. Animal-shaped measures such as those shown in Figure 22-3 are also helpful in enticing reluctant toddlers to take necessary medications. In each instance, the goal is to ensure that the infant or child actually swallows the total dosage.

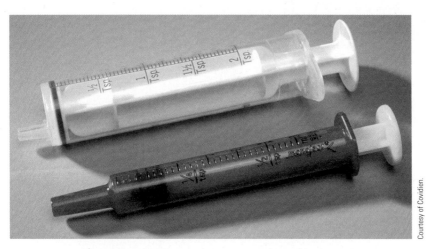

▲ **FIGURE 22-1** Oral syringes.

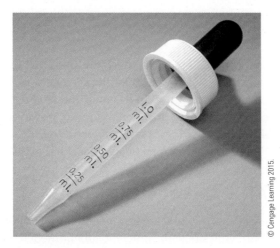

▲ **FIGURE 22-2** Calibrated dropper.

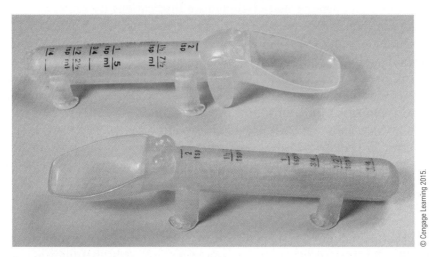

▲ **FIGURE 22-3** Animal-shaped measures.

Care must be taken with liquid oral drugs to identify those prepared as **suspensions**. A **suspension consists of an insoluble drug in a liquid base**; for example, the cefaclor oral suspension in Figure 22-4. The drug in a suspension settles to the bottom of the bottle between uses, and **thorough mixing immediately prior to pouring** is mandatory. Suspensions must also be administered to the child promptly after measurement to prevent the drug from settling out again and an incomplete dosage being administered.

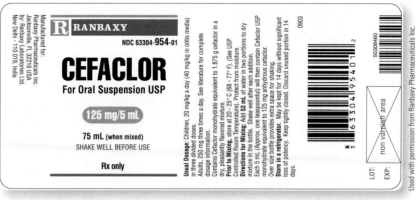

▲ FIGURE 22-4

 KEY_point:_ Suspensions must be thoroughly mixed before measurement and promptly administered to prevent the settling out of their insoluble drugs.

When a tablet or capsule is administered, the child's mouth must be checked to be certain the medication has actually been swallowed. If swallowing is a problem, some tablets can be crushed and given in a small amount of applesauce, ice cream, or juice if the child has no dietary restrictions to contraindicate this. Keep in mind, however, that **enteric-coated and timed-release tablets or capsules cannot be crushed** because this would destroy the coating that allows them to function on a delayed-action basis.

INTRAMUSCULAR AND SUBCUTANEOUS MEDICATIONS

The drugs most often given subcutaneously are insulin and immunizations that specifically require the subcutaneous route. Any site with sufficient subcutaneous tissue may be used, with the upper arm being the site of choice for immunizations. The intramuscular route is used most frequently for preoperative and postoperative medications for sedation and pain, and for immunizations such as DPT (diphtheria, pertussis, tetanus), which must be administered deep IM. The intramuscular site of choice for infants and small children is the vastus lateralis or rectus femoris of the thigh because the gluteal muscles do not develop until a child has learned to walk. Usually, not more than 1 mL is injected per site, and sites are rotated regularly.

Dosage calculation is the same as for adults, except **dosages are sometimes calculated to the nearest hundredth and measured using a tuberculin syringe** (refer to Chapter 8 if you need to review the calibrations and use of a TB syringe). There is less margin for error in pediatric dosages, and calculations and measurements are carefully double-checked.

Summary

This concludes the introduction to pediatric oral, IM, and subcutaneous medication administration. The important points to remember from this chapter are:

▽ Care must be taken when administering oral drugs to ensure that the child has actually swallowed the dosage.

▽ If liquid medications are prepared as suspensions, mix thoroughly prior to measurement, and administer promptly to prevent the settling out of their insoluble drugs.

▼ Care must be taken not to confuse oral syringes, which are unsterile, with hypodermic syringes, which are sterile.

▼ The IM site of choice for infants and small children is the vastus lateralis or rectus femoris of the thigh.

▼ Usually not more than 1 mL is injected per IM or subcutaneous site, and sites are rotated regularly.

▼ Pediatric parenteral dosages are frequently calculated to the nearest hundredth and measured using a TB syringe.

Summary Self-Test

For Part I, use the pediatric medication labels provided to measure the following oral dosages. Indicate in the second column if the medication is a suspension.

PART I

	mL	Suspension
1. Prepare a 10 mg dosage of oxycodone.	_____	_____
2. Prepare a 125 mg dosage of penicillin V potassium.	_____	_____

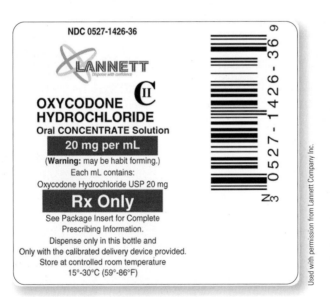

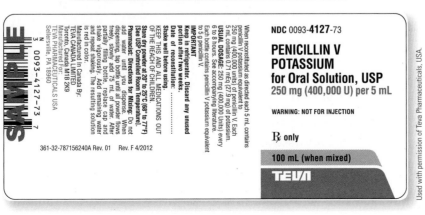

	mL	Suspension
3. Prepare 100 mg of amoxicillin.	_____	_____
4. Prepare 100 mg of Vantin®.	_____	_____
5. Prepare 5 mg of Lomotil®.	_____	_____
6. Prepare cefpodoxime proxetil 60 mg.	_____	_____
7. Prepare Depakene® 150 mg.	_____	_____
8. Prepare 120 mg of acetaminophen.	_____	_____
9. Prepare 187 mg of cefaclor.	_____	_____

CEFACLOR
For Oral Suspension USP

NDC 63304-955-04

RANBAXY

187 mg/5 mL

100 mL (when mixed)
SHAKE WELL BEFORE USE

Rx only

Used with permission from Ranbaxy Pharmaceuticals Inc.

Store dry powder at room temperature. Keep tightly closed. Shake well before using. Refrigeration preferable but not required. Discard suspension after 14 days.
Directions for mixing: Add 23 mL of water. Shake vigorously. Each mL will then contain amoxicillin trihydrate equivalent to 50 mg amoxicillin.

NDC 0000-0000-00

AMOXICILLIN

50 mg/mL
PEDIATRIC DROPS
FOR ORAL SUSPENSION

Rx only

30 mL (when reconstituted)

CL Cengage Learning
For Educational Purposes Only

Dosage: 20 to 40 mg/kg/day in divided doses every 8 hours depending on age, weight, and infection severity. See accompanying prescribing information.
Net contents: Equivalent to 1.5 grams amoxicillin as the trihydrate.

Lot:
Exp. Date:

0000-0000-00

© Cengage Learning 2015.

NDC 0087-0730-01

DROPS

TEMPRA®
ACETAMINOPHEN

ANALGESIC
1/2 FL. OZ. (15 mL.)

10% SOLUTION

Mead Johnson

TO RELIEVE DISCOMFORT DUE TO COLDS, SIMPLE HEADACHES, MINOR ACHES AND PAINS.
Each 0.6 mL of TEMPRA® drops contains 60 mg. (1 grain) of acetaminophen and 10% alcohol.
Your physician is the best source of counsel and guidance in illness when pain or fever is present.
KEEP THIS AND ALL MEDICATIONS OUT OF THE REACH OF CHILDREN.
Made in U.S.A. ●M.J.& Co.

MEAD JOHNSON NUTRITIONAL DIVISION
Mead Johnson & Company • Evansville, Indiana 47721 U.S.A.

P 7698-03

Used with permission from Bristol-Myers Squibb Company.

Do not accept if band on cap is broken or missing.

Each 5 mL contains equivalent to 250 mg valproic acid as the sodium salt.

See enclosure for prescribing information.

©Abbott

Abbott Laboratories
North Chicago, IL60064, U.S.A.

Exp.

Lot

NDC 0074-5682-16
16 fl oz Syrup

DEPAKENE®

VALPROIC ACID
SYRUP, USP

**250 mg
per 5 mL**

Caution: Federal (U.S.A.) law prohibits dispensing without prescription.

6505-01-094-9241

Dispense in the original container or a glass, USP tight container.

Store below 86°F (30°C).

0074568216

02-7538-2/R12

Used with permission from Abbott Laboratories.

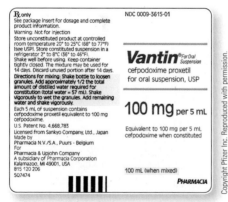

Rx only
See package insert for dosage and complete product information.
Warning: Not for injection
Store unconstituted product at controlled room temperature 20° to 25°C (68° to 77°F) [see USP]. Store constituted suspension in a refrigerator 2° to 8°C (36° to 46°F). Shake well before using. Keep container tightly closed. The mixture may be used for 14 days. Discard unused portion after 14 days.
Directions for mixing: Shake bottle to loosen granules. Add approximately 1/2 the total amount of distilled water required for constitution (total water = 57 mL). Shake vigorously to wet the granules. Add remaining water and shake vigorously.
Each 5 mL of suspension contains cefpodoxime proxetil equivalent to 100 mg cefpodoxime.
U.S. Patent No. 4,668,783
Licensed from Sankyo Company, Ltd., Japan
Made by
Pharmacia N.V./S.A., Puurs - Belgium
For
Pharmacia & Upjohn Company
A subsidiary of Pharmacia Corporation
Kalamazoo, MI 49001, USA
815 120 206
5Q7474

NDC 0009-3615-01

Vantin® For Oral Suspension
cefpodoxime proxetil
for oral suspension, USP

100 mg per 5 mL

Equivalent to 100 mg per 5 mL cefpodoxime when constituted

100 mL (when mixed)

PHARMACIA

Copyright Pfizer Inc. Reproduced with permission.

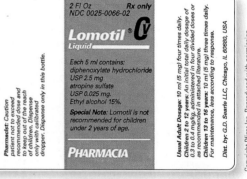

2 Fl Oz
NDC 0025-0066-02

Rx only

Lomotil®
Liquid

C V

Each 5 ml contains:
diphenoxylate hydrochloride USP 2.5 mg
atropine sulfate USP 0.025 mg.
Ethyl alcohol 15%.

Special Note: Lomotil is not recommended for children under 2 years of age.

PHARMACIA

Store below 77°F (25°C).

Pharmacist: Caution patient not to exceed recommended dose and to keep out of the reach of children. Dispense only with calibrated dropper. Dispense only in this bottle.

Usual Adult Dosage: 10 ml (5 mg) four times daily.
Children 2 to 12 years: An initial total daily dosage of 0.3 to 0.4 mg/kg, administered in four divided doses or as recommended in attached literature.
Children 13 to 16 years: 10 ml (5 mg) three times daily. For maintenance, less according to response.

Dist. by: G.D. Searle LLC, Chicago, IL 60680, USA

Copyright Pfizer Inc. Reproduced with permission.

CHAPTER 22

Use the labels provided to calculate the dosages for Parts II and III. Calculate all dosages to hundredths.

PART II

10. Prepare a 20 mg dosage of meperidine.   _____

11. A dosage of morphine 10 mg has been ordered.   _____

12. Draw up a 100 mg dosage of clindamycin.   _____

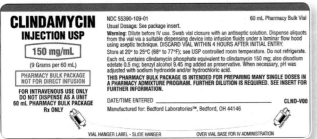

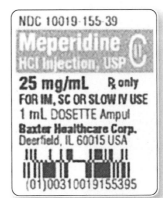

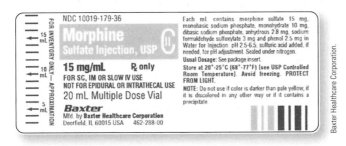

PART III

13. Prepare a 40 mg dosage of meperidine.   _____

14. A dosage of Dilantin® 50 mg has been ordered.   _____

15. Prepare a 6 mg dosage of morphine.   _____

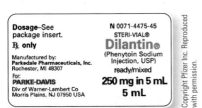

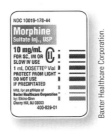

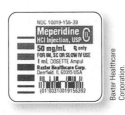

Answers			
1. 0.5 mL; no	**4.** 5 mL; suspension	**8.** 1.2 mL; no	**12.** 0.67 mL
2. 2.5 mL; no	**5.** 10 mL; no	**9.** 5 mL; suspension	**13.** 0.8 mL
3. 2 mL; suspension	**6.** 3 mL; suspension	**10.** 0.8 mL	**14.** 1 mL
	7. 3 mL; no	**11.** 0.67 mL	**15.** 0.6 mL

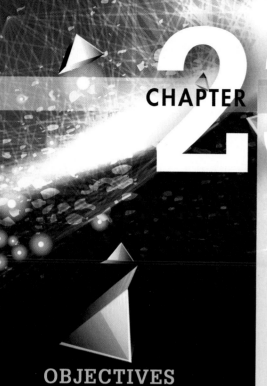

23 PEDIATRIC INTRAVENOUS MEDICATIONS

OBJECTIVES

The learner will:

1. list the steps in preparing and administering IV medications from a solution bag.

2. list the steps in preparing and administering IV medications using a calibrated burette.

3. explain why a flush is included in IV medication administration.

4. calculate flow rates for the administration of pediatric IV medications.

5. use normal daily and hourly dosage ranges to calculate and assess dosages ordered.

PREREQUISITES

Chapters 15–18

Pediatric IV medication administration involves a challenge and a responsibility that is multifaceted. Infants and children, particularly under the age of 4, are incompletely developed physiologically, and drug tolerance, absorption, and excretion are ongoing concerns. In addition, infants and acutely ill children can tolerate only a narrow range of hydration, making administration of IV drugs, which are diluted for administration, a critical and exact skill. Drug dilution protocols may specify a range for dilution, and on many occasions the smallest possible volume may have to be used in order to not overhydrate a child. Dosage and dilution decisions may have to be made on a day-to-day or even a dose-to-dose basis and will involve the team effort of nurse, physician, and pharmacist. In addition, the suitability of any flow rate calculated for administration must be made on an individual basis. For example, a calculated flow rate of 100 gtt/min for a 2-year-old child is too high a rate to administer.

The fragility of infants' and children's veins, and the irritating nature of many medications, mandate careful site inspection for signs of inflammation and infiltration. This should be done immediately before, during, and after each infusion. Signs of inflammation include redness, heat, swelling, and tenderness. Signs of infiltration include swelling, coldness, pain, and lack of blood return in the IV tubing. Either complication necessitates discontinuance of the IV and a restart at a new site.

IV medication guidelines are always used to determine drug dosages, dilutions, and administration rates.

Let's start by looking at the different methods of IV medication administration.

METHODS OF IV MEDICATION ADMINISTRATION

Intravenous medications may be administered over a period of several hours or on an **intermittent** basis involving several dosages in a 24-hour period. When ordered to infuse over several hours, medications are usually added to an IV solution bag. Adding the drug to the IV bag may be a hospital pharmacy or nurse responsibility. The steps for adding the drug to the solution are as follows:

STEP 1 Locate the type and volume of IV solution ordered.

STEP 2 Measure the dosage of drug to be added.

STEP 3 Use strict aseptic technique to add the drug to the solution bag through the medication port.

STEP 4 Mix the drug thoroughly in the solution.

STEP 5 Label the IV solution bag with the name and dosage of the drug added.

STEP 6 Add your initials and the time and date you added the drug.

STEP 7 Hang the IV and then set the flow rate for the infusion. Chart the administration when it has completed.

For intermittent administrations, the medication may also be prepared in small-volume solution bags, or using a calibrated burette such as the one illustrated in Figure 23-1. Because the total capacity of burettes is between 100 and 150 mL, calibrated in 1 mL increments, the exact measurement of small volumes is possible.

Regardless of the method of intermittent administration, the medication infusion is **routinely followed by a flush** to make sure the medication has cleared the tubing and that the total dosage has been administered. The volume of the flush will vary depending on the length of IV tubing from the medication source—that is, the burette or syringe—to the infusion site. If a primary line exists, the medication may be administered by IVPB (IV piggyback) via a secondary line. If no IV is infusing, a saline or heparin lock (heplock) is frequently in place and used for intermittent administration.

When IV medications are diluted for administration, it is necessary to determine hospital policy on **inclusion of the medication volume as part of the volume specified for dilution.** For example, if 20 mg has a volume of 2 mL, and it is to be diluted in 30 mL, does this mean you must add 28 mL of diluent to the burette or 30 mL?

Hospital policies may vary, but in all examples and problems in this chapter **the drug volume will be treated as part of the total diluent volume.** The sequencing of medication and flush administration covered next for burette use is also representative of the procedure that might be followed for IVPB administrations.

MEDICATION ADMINISTRATION VIA BURETTE

When a burette is used for medication administration, the entire preparation is usually done by nurses. Volumetric and syringe pumps are used extensively to administer intermittent IV medications to infants and children. When these are used, the alarm will sound each time the burette or syringe empties to signal when each successive step is necessary. For example, it will alarm when the medication has infused and the flush must be started and again when the flush is completed.

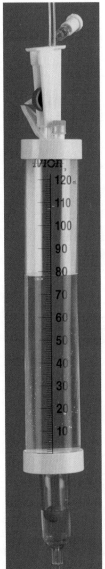

▲ **FIGURE 23-1**
Calibrated burette.

SECTION 7

Let's look at some sample orders and go step by step through one procedure that may be used.

EXAMPLE 1 ▸ A dosage of **250 mg** in **15 mL** of D5 ½ NS is to be infused in **30 minutes**. It is to be followed with a **5 mL** D5 ½ NS flush. A volumetric pump will be used, and the tubing is a **microdrip** burette.

STEP 1 ▸ Read the drug label to determine what volume the 250 mg dosage is contained in. Let's assume this is 1 mL.

STEP 2 ▸ The dilution is to be 15 mL. Run a total of 14 mL of D5 ½ NS into the burette, then add the 1 mL containing the medication dosage of 250 mg. This gives the ordered volume of 15 mL. Roll the burette between your hands to mix the drug thoroughly with the solution.

STEP 3 ▸ Calculate the flow rate for this microdrip.

Total volume = **15 mL** Infusion time = **30 min**

Using Ratio and Proportion

$$\frac{15\ \text{mL}}{30\ \text{min}} = \frac{X\ \text{mL}}{60\ \text{min}} \quad \text{or} \quad 15\ \text{mL} : 30\ \text{min} = X\ \text{mL} : 60\ \text{min}$$

$$X = \textbf{30 mL/hr} \qquad\qquad 30X = 60 \times 15$$

$$X = \textbf{30 mL/hr}$$

Using Dimensional Analysis

$$\frac{\text{mL}}{\text{hr}} = \frac{15\ \text{mL}}{30\ \text{min}} \times \frac{60\ \text{min}}{1\ \text{hr}} = \textbf{30 mL/hr}$$

STEP 4 ▸ Set the pump to infuse 30 mL/hr.

STEP 5 ▸ Label the burette to identify the drug and dosage added. Attach a label that states "medication infusing." This makes it possible for others to know the status of the administration if you are not present when the infusion is complete and the pump alarms.

STEP 6 ▸ When the medication has infused, add the 5 mL D5 ½ NS flush. Remove the "medication infusing" label and attach a "flush infusing" label. Continue to infuse at the 30 mL/hr rate until the burette empties for the second time.

STEP 7 ▸ When the flush has been completed, restart the primary IV or disconnect from the saline/heparin lock. Remove the "flush infusing" label. Chart the dosage and time.

EXAMPLE 2 ▸ An antibiotic dosage of **125 mg in 1 mL** is to be **diluted in 20 mL** of D5 ¼ NS and infused over **30 min**. A **flush of 15 mL** D5 ¼ NS is to follow. A volumetric pump will be used.

STEP 1 ▸ 125 mg has a volume of 1 mL. Add 19 mL of D5 ¼ NS to the burette, add the 1 mL of medication, and mix thoroughly.

STEP 2   **Calculate the mL/hr flow rate.**

Total volume = **20 mL**   Infusion time = **30 min**

Using Ratio and Proportion

$$\frac{20\ \text{mL}}{30\ \text{min}} = \frac{X\ \text{mL}}{60\ \text{min}} \quad \text{or} \quad 20\ \text{mL} : 30\ \text{min} = X\ \text{mL} : 60\ \text{min}$$

$$30X = 60 \times 20$$

$$X = \textbf{40 mL/hr} \qquad\qquad X = \textbf{40 mL/hr}$$

Using Dimensional Analysis

$$\frac{\text{mL}}{\text{hr}} = \frac{20\ \text{mL}}{30\ \text{min}} \times \frac{60\ \text{min}}{1\ \text{hr}} = \textbf{40 mL/hr}$$

STEP 3   **Set the pump to infuse 40 mL/hr.**

STEP 4   **Label the burette with the drug and dosage, and attach a "medication infusing" label.**

STEP 5   **When the medication has infused, start the 15 mL flush. Remove the "medication infusing" label and add the "flush infusing" label.**

STEP 6   **When the flush has completed, restart the primary IV or disconnect from the saline lock. Remove the "flush infusing" label. Chart the dosage and time.**

 KEY*point:* If a 60 gtt/mL calibrated burette is used without a pump, the gtt/min rate will be the same as the mL/hr rate.

EXAMPLE 3   An antibiotic dosage of **50 mg** has been ordered diluted in **20 mL** of D5W to infuse over **20 min**. A **15 mL flush** of D5W is to follow. A **microdrip** will be used, but an infusion control device will not be used.

STEP 1   **Read the medication label to determine what volume contains 50 mg. You determine that 50 mg is contained in 2 mL.**

STEP 2   **Run 18 mL of D5W into the burette and add the 2 mL containing 50 mg of drug. Roll between your hands to mix thoroughly.**

STEP 3   **Calculate the flow rate in gtt/min necessary to deliver the medication.**

Total volume = **20 mL**   Infusion time = **20 min**

Using Ratio and Proportion

$$\frac{20\ \text{mL}}{20\ \text{min}} = \frac{X\ \text{mL}}{60\ \text{min}} \quad \text{or} \quad 20\ \text{mL} : 20\ \text{min} = X\ \text{mL} : 60\ \text{min}$$

$$20X = 20 \times 60$$

$$X = \textbf{60 mL/hr} \qquad\qquad X = \textbf{60 mL/hr}$$

Using Dimensional Analysis

$$\frac{\text{gtt}}{\text{min}} = \frac{60 \text{ gtt}}{1 \text{ mL}} \times \frac{20 \text{ mL}}{20 \text{ min}} = \textbf{60 gtt/min}$$

STEP 4 The mL/hr and gtt/min rates are identical for a microdrip. Set the rate at 60 gtt/min.

STEP 5 Label the burette with drug name and dosage, and attach a "medication infusing" label.

STEP 6 When the medication has cleared the burette, add the 15 mL D5W flush. Continue to run at 60 gtt/min. Remove the "medication infusing" label and replace with a "flush infusing" label.

STEP 7 When the burette empties for the second time, restart the primary IV or disconnect from the saline lock. Remove the "flush infusing" label. Chart the dosage and time administered.

EXAMPLE 4 An IV medication dosage of **100 mcg** has been ordered diluted in **35 mL** of NS and infused in **50 min**. A **10 mL** flush is to follow. A **microdrip** burette will be used.

STEP 1 Read the medication label to determine what volume contains 100 mcg: 100 mcg = 1.5 mL.

STEP 2 Run 33.5 mL of NS into the burette, and add the 1.5 mL of medication. Roll the burette between your hands to mix thoroughly.

STEP 3 Calculate the gtt/min flow rate.

Using Ratio and Proportion

Total volume = **35 mL**   Infusion time = **50 min**

$$\frac{35 \text{ mL}}{50 \text{ min}} = \frac{X \text{ mL}}{60 \text{ min}} \quad \text{or} \quad 35 \text{ mL} : 50 \text{ min} = X \text{ mL} : 60 \text{ min}$$

$$50X = 35 \times 60$$

$$X = \textbf{42 mL/hr} \qquad\qquad X = \textbf{42 mL/hr}$$

$$= \textbf{42 gtt/min} \qquad\qquad = \textbf{42 gtt/min}$$

USING DIMENSIONAL ANALYSIS

$$\frac{\text{gtt}}{\text{min}} = \frac{60 \text{ gtt}}{1 \text{ mL}} \times \frac{35 \text{ mL}}{50 \text{ min}} = \textbf{42 gtt/min}$$

STEP 4 Set the flow rate at 42 gtt/min.

STEP 5 Label the burette with the drug name and dosage and "medication infusing" label.

STEP 6 When the medication has cleared the burette, add the 10 mL flush. Continue to run at 42 gtt/min. Replace the "medication infusing" label with the "flush infusing" label.

STEP 7 When the burette empties of the flush solution, restart the primary IV or disconnect from the saline lock. Remove the "flush infusing" label, and chart the dosage and time administered.

▶▶▶ PROBLEMS 23.1

Determine the volume of solution that must be added to a burette to mix the following IV drugs. Then, calculate the flow rate in gtt/min for each administration using a microdrip, and indicate the mL/hr setting for a pump.

1. An IV medication of 75 mg in 3 mL is ordered diluted to 55 mL to infuse over 45 min.

    Dilution volume _____ gtt/min _____ mL/hr_____

2. A dosage of 100 mg in 2 mL is diluted to 30 mL of D5W to infuse in 20 min.

    Dilution volume _____ gtt/min _____ mL/hr_____

3. The volume of a 10 mg dosage of medication is 1 mL.

    Dilute to 40 mL and administer over 50 min.

    Dilution volume _____ gtt/min _____ mL/hr_____

4. A dosage of 15 mg with a volume of 3 mL is to be diluted to 70 mL and administered in 50 min.

    Dilution volume _____ gtt/min _____ mL/hr_____

5. A medication of 1 g in 4 mL is to be diluted to 60 mL and infused over 90 min.

    Dilution volume _____ gtt/min _____ mL/hr_____

Answers 1. 52 mL; 73 gtt/min; 73 mL/hr **2.** 28 mL; 90 gtt/min; 90 mL/hr **3.** 39 mL; 48 gtt/min; 48 mL/hr **4.** 67 mL; 84 gtt/min; 84 mL/hr **5.** 56 mL; 40 gtt/min; 40 mL/hr

COMPARING IV DOSAGES ORDERED WITH AVERAGE DOSAGES

Knowing how to compare dosages ordered with average dosages for a particular medication is a nursing responsibility.

KEYpoint: Dosages of IV medications are calculated on the basis of body weight, or BSA.

Average dosages may be listed in terms of mg, mcg, or units per day or per hour. BSA in m^2 is most often used to calculate chemotherapeutic drugs, which are administered only by certified nursing staff. The following examples will demonstrate how to use average dosage to check dosages ordered.

EXAMPLE 1 A child weighing **22.6 kg** has an order for **500 mg** of medication in **100 mL** of D5W **every 12 hours**. The normal dosage range is **40–50 mg/kg/day**. Determine if the dosage ordered is within the normal range.

STEP 1 Calculate the normal daily dosage range for this child.

40 mg/day $\times$ 22.6 kg = **904 mg**

50 mg/day $\times$ 22.6 kg = **1130 mg**

STEP 2 Calculate the dosage infusing in 24 hr.

500 mg in 12 hr = **1000 mg in 24 hr**

STEP 3 Assess the accuracy of the dosage ordered.

The 500 mg in 12 hr, or 1000 mg in 24 hr, is within the 904–1130 mg/day dosage range.

EXAMPLE 2 A child with a body weight of **18.4 kg** is to receive a medication with a dosage range of **100–150 mg/kg/day**. The order is for **600 mg** in **75 mL** of D5W **every 6 hours**. Determine if the dosage is within normal range.

STEP 1 Calculate the normal daily dosage range.

100 mg/day $\times$ 18.4 kg = **1840 mg/day**

150 mg/day $\times$ 18.4 kg = **2760 mg/day**

STEP 2 Calculate the daily dosage ordered.

The dosage ordered is 600 mg every 6 hours (4 doses/24 hours)

600 mg $\times$ 4 = **2400 mg/day**

STEP 3 Assess the accuracy of the dosage ordered.

The dosage ordered, 2400 mg/day, is within the normal range of 1840–2760 mg/day.

EXAMPLE 3 A child weighing **17.7 kg** is receiving an IV of **250 mL** of D5W containing **2000 units** of medication, which is to infuse at **50 mL/hr**. The dosage range is **10–25 units/kg/hr**. Assess the accuracy of this dosage.

STEP 1 Calculate the dosage range per hour.

10 units/kg/hr $\times$ 17.7 kg = **177 units/hr**

25 units/kg/hr $\times$ 17.7 kg = **442.5 units/hr**

STEP 2 Calculate the dosage infusing per hour.

Using Ratio and Proportion

$$\frac{2000 \text{ units}}{250 \text{ mL}} = \frac{X \text{ units}}{50 \text{ mL}} \qquad \text{or} \qquad 2000 \text{ units} : 250 \text{ mL} = X \text{ units} : 50 \text{ mL}$$

$$250X = 2000 \times 50$$

$$X = \textbf{400 units/hr} \qquad\qquad\qquad X = \textbf{400 units/hr}$$

Using Dimensional Analysis

$$\frac{\text{units}}{\text{hr}} = \frac{2000 \text{ units}}{250 \text{ mL}} \times \frac{50 \text{ mL}}{1 \text{ hr}} = \textbf{400 units/hr}$$

STEP 3 **Assess the accuracy of the dosage ordered.**

The IV is infusing at a rate of 50 mL per hour, which is 400 units/hr.
The normal dosage range is 177–442.5 units/hr. The dosage is within the
normal range.

EXAMPLE 4 A child weighing **32.7 kg** has an IV of **250 mL** of D5 ¼ S containing
400 mcg of medication to infuse in **5 hours**. The normal range for
this drug is **1–3 mcg/kg/hr**. Determine if this dosage is within the
normal dosage range.

STEP 1 **Calculate the hourly dosage range.**

1 mcg/kg/hr × 32.7 kg = **32.7 mcg/hr**

3 mcg/kg/hr × 32.7 kg = **98.1 mcg/hr**

STEP 2 **Calculate the dosage infusing per hour.**

400 mcg ÷ 5 hr = **80 mcg/hr**

STEP 3 **Assess the accuracy of the dosage ordered.**
The dosage of 80 mcg/hr infusing is within the normal range of
32.7–98.1 mcg/hr.

▶▶▶ PROBLEMS 23.2

Calculate the normal dosage range to the nearest tenth and the dosage being
administered for the following medications. Assess the dosages ordered.

1. A child weighing 24.4 kg has an IV of 250 mL of D5W containing 2500 units of a drug.
   The dosage range for this drug is 15–25 units/kg/hr. The pump is set to deliver
   50 mL/hr.

   Dosage range per hr _____   Dosage infusing per hr _____

                                            Assessment _____

2. A solution of D5W containing 25 mg of a drug is to infuse in 30 min. The dosage range
   is 4–8 mg/kg/day every 6 hours. The child weighs 18.7 kg.

   Dosage range per day _____   Daily dosage ordered _____

                                            Assessment _____

3. An IV solution containing 125 mg of medication is infusing. The dosage range
   is 5–10 mg/kg/dose, and the child weighs 14.2 kg.

   Dosage range per dose _____   Assessment _____

4. A child weighing 14.3 kg is to receive an IV drug with a dosage range of
   50–100 mcg/kg/day in two divided doses. An infusion of 50 mL of D5W
   containing 400 mcg to run 30 min has been ordered.

   Daily dosage range _____   Daily dosage ordered _____

                                            Assessment _____

5. A dosage of 4 mg (4000 mcg) of drug in 500 mL of D5 ½ S is to infuse in 4 hours. The dosage range of the drug is 24–120 mcg/kg/hr, and the child weighs 16.1 kg.

Dosage range per hr _____   Dosage infusing per hr _____

Assessment _____

6. A child weighing 20.9 kg is to receive a medication with a normal dosage range of 80–160 mg/kg/day in divided doses every 6 hours. The IV ordered contains 500 mg.

Dosage range per day _____   Daily dosage ordered _____

Assessment _____

7. A child weighing 22.3 kg is to receive 750 mL of D5 ¼ S containing 6 g of a drug, which is to run for 24 hours. The dosage range of the drug is 200–300 mg/kg/day.

Dosage range per day _____   Assessment _____

8. An IV of 50 mL of D5W containing 55 mcg of a drug is infusing in a 30-min period. The child weighs 14.9 kg and the dosage range is 6–8 mcg/kg/day, every 12 hours.

Dosage range per day _____   Daily dosage ordered _____

Assessment _____

9. A child weighing 27.1 kg is to receive a medication with a normal range of 0.5–1 mg/kg/dose. An IV containing 20 mg of medication has been ordered.

Dosage per dose _____   Assessment _____

10. An IV medication of 60 mcg in 200 mL is ordered to infuse in 2 hr. The normal dosage range is 1.5–3 mcg/kg/hr. The child weighs 16.7 kg.

Dosage range per hr _____   Dosage infusing per hr _____

Assessment _____

Answers 1. 366–610 units/hr; 500 units/hr; normal range 2. 74.8–149.6 mg/day; 100 mg/day; normal range 3. 71–142 mg/dose; normal range 4. 715–1430 mcg/day; 800 mcg; normal range 5. 386.4–1932 mcg/hr; 1000 mcg; normal range 6. 1672–3344 mg/day; 2000 mg; normal range 7. 4460–6690 mg/day; normal range 8. 89.4–119.2 mcg/day; 110 mcg; normal range 9. 13.6–27.1 mg/dose; normal range 10. 25.1–50.1 mcg/hr; 30 mcg; normal range

Summary

This concludes the chapter on administration of IV drugs to infants and children. The important points to remember from this chapter are:

▼ IV medications may be ordered to infuse in several hours or minutes.

▼ IV medications are diluted for administration, and it is important to determine hospital policy on inclusion of the medication volume as part of the total dilution volume.

▼ A flush is used following medication administration to make sure the medication has cleared the tubing and the total dosage has been administered.

▼ The volume of flush solution on intermittent infusions will vary depending on the amount needed to clear the infusion line.

▼ Average dosage ranges are used to assess dosages ordered.

▼ Pediatric IV medication administration requires constant assessment of the child's ability to tolerate dosage, dilution, and rate of administration.

▼ Children's veins are very fragile, and intravenous sites must be checked for inflammation and infiltration immediately before, during, and after each medication administration.

Summary Self-Test

Determine the volume of solution that must be added to a calibrated burette to mix the following IV drugs. The medication volume is included in the total dilution volume. Calculate the flow rate in gtt/min for each infusion. A microdrip with a calibration of 60 gtt/mL is used.

	Volume of diluent	gtt/min rate
1. An IV antibiotic of 750 mg in 3 mL has been ordered diluted to a total of 25 mL of D5W to infuse in 40 minutes.	_____	_____
2. A dosage of 500,000 units of a penicillin preparation with a volume of 4 mL has been ordered diluted to 50 mL D5 ½ NS to infuse in 60 min.	_____	_____
3. A dosage of 1.5 g/2 mL of an antibiotic is to be diluted to a total of 40 mL of D5W and administered in 40 min.	_____	_____
4. An antibiotic dosage of 200 mg in 4 mL is to be diluted to 50 mL and administered in 70 min.	_____	_____
5. A dosage of 20 mg in 2 mL has been ordered diluted to 30 mL to be infused in 35 min.	_____	_____
6. A dosage of 25 mg in 5 mL has been ordered diluted to 40 mL and administered in 50 min.	_____	_____
7. A 10 mg in 2 mL dosage has been ordered diluted to 20 mL to infuse in 30 min.	_____	_____
8. A medication dosage of 800 mg in 4 mL is to be diluted to 60 mL and infused in 80 min.	_____	_____
9. A dosage of 0.5 g in 2 mL is to be diluted to 40 mL and run in 30 min.	_____	_____
10. A medication of 1000 mg in 1 mL is to be diluted to 15 mL and administered in 20 min.	_____	_____

The following IV drugs are to be administered using a volumetric or syringe pump. Determine the amount of diluent to be added and the flow rate in mL/hr to set the pumps.

	Volume of diluent	mL/hr rate
11. A dosage of 40 mg in 4 mL is to be diluted to 50 mL and administered in 90 min.	_____	_____
12. A 2 g in 5 mL dosage has been ordered diluted to a total of 90 mL and administered in 45 min.	_____	_____

13. An 80 mg dosage with a volume of 2 mL is to be diluted to 80 mL and administered in 60 min.   _____ _____

14. A 60 mg dosage with a volume of 4 mL is ordered diluted to 30 mL and run in 20 min.   _____ _____

15. A 5 mg per 2 mL dosage is to be diluted to 80 mL and administered in 50 min.   _____ _____

16. The dosage ordered is 0.75 g in 3 mL to be diluted to 30 mL and infused in 40 min.   _____ _____

17. A medication of 100 mg in 2 mL is ordered diluted to 30 mL and run in 25 min.   _____ _____

18. The dosage ordered is 100 mg in 1 mL to be diluted to 50 mL and infused in 45 min.   _____ _____

19. A 30 mg dosage in 1 mL has been ordered diluted to 10 mL to infuse in 10 min.   _____ _____

20. A dosage of 250 mg in 5 mL has been ordered diluted to 40 mL and infused in 60 min.   _____ _____

Calculate the normal dosage range to the nearest tenth and the dosage being administered for the following medications. Assess the dosages ordered.

21. A child weighing 15.4 kg is to receive a dosage with a range of 5–7.5 mg/kg/dose. The solution bag is labeled 100 mg.

Dosage range _____   Assessment_____

22. The order is for 200 units in 75 mL. The child weighs 13.1 kg, and the dosage range is 15–20 units/kg per dose.

Dosage range _____   Assessment_____

23. A dosage of 1.5 mg in 20 mL has been ordered. The normal dosage range is 0.1–0.3 mg/kg/day in two divided doses. The child's weight is 12.4 kg.   Dosage range per day _____

Daily dosage ordered _____   Assessment _____

24. A dosage of 400 mg in 75 mL of medication is to be infused every 8 hours. The normal range is 15–45 mg/kg/day, and the child weighs 27.9 kg.   Dosage range per day _____

Daily dosage ordered _____   Assessment _____

25. A child weighing 15.7 kg is to receive a medication with a normal hourly range of 3–7 mcg/kg. A 250 mL solution bag containing 350 mcg is infusing at a rate of 50 mL/hr.

Dosage range per hr _____   Dosage infusing per hr _____

Assessment _____

26. A child weighing 19.6 kg is to receive a medication with a normal dosage range of 60–80 mg/kg/day. A 90 mL infusion containing 375 mg has been ordered every 6 hours.

Dosage range per day _____   Daily dosage ordered _____

Assessment _____

27. Two infusions of 250 mL, each containing 300 mg of medication, are to infuse continuously over a 24 hr period. The child receiving the infusion weighs 11.7 kg, and the normal dosage range of the drug is 50–100 mg/kg/day.

    Dosage range per day _____   Daily dosage ordered _____

    Assessment _____

28. The order is for 100 mL of D5W containing 150 mg of medication to infuse every 8 hours. The normal dosage range is 3–12 mg/kg/day, and the child weighs 40.1 kg.   Dosage range per day _____

    Daily dosage ordered _____   Assessment _____

29. A child has an infusion of 250 mL containing 500 units of medication to run at 50 mL/hr. The normal dosage range is 10–25 units/kg/hr. The child weighs 10.3 kg.   Dosage range per hr _____

    Dosage infusing per hr _____   Assessment _____

30. The normal dosage range of a drug is 0.5–1.5 units/kg/hr. A child weighing 10.7 kg has a 150 mL volume of solution containing 45 units infusing at a rate of 20 mL/hr.

    Normal dosage range per hr _____

    Dosage infusing per hr _____   Assessment _____

31. A child weighing 12.5 kg is receiving an IV of 2500 units of medication in 250 mL of D5W at 40 mL/hr. The normal dosage range is 10–25 units/kg/hr.   Normal dosage range per hr _____

    Dosage infusing per hr _____   Assessment _____

32. A child with a weight of 10 kg is to receive a medication with a normal dosage range of 60–80 mg/kg/day. The order is for 200 mg every 6 hours.   Normal dosage range per hr _____

    Daily dosage ordered _____   Assessment _____

33. The order is for 0.5 g in 100 mL of D5W every 6 hours. The normal dosage range is 100–200 mg/kg/day. The child weighs 15 kg.

    Normal dosage range per hr _____

    Daily dosage ordered _____   Assessment _____

34. A continuous IV of 500 mL with 20 mEq KCl is infusing at 30 mL/hr. The dosage for potassium chloride is not to exceed 40 mEq/day.

    Dosage infusing per hr _____

    Dosage infusing per day _____   Assessment _____

35. A 24 kg child is receiving 116 mg of medication via IV 3 times each day (every 8 hours). Dosage range for this drug is 10–20 mg/kg/day.

    Normal dosage range per day _____

    Dosage received after 3 doses _____   Assessment _____

36. A child weighing 15 kg has an order for 40 mcg of medication in 75 mL D5W to infuse every 12 hours. The normal dosage range is 8–10 mcg/kg/day.

    Normal dosage per day _____   Dosage ordered _____

    Assessment _____

37. The usual dosage for children is 50 mg/kg/24 hr in equally divided doses. The order is to infuse 50 mL with 290 mg every 6 hours. The child weighs 51 lb.

Normal dosage per day _____   Daily dosage ordered _____

Assessment _____

38. Order: 500 mL D5RL with 30 mEq KCl to infuse at 40 mL/hr. A maximum of 10 mEq/hr of KCl should not be exceeded, and the total 24 hr dosage should not exceed 40 mEq/day.

Dosage infusing per hr _____   Dosage infusing per day _____

Assessment _____

39. A child weighing 30 kg has an IV of 100 mL of D5W containing 600 mcg of medication to infuse in 2 hours. The normal range for this drug is 2–4 mcg/kg/hr.

Normal dosage range per hr _____

Dosage infusing per hr _____   Assessment _____

40. 150 mL with 18 mg of medication is ordered to infuse in 10 hours. The normal range for this drug is 0.2–0.6 mg/kg/hr. The child weighs 9 kg.

Normal dosage range per hr _____

Dosage infusing per hr _____   Assessment _____

Answers
1. 22 mL; 38 gtt/min
2. 46 mL; 50 gtt/min
3. 38 mL; 60 gtt/min
4. 46 mL; 43 gtt/min
5. 28 mL; 51 gtt/min
6. 35 mL; 48 gtt/min
7. 18 mL; 40 gtt/min
8. 56 mL; 45 gtt/min
9. 38 mL; 80 gtt/min
10. 14 mL; 45 gtt/min
11. 46 mL; 33 mL/hr
12. 85 mL; 120 mL/hr
13. 78 mL; 80 mL/hr
14. 26 mL; 90 mL/hr
15. 78 mL; 96 mL/hr
16. 27 mL; 45 mL/hr
17. 28 mL; 72 mL/hr
18. 49 mL; 67 mL/hr
19. 9 mL; 60 mL/hr
20. 35 mL; 40 mL/hr

21. 77–115.5 mg/dose; normal
22. 196.5–262 units/dose; normal
23. 1.2–3.7 mg/day; 3 mg; normal
24. 418.5–1255.5 mg/day; 1200 mg; normal
25. 47.1–109.9 mcg/hr; 70 mcg; normal
26. 1176–1568 mg/day; 1500 mg; normal
27. 585–1170 mg/day; 600 mg; normal
28. 120.3–481.2 mg/day; 450 mg; normal
29. 103–257.5 units/hr; 100 units/hr; too low
30. 5.4–16.1 units/hr; 6 units/hr; normal

31. 125–312.5 units/hr; 400 units/hr; too high
32. 600–800 mg/day; 800 mg; normal
33. 1500–3000 mg/day; 2000 mg; normal
34. 1.2 mEq/hr; 28.8 mEq/day; normal
35. 240–480 mg/day; 348 mg; normal
36. 120–150 mcg/day; 80 mcg/day; too low
37. 1160 mg/day; 1160 mg; normal
38. 2.4 mEq/hr; 58 mEq/day; too high
39. 60–120 mcg/hr; 300 mcg; too high
40. 1.8–5.4 mg/hr; 1.8 mg; normal

APOTHECARY MEASURES

The ancient and now extinct apothecary system was based on the weight of a grain of wheat, which immediately points out its inaccuracy. Thus the basic unit of measure was named a **grain** (gr). Liquid measures in the system were based on a **drop**; liquid measures included **minim** (min), **dram** (dr, or ʒ), and **ounce** (oz, or ℥). Metric measures started to displace apothecary use in the 1950s, but some physicians continued to use it apothecary notations, necessitating a conversion chart from apothecary to metric measures (see below). While these charts still appear occasionally in literature, they are rapidly disappearing. The oz and dr measures still appear on some disposable medication cups as part of the household system of measures, necessitating careful distinction when using medication cups for liquid metric measures.

The apothecary measures and their abbreviations were as follows:

WEIGHT		VOLUME		
grain	gr	minim	m	min
		dram	dr	fluid dram ʒ (4 mL)
		ounce	oz	fluid ounce ℥ (30 mL)

APOTHECARY/ HOUSEHOLD/ METRIC EQUIVALENTS							
Liquid				**Weight**			
oz	mL	min	mL	gr	mg	gr	mg
1 = 30		45 = 3		15 = 1000		1/4 = 15	
½ = 15		30 = 2		10 = 600		1/6 = 10	
		15 = 1		7½ = 500		1/8 = 7.5	
dr	mL	12 = 0.75		5 = 300		1/10 = 6	
2½ = 10		10 = 0.6		4 = 250		1/15 = 4	
2 = 8		8 = 0.5		3 = 200		1/20 = 3	
1¼ = 5		5 = 0.3		2½ = 150		1/30 = 2	
1 = 4		4 = 0.25		2 = 120		1/40 = 1.5	
		3 = 0.2		1½ = 100		1/60 = 1	
1 min = 1 gtt		1½ = 0.1		1 = 60		1/100 = 0.6	
1T = 15 mL		1 = 0.06		¾ = 45		1/120 = 0.5	
1t = 5 mL		¾ = 0.05		½ = 30		1/150 = 0.4	
		½ = 0.03		⅓ = 20		1/200 = 0.3	
						1/250 = 0.25	

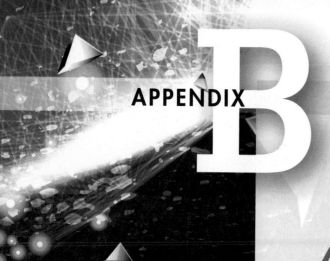

B

ISMP's LIST OF ERROR-PRONE ABBREVIATIONS, SYMBOLS, AND *DOSE* DESIGNATIONS

ISMP's List of *Error-Prone Abbreviations, Symbols, and Dose Designations*

The abbreviations, symbols, and dose designations found in this table have been reported to ISMP through the ISMP National Medication Errors Reporting Program (ISMP MERP) as being frequently misinterpreted and involved in harmful medication errors. They should **NEVER** be used when communicating medical information. This includes internal communications, telephone/verbal prescriptions, computer-generated labels, labels for drug storage bins, medication administration records, as well as pharmacy and prescriber computer order entry screens.

Abbreviations	Intended Meaning	Misinterpretation	Correction
μg	Microgram	Mistaken as "mg"	Use "mcg"
AD, AS, AU	Right ear, left ear, each ear	Mistaken as OD, OS, OU (right eye, left eye, each eye)	Use "right ear," "left ear," or "each ear"
OD, OS, OU	Right eye, left eye, each eye	Mistaken as AD, AS, AU (right ear, left ear, each ear)	Use "right eye," "left eye," or "each eye"
BT	Bedtime	Mistaken as "BID" (twice daily)	Use "bedtime"
cc	Cubic centimeters	Mistaken as "u" (units)	Use "mL"
D/C	Discharge or discontinue	Premature discontinuation of medications if D/C (intended to mean "discharge") has been misinterpreted as "discontinued" when followed by a list of discharge medications	Use "discharge" and "discontinue"
IJ	Injection	Mistaken as "IV" or "intrajugular"	Use "injection"
IN	Intranasal	Mistaken as "IM" or "IV"	Use "intranasal" or "NAS"
HS	Half-strength	Mistaken as bedtime	Use "half-strength" or "bedtime"
hs	At bedtime, hours of sleep	Mistaken as half-strength	
IU**	International unit	Mistaken as IV (intravenous) or 10 (ten)	Use "units"
o.d. or OD	Once daily	Mistaken as "right eye" (OD-oculus dexter), leading to oral liquid medications administered in the eye	Use "daily"
OJ	Orange juice	Mistaken as OD or OS (right or left eye); drugs meant to be diluted in orange juice may be given in the eye	Use "orange juice"
Per os	By mouth, orally	The "os" can be mistaken as "left eye" (OS-oculus sinister)	Use "PO," "by mouth," or "orally"
q.d. or QD**	Every day	Mistaken as q.i.d., especially if the period after the "q" or the tail of the "q" is misunderstood as an "i"	Use "daily"
qhs	Nightly at bedtime	Mistaken as "qhr" or every hour	Use "nightly"
qn	Nightly or at bedtime	Mistaken as "qh" (every hour)	Use "nightly" or "at bedtime"
q.o.d. or QOD**	Every other day	Mistaken as "q.d." (daily) or "q.i.d. (four times daily) if the "o" is poorly written	Use "every other day"
q1d	Daily	Mistaken as q.i.d. (four times daily)	Use "daily"
q6PM, etc.	Every evening at 6 PM	Mistaken as every 6 hours	Use "daily at 6 PM" or "6 PM daily"
SC, SQ, sub q	Subcutaneous	SC mistaken as SL (sublingual); SQ mistaken as "5 every;" the "q" in "sub q" has been mistaken as "every" (e.g., a heparin dose ordered "sub q 2 hours before surgery" misunderstood as every 2 hours before surgery)	Use "subcut" or "subcutaneously"
ss	Sliding scale (insulin) or ½ (apothecary)	Mistaken as "55"	Spell out "sliding scale;" use "one-half" or "½"
SSRI	Sliding scale regular insulin	Mistaken as selective-serotonin reuptake inhibitor	Spell out "sliding scale (insulin)"
SSI	Sliding scale insulin	Mistaken as Strong Solution of Iodine (Lugol's)	
i/d	One daily	Mistaken as "tid"	Use "1 daily"
TIW or tiw	3 times a week	Mistaken as "3 times a day" or "twice in a week"	Use "3 times weekly"
U or u**	Unit	Mistaken as the number 0 or 4, causing a 10-fold overdose or greater (e.g., 4U seen as "40" or 4u seen as "44"); mistaken as "cc" so dose given in volume instead of units (e.g., 4u seen as 4cc)	Use "unit"
UD	As directed ("ut dictum")	Mistaken as unit dose (e.g., diltiazem 125 mg IV infusion "UD" misinterpreted as meaning to give the entire infusion as a unit [bolus] dose)	Use "as directed"

Dose Designations and Other Information	Intended Meaning	Misinterpretation	Correction
Trailing zero after decimal point (e.g., 1.0 mg)**	1 mg	Mistaken as 10 mg if the decimal point is not seen	Do not use trailing zeros for doses expressed in whole numbers
"Naked" decimal point (e.g., .5 mg)**	0.5 mg	Mistaken as 5 mg if the decimal point is not seen	Use zero before a decimal point when the dose is less than a whole unit
Abbreviations such as mg. or mL. with a period following the abbreviation	mg	The period is unnecessary and could be mistaken as the number 1 if written poorly	Use mg, mL, etc. without a terminal period
	mL		

(continues)

APPENDIX B

ISMP's **List of** *Error-Prone Abbreviations, Symbols, and Dose Designations* (continued)

Dose Designations and Other Information	Intended Meaning	Misinterpretation	Correction
Drug name and dose run together (especially problematic for drug names that end in "l" such as Inderal40 mg; Tegretol300 mg)	Inderal 40 mg Tegretol 300 mg	Mistaken as Inderal 140 mg Mistaken as Tegretol 1300 mg	Place adequate space between the drug name, dose, and unit of measure
Numerical dose and unit of measure run together (e.g., 10mg, 100mL)	10 mg 100 mL	The "m" is sometimes mistaken as a zero or two zeros, risking a 10- to 100-fold overdose	Place adequate space between the dose and unit of measure
Large doses without properly placed commas (e.g., 100000 units; 1000000 units)	100,000 units 1,000,000 units	100000 has been mistaken as 10,000 or 1,000,000; 1000000 has been mistaken as 100,000	Use commas for dosing units at or above 1,000, or use words such as 100 "thousand" or 1 "million" to improve readability

Drug Name Abbreviations	Intended Meaning	Misinterpretation	Correction
To avoid confusion, do not abbreviate drug names when communicating medical information. Examples of drug name abbreviations involved in medication errors include:			
APAP	acetaminophen	Not recognized as acetaminophen	Use complete drug name
ARA A	vidarabine	Mistaken as cytarabine (ARA C)	Use complete drug name
AZT	zidovudine (Retrovir)	Mistaken as azathioprine or aztreonam	Use complete drug name
CPZ	Compazine (prochlorperazine)	Mistaken as chlorpromazine	Use complete drug name
DPT	Demerol-Phenergan-Thorazine	Mistaken as diphtheria-pertussis-tetanus (vaccine)	Use complete drug name
DTO	Diluted tincture of opium, or deodorized tincture of opium (Paregoric)	Mistaken as tincture of opium	Use complete drug name
HCl	hydrochloric acid or hydrochloride	Mistaken as potassium chloride (The "H" is misinterpreted as "K")	Use complete drug name unless expressed as a salt of a drug
HCT	hydrocortisone	Mistaken as hydrochlorothiazide	Use complete drug name
HCTZ	hydrochlorothiazide	Mistaken as hydrocortisone (seen as HCT250 mg)	Use complete drug name
MgSO4**	magnesium sulfate	Mistaken as morphine sulfate	Use complete drug name
MS, MSO4**	morphine sulfate	Mistaken as magnesium sulfate	Use complete drug name
MTX	methotrexate	Mistaken as mitoxantrone	Use complete drug name
PCA	procainamide	Mistaken as patient controlled analgesia	Use complete drug name
PTU	propylthiouracil	Mistaken as mercaptopurine	Use complete drug name
T3	Tylenol with codeine No. 3	Mistaken as liothyronine	Use complete drug name
TAC	triamcinolone	Mistaken as tetracaine, Adrenalin, cocaine	Use complete drug name
TNK	TNKase	Mistaken as "TPA"	Use complete drug name
ZnSO4	zinc sulfate	Mistaken as morphine sulfate	Use complete drug name

Stemmed Drug Names	Intended Meaning	Misinterpretation	Correction
"Nitro" drip	nitroglycerin infusion	Mistaken as sodium nitroprusside infusion	Use complete drug name
"Norflox"	norfloxacin	Mistaken as Norflex	Use complete drug name
"IV Vanc"	intravenous vancomycin	Mistaken as Invanz	Use complete drug name

Symbols	Intended Meaning	Misinterpretation	Correction
℥	Dram	Symbol for dram mistaken as "3"	Use the metric system
♏	Minim	Symbol for minim mistaken as "mL"	
x3d	For three days	Mistaken as "3 doses"	Use "for three days"
> and <	Greater than and less than	Mistaken as opposite of intended; mistakenly use incorrect symbol; "< 10" mistaken as "40"	Use "greater than" or "less than"
/ (slash mark)	Separates two doses or indicates "per"	Mistaken as the number 1 (e.g., "25 units/10 units" misread as "25 units and 110 units")	Use "per" rather than a slash mark to separate doses
@	At	Mistaken as "2"	Use "at"
&	And	Mistaken as "2"	Use "and"
+	Plus or and	Mistaken as "4"	Use "and"
°	Hour	Mistaken as a zero (e.g., q2° seen as q 20)	Use "hr," "h," or "hour"
Φ or ⌀	zero, null sign	Mistaken as numerals 4, 6, 8, and 9	Use 0 or zero, or describe intent using whole words

**These abbreviations are included on The Joint Commission's "minimum list" of dangerous abbreviations, acronyms, and symbols that must be included on an organization's "Do Not Use" list, effective January 1, 2004. Visit www.jointcommission.org for more information about this Joint Commission requirement.

ISMP
INSTITUTE FOR SAFE MEDICATION PRACTICES
www.ismp.org

INDEX